Update on

MDR Tuberculosis

Update on
MDR Tuberculosis

The Tuberculosis Association of India

Editors

VK Arora Diploma in Chest Diseases(DCD)
MD(Tuberculosis and Respiratory Diseases/Medicine) MBBS
Tuberculous and Chest Diseases Specialist
Chairman, TB Association of India
Executive Editor of Indian Journal of Tuberculosis
New Delhi, India

Kamal Chopra MBBS MD(Chest and TB)
DTCE(Diploma in TB control and Eradication) Tokyo
Consultant and Former Director
New Delhi Tuberculosis Center
Academic Editor, PLoS One
Associate Executive Editor of Indian Journal of Tuberculosis
New Delhi, India

Foreword

Vishwa Mohan Katoch

JAYPEE

JAYPEE BROTHERS MEDICAL PUBLISHERS

The Health Sciences Publisher

New Delhi | London

Jaypee Brothers Medical Publishers (P) Ltd

Headquarters
EMCA House
23/23-B, Ansari Road, Daryaganj
New Delhi 110 002, India
Landline: +91-11-23272143, +91-11-23272703
+91-11-23282021, +91-11-23245672
E-mail: jaypee@jaypeebrothers.com

Corporate Office
Jaypee Brothers Medical Publishers (P) Ltd.
4838/24, Ansari Road, Daryaganj
New Delhi 110 002, India
Phone: +91-11-43574357
Fax: +91-11-43574314
E-mail: jaypee@jaypeebrothers.com

Overseas Office
JP Medical Ltd.
83, Victoria Street, London
SW1H 0HW (UK)
Phone: +44-20 3170 8910
Fax: +44(0)20 3008 6180
E-mail: info@jpmedpub.com

Website: www.jaypeebrothers.com
Website: www.jaypeedigital.com

Update on MDR Tuberculosis / VK Arora, Kamal Chopra

First Edition: **2025**

ISBN: 978-93-6616-242-3

Printed in India

Dedication

To Dr Robert Koch,
the discoverer of Mycobacterium tuberculosis.

To our parents for their blessings and wife and children
for their constant support.

VK Arora
Kamal Chopra

Contributors

Aastha Gupta MBA
Director Market Access
TB Alliance
New Delhi Tuberculosis Centre
New Delhi, India

Ajantha Panneerselvam DNB(TB and Respiratory Diseases)
Medical Officer
Department of TB and Chest
National Institute of Tuberculosis and Respiratory Diseases
New Delhi, India

Ashish Ranjan DNB(TB and Respiratory Diseases)
Specialist
Department of TB and Chest
National Institute of Tuberculosis and Respiratory Diseases
New Delhi, India

Ankita Anand MBBS MD(Microbiology)
Bacteriologist
Department of Microbiology, Tuberculosis, Serology, Immunology, Mycology
New Delhi Tuberculosis Centre
New Delhi, India

Ankit Kumar MD(Respiratory Medicine)
Assistant Professor
Department of Respiratory Medicine
King George's Medical University
Lucknow, Uttar Pradesh, India

Ankur Gupta DNB
Senior Medical Officer, Nodal DRTB Centre
Department of Respiratory Medicine and Tuberculosis
JLN Medical College
Ajmer, Rajasthan, India

Arun Sampath MD DNB EDARM FRCP(Glasgow) FCCP FAPSR
Senior Consultant Pulmonologist
Department of Pulmonary and Sleep Medicine
MIOT International
Chennai, Tamil Nadu, India

Alex Anthony MD ACMDC AFIH FAM(Palliative Care, Bioethics)
Speciality Doctor Geriatric Medicine
Departments of Geriatric Medicine
Royal Lancaster Infirmary
University Hospitals of Morecambe Bay Trust (UHMBT)
Lancaster, United Kingdom

Banurekha V Velayutham MBBS MPH PGDBE
Public Heath, Bioethics; Scientist
Department of Clinical Research
ICMR National Institute for Research in Tuberculosis
Chennai, Tamil Nadu, India

Bineeta Kashyap MBBS MD(Microbiology)
Director Professor
Department of Microbiology
University College of Medical Sciences
and Guru Teg Bahadur Hospital
New Delhi, India

Chaitali Nikam PhD MPH
Consultant
Director Haystack Analytics
IIT Bombay, Thyrocare Technologies Limited
Mumbai, Maharashtra, India

Chandragiri Pranay Sai MD DM
Senior Resident
Department of Pulmonary, Critical Care and Sleep Medicine
All India Institute of Medical Sciences
New Delhi, India

D Bhima Sankar MBBS MD
Associate Professor
Department of Respiratory Medicine
KIMS Medical College
Amalapuram, Andhra Pradesh, India

Eugene Sun MD
Senior Vice President
Head of Research and Development
TB Alliance
New York, USA

Gyanshankar Mishra MBBS MD(Respiratory Medicine) DNB(Respiratory Diseases) MNAMS FNCCP(I)
Associate Professor
Department of Respiratory Medicine
Indira Gandhi Government Medical
Nagpur, Maharashtra, India

Jaya Lalwani MD(Microbiology)
Associate Professor
Department of Microbiology
Gandhi Medical College
Bhopal, Madhya Pradesh, India

Judo J Vachaparambil MBBS MD Chest(JIPMER) FCCP USA
Chief Consultant Pulmonologist and Medical Superintendent
Sun Medical and Research Centre
Thrissur, Kerala, India

Kalpana Chandra MD(Internal Medicine) PhD(TB and Chest Diseases) WHO Fellow in Anti-Microbial Resistance(Sweden) FIACM
Medical Officer Incharge
Delhi Jal Board
Government of NCT of Delhi
New Delhi, India

Karthikasri K MTech(Biotechnology)
Clinical SAS Programmer
Department of Biotechnology
PSG College of Technology
Coimbatore, Tamil Nadu, India

Karthikeyan Sundaram MSc
Assistant Professor
Department of Microbiology
Mohamed Sathak College of Arts and Science
Research Scholar
SRM Medical College Hospital and Research Centre Kattangulathur
Chennai, Tamil Nadu, India

Kaushal Kumar Dwivedi PhD(Microbiology)
Microbiologist
Intermediate Reference Laboratory
New Delhi Tuberculosis Centre
New Delhi, India

KB Gupta MD(Respiratory Medicine) FICS FIAB FNCCP FICAAI
Professor and Head
Department of Respiratory Medicine
Era Medical College and Hospital
Lucknow, Uttar Pradesh, India

Kamal Chopra MBBS MD(Chest and TB) DTCE (Diploma in TB control and Eradication) Tokyo
Consultant and Former Director
New Delhi Tuberculosis Center
Academic Editor, PLoS One
Associate Executive Editor of Indian Journal of Tuberculosis
New Delhi, India

Kranti Garg MBBS MD(Pulmonary Medicine)
Associate Professor
Department of Pulmonary Medicine
Government Medical College
Patiala, Punjab, India

Leela Kagithakara Vajravelu MD(Microbiology) DGO
Professor and Head
Department of Microbiology
SRM Medical College Hospital and Research Centre
Chennai, Tamil Nadu, India

Lokender Kumar MBBS MD
Chest Physician (SAG)
National Institute of Tuberculosis and Respiratory Diseases
New Delhi, India

MM Puri MBBS MD
Consultant Chest Physician
National Institute of Tuberculosis and Respiratory Diseases
New Delhi, India

Maria Diachenko PhD
Senior Manager, Market Access
TB Alliance
New Delhi Tuberculosis Centre
New Delhi, India

N Meenakshi MD(TB and Respiratory Medicine) DTCD DEAN(Pulmonology)
Professor and Head
Department of Respiratory Medicine
Chettinad Hospital and Research Institute
Kelambakkam, Tamil Nadu, India

Mina Chandra DNB Psychiatry(Gold medalist) PhD(Neurology) MNAMS WHO Fellow in Drug and Alcohol Medicine(Australia, FIPS)
Head
Department of Psychiatry
Head of Centre of Excellence in Mental Health
ABVIMS and RML Hospital
New Delhi, India

MVNL Chaitanya PhD
Professor
School of Pharmaceutical Sciences
Lovely Professional University
Phagwara, Punjab, India

Nagraj Perumal MSc(Medical Microbiology) PhD(Medical Microbiology)
Scientist
Department of Infectious Diseases
B, State Virology Laboratory
Gandhi Medical College
Bhopal, Madhya Pradesh, India

Namita Chopra MBBS MD
Consultant
Department of Gynecology and Obstetrics
ABVIMS and RML Hospital
New Delhi, India

Nibedita Rath PhD
Scientific Director
Open Source Pharma Foundation
Vice President (2022–2024)
The Union Lung Health
South East Asia Region
Open Source Pharma Foundation
Manyata Tech Park
Bengaluru, Karnataka, India

Nishi Aggarwal PhD(Statistics)
Statistician
New Delhi Tuberculosis Centre
New Delhi, India

Niti Singh PhD
Consultant Microbiologist
National Institute of Tuberculosis and Respiratory Diseases
New Delhi, India

Pallavi Purwar Doctracte(Thoracic Surgery)
Consultant Thoracic Surgeoan
Holy Family Hospital
New Delhi, India

Prabhpreet Sethi MBBS MD
Chest Physician (SAG)
National Institute of Tuberculosis and Respiratory Diseases
New Delhi, India

Pratibha Narang MD(Microbiology)
Advisor in Microbiology and TB research
Recipient of Dr BC Roy National Award
Department of Microbiology
Mahatma Gandhi Institute of Medical Sciences Sevagram
Wardha, Maharashtra, India

Priya Rajendran PhD(Medical Microbiology)
Scientist D
Department of Bacteriology
ICMR National Institute for Research in Tuberculosis
Chennai, Tamil Nadu, India

PS Sarma MBBS DAEF FCGP
Konaseema Institute of Medical Sciences and Research Foundation Hospital
Amalapuram, Andhra Pradesh, India

R Sridhar MD
Vice Chancellor
Department of TB and Respiratory Medicine
Chettinad Academy of Research and Education
Kelambakkam, Tamil Nadu, India

Radha Munje MBBS MD(Medicine) DTCD FICS
Professor and Head
Department of Respiratory Medicine
Indira Gandhi Government Medical College
Nagpur, Maharashtra, India

Rajat Jhamb MBBS MD
Director Professor
Department of Medicine
University College of Medical Sciences and Guru Teg Bahadur Hospital
New Delhi, India

Rajnish Gupta MD(TB and Chest)
Head
Department of Respiratory Critical Care and Incharge Sleep Lab
National Institute of Tuberculosis and Respiratory Diseases
New Delhi, India

Ramakant Dixit MBBS MD
Senior Professor and Head
Department of Respiratory Medicine and Tuberculosis
JLN Medical College
Ajmer, Rajasthan, India

Rashmi Saxena Pal PhD
Professor
School of Pharmaceutical Sciences
Lovely Professional University
Phagwara, Punjab, India

Rishabh Kacker MBBS MD(Respiratory Medicine)
Assistant Professor
Department of Respiratory Medicine
Era Medical college and Hospital
Lucknow, Uttar Pradesh, India

Ritu Singhal MBBS MD(Microbiology)
Specialist (Senior Administrative Grade)
National Reference Laboratory and Center of Excellence (TB) WHO
Department of Microbiology
National Institute of Tuberculosis and Respiratory Diseases
New Delhi, India

Salah Foraida MD, MS
Senior Medical Director
TB Alliance
New York, USA

Salil Bhargava MBBS MD(Medicine) DTCD DNB(Respiratory Medicine) Pulmonary Medicine
Professor and Head
Department of Respiratory Medicine
Mahatma Gandhi Memorial Medical College
Indore, Madhya Pradesh, India

Sandeep Juneja MBA MD DM
Senior Vice President
Department of Pulmonary, Critical Care and Sleep Medicine
Senior Resident
All India Institute of Medical Sciences
New Delhi, India

Sandeep Katiyar DNB(Respiratory Medicine) MNAMS EDRM
Director
Katiyar Chest Centre
Consultant Pulmonologist and Interventionist
Apollo Spectra Hospital
Kanpur, Uttar Pradesh, India

Sangeeta Sharma MD MNAMS FNCCP(I)
Pediatric Pulmonologist and Pediatric TB/DRTB Expert
Consultant Pediatrics
Former Director
National Institute of TB and Respiratory Diseases
New Delhi, India

Sanjay Rajpal MBBS DTCD
Director
Department of TB and Chest Diseases
New Delhi Tuberculosis Centre
New Delhi, India

Sarman Singh MD FRCP FRSC FAMS
Director
Department of Infectious Diseases
Medical Research, AVMC&H, VMRF (Deemed University)
Puducherry, India

Shikha Dhawan PGDM(Biotechnology Business Management) PhD(Molecular Biology Microbiology, Public Health)
Managing Director
Abhya Life Foundation
New Delhi, India

Shanker Matta MBBS MD
Epidemiologist
Head Epidemiology Section
New Delhi Tuberculosis Centre
New Delhi, India

Sivakumar Shanmugam PhD(Molecular Biology and Immunology)
Scientist E and Head
Department of Bacteriology
ICMR National Institute for Research in Tuberculosis
Chennai, Tamil Nadu, India

Shivani Pawar MBBS DTCD
Medical Officer
New Delhi Tuberculosis Centre
New Delhi, India

Shobana S PhD(Biotechnology)
Assistant Professor
Department of Biotechnology
PSG College of Technology Coimbatore, Tamil Nadu, India

SK Katiyar DNB(Respiratory Medicine) MNAMS MNCCP
Director
Katiyar Chest Centre
Professor and Head
Department of Tuberculosis and Respiratory Diseases
Principal and Dean
GSUM Medical College, CSJM University
Kanpur, Uttar Pradesh, India

Sunil Khaparde MBBS MD
EX-Deputy Director General (TB)
Senior Advisor
TB Alliance
New York, USA

Surya Kant MD(Gold Medalist) DSc(Honoris Causa) FCCP(USA) FACP(USA) FRCP(London) FRCP(Glasgow) FGAPIO FAPSR FISEB FGSI FAMS FIAMS FNCCP FCAI FIMSA FIAB FICS FUPDA FIACM FICP FCGP FISC FUAPMI FISH
Professor and Head
Department of Respiratory Medicine
King George's Medical University
Lucknow, Uttar Pradesh, India

T Pratyusha MD
Associate Professor
Department of Respiratory Medicine
Konaseema Institute of Medical Sciences and Research Foundation Hospital
Amalapuram, Andhra Pradesh, India

Tejas Menon Suri MD DM
Pulmonalogist
Department of Pulmonary, Critical Care and Sleep Medicine
All India Institute of Medical Sciences
New Delhi, India

Thomas Vadakkan Devassy MBBS MD(JIPMER) DRCP(UK) FCCS
Professor
Department of Pulmonary Medicine
Amala Institute of Medical Sciences
Thrissur, Kerala, India

Varsha Reddy J MD ACMDC AFIH FAM (Palliative Care, Bioethics)
Speciality Doctor Geriatric Medicine
Royal Lancaster Infirmary
University Hospitals of Morecambe Bay Trust (UHMBT)
Lancaster, United Kingdom

VK Arora Diploma in Chest Diseases(DCD) MD(Tuberculosis and Respiratory Diseases/ Medicine) MBBS
Tuberculous and Chest Diseases Specialist
Chairman, TB Association of India
Executive Editor of Indian Journal of Tuberculosis
New Delhi, India

Zaid Tanvir MS
Preclinical Project Manager
TB Alliance
New York, USA

Zeeshan Sidiq PhD(Microbiology) PGP(Epidemiology)
Microbiologist
Department of Microbiology
New Delhi Tuberculosis Centre
New Delhi, India

Foreword

Drug resistance in tuberculosis is an old, well-known problem whose consequences have been devastating. The solutions to manage drug resistance have also been difficult. Clinicians and public health experts have witnessed a worsening situation for a long time. However, during the recent years the situation has been turning for better with the availability of several effective drugs to treat drug-resistant tuberculosis, choice of new molecular methods, some of which are easily accessible even at the microscopy center level, better imaging methods, and new emerging technologies based on artificial intelligence and machine-learning approaches.

Professor VK Arora, a stalwart with an experience of over 50 years in tuberculosis, and Dr Kamal Chopra, another well-known clinician and academician, have edited this book "*Update on MDR Tuberculosis*" that has contributions from more than 40 authors—clinicians, public health experts, and laboratory and other professionals. This book is a unique compilation of 43 chapters on all important aspects of multidrug resistance (MDR)/drug resistance in tuberculosis. This reflects the vast experience of contributors and their in-depth analysis of the current knowledge about different aspects of drug-resistant tuberculosis. There are chapters on "General" aspects including burden, trends, impact of MDR tuberculosis as well as barriers in the development of specific drug testing. There are important chapters related to "Diagnostic" aspects which provide valuable latest information about the genetic basis of drug resistance in tuberculosis and technologies to detect the same. Chapters on "Clinical" aspects deal with fundamental issues such as adherence, gaps in implementation of evidence-based treatment strategies, and therapeutic drug monitoring. Chapters on "Treatment" deal with new molecules, new regimens, and other advances in the medical and surgical management of tuberculosis. There are many important chapters on other relevant aspects such as MDR and pregnancy, diabetes, and mental health as well as programmatic implementation. Due attention has been given to "Prevention" by contributions from various authors on transmission, contact tracing, vaccination, and role of conventional approaches. Chapters on use of artificial intelligence, fingerprinting, epigenetics, phenotypic drug resistance, and functional characterization of the toxin–antitoxin system in *Mycobacterium tuberculosis* would stimulate the readers to look ahead and explore newer opportunities offered by these approaches.

I am sure that this book being published by Jaypee Brothers Medical Publishers under the aegis of Tuberculosis Association of India (TAI) will be very useful to clinicians, public health experts, and researchers involved/interested in the diagnosis and management of drug-resistant tuberculosis. I am optimistic that this will be equally popular among students, established professionals, and scientists.

Vishwa Mohan Katoch MD FNASc FASc FAMS FNA
President, Tuberculosis Association of India
Editor, Indian Journal of Leprosy
Former President, JIPMER, Puducherry
Former Chairman, LEPRA Society
Former Secretary, Department of Health Research, Government of India
Director-General, Indian Council of Medical Research and
Former NASI-ICMR Chair on Public Health Research
Rajasthan University of Health Sciences (RUHS)
Jaipur, Rajasthan, India
E-mail: vishwamohankatoch18@gmail.com

Preface

Multidrug-resistant tuberculosis (MDR-TB) is a life-threatening disease that poses significant diagnostic and therapeutic challenges. The advent of molecular laboratory tests has facilitated rapid diagnosis, but interpreting these tests requires specialized expertise. Use of artificial intelligence (AI) in TB control has added new dimension.

Treating MDR-TB is equally complex, and managing such cases is not straight-forward for every physician. Furthermore, National TB Control Programme guidelines are constantly evolving due to emerging clinical evidence, in making early diagnosis and discovery of new drugs, making it difficult for physicians, especially in the private sector, to stay updated.

Additionally, MDR-TB often coexists with other conditions like pregnancy, liver disease, and renal diseases, requiring meticulous management of comorbidities.

To address these challenges, we have compiled a comprehensive, multiauthor book on MDR-TB, covering all aspects of diagnosis and management. Our expert authors, selected for their specialty and experience, have crafted engaging chapters using flowcharts, tables, and pictures.

Each chapter includes five to seven recent references for further reading. Authors have ensured that the information is authentic and aligned with National TB Programme guidelines.

VK Arora
Kamal Chopra

Acknowledgments

We acknowledge all the worthy authors for contributing updated information in their respective chapters for their sincere efforts and hard work.

We are thankful to Jaypee Brothers Medical Publishers (especially Mr Ashish Kumar and Mr Piyush Mohan Bhatnagar) for timely publishing the book and also assisting the authors in bringing the chapters in final shape.

We sincerely acknowledge the support of Dr Ashwani Khanna (Vice Chairman), Sh Tejinder Ahluwalia (Honorary Treasurer), Mr Vikram Malhotra (Secretary General), Mr Satish Kumar Saini (Accounts Consultant), Mr Raman Kwatra (Admin Consultant), Ms Priti Kaushik (Journal Coordinator) of TB Association of India, and Mrs Sulekha Chakrawarti (Administrative Officer, New Delhi TB Centre) for coordinating with authors to bring out uniformity in chapters.

VK Arora
Kamal Chopra

Acknowledgements

Contents

Section 1: General

Section 2: Diagnostic

Section 7: Newer Initiatives

PLATE 1

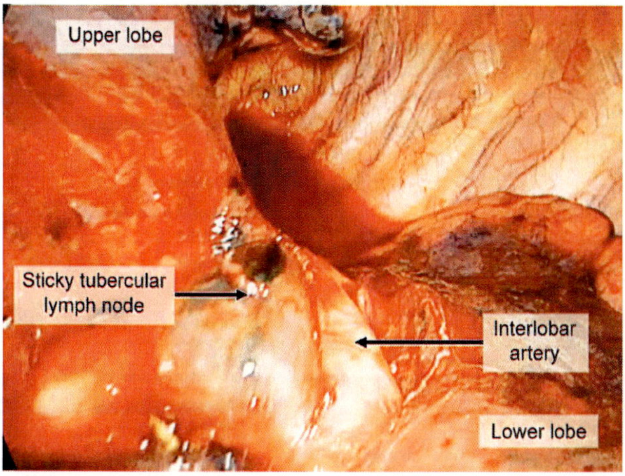

FIG. 1: Adherent sticky lymph node on the interlobar artery ***(Chapter 22)***.

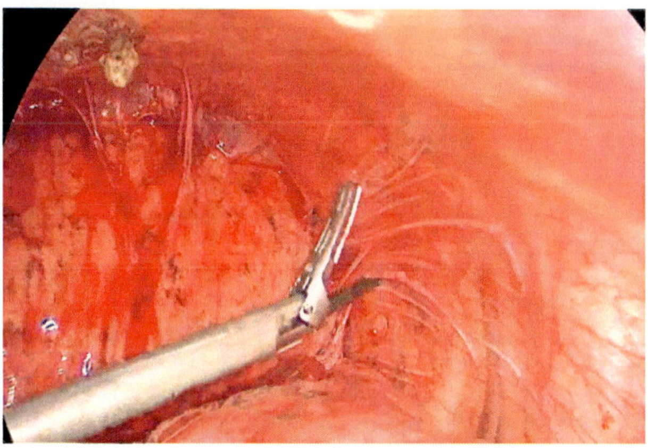

FIG. 2: Adhesions in tuberculosis surgery ***(Chapter 22)***.

PLATE 2

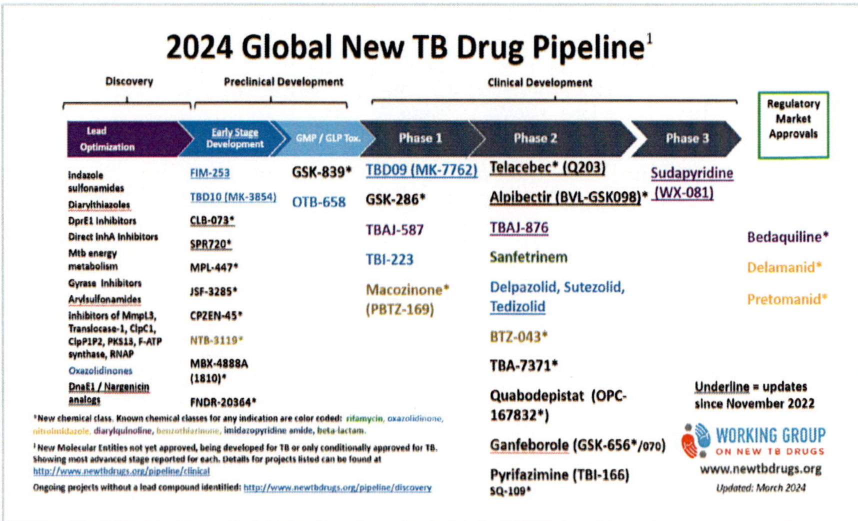

FIG. 1: New chemical entities being evaluated globally for TB treatment ***(Chapter 24)***.

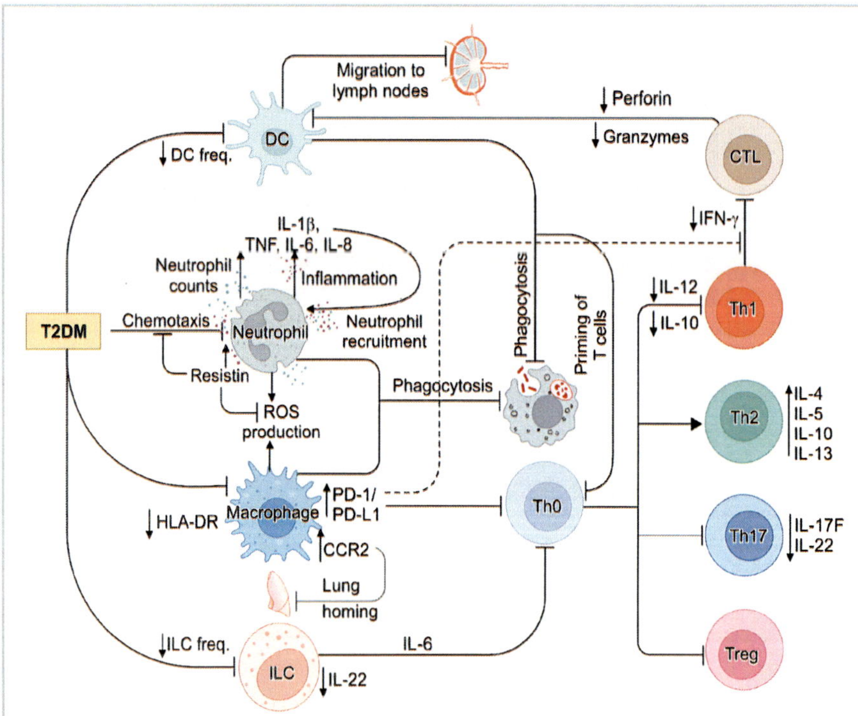

FIG. 1: TB and T2DM immunological dysregulation. Effects of T2DM on the various innate (DC, neutrophil, macrophage, and ILC) and adaptive (CTL, Th1, Th2, Th17, and Tregs) immune cells ***(Chapter 28)***.

(DC: dendritic cell; ILC: innate lymphoid cell; TB: tuberculosis; T2DM: type 2 diabetes mellitus)

PLATE 3

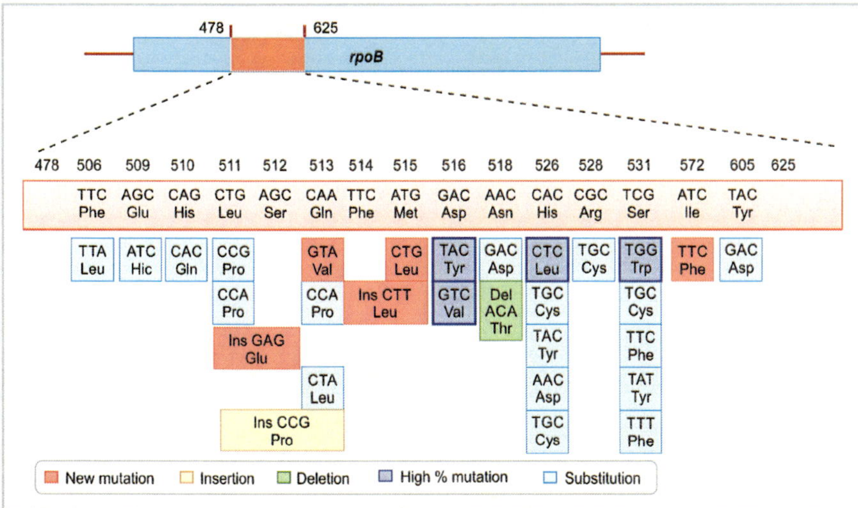

FIG. 1: The hotspot region (HSR) (red) of the *rpoB* gene which depicts that any mutation in this area is likely to confer high level RIF resistance. The flanking blue regions indicates mutation in these areas are associated with low-level resistance.[4] ***(Chapter 31)***

Section 1: General

CHAPTER

1

Impact of Higher Prevalence in Countries with Evolving Healthcare Systems and High Multidrug-resistant Tuberculosis Burden

Radha Munje, Gyanshankar Mishra

Abstract

Managing tuberculosis (TB), particularly multidrug-resistant TB (MDR-TB), is highly challenging in regions with weak healthcare systems. Over 80% of TB cases and deaths occur in low- and middle-income countries, where inadequate healthcare infrastructure exacerbates the problem. Key contributors are diagnostic delays, treatment interruptions, and socioeconomic factors like poverty and malnutrition. Public health policies and cultural influences further complicate control efforts, highlighting the urgent need to strengthen healthcare systems. While molecular tests and universal drug susceptibility testing (UDST) are available, a comprehensive strategy integrating medical and socioeconomic approaches is crucial for addressing TB and MDR-TB in high-burden regions.

Keywords: Multidrug-resistant tuberculosis (MDR-TB), weak healthcare systems, tuberculosis management, diagnostic challenges, socio-economic factors in TB

INTRODUCTION

Multidrug-resistant tuberculosis (MDR-TB) is primarily a man-made phenomenon, mainly resulting from inadequate treatment of drug-sensitive TB (DSTB) and presents a significant challenge in its management. Thus, previous TB treatment is the strongest risk factor for MDR-TB, reflecting the effectiveness of TB control programs.[1] In 2022, 410,000 people developed MDR-TB, yet less than half received proper diagnosis and treatment, highlighting the need for enhanced capacities.[2] MDR-TB is concentrated in regions like India, China, and Pakistan, with Sub-Saharan Africa, particularly Somalia, bearing a high burden relative to its population.[3] Economic challenges, undernutrition, and ineffective TB control programs primarily drive this. The Industrial Revolution, which improved living conditions and reduced TB mortality in the West, underscores the critical link between socioeconomic progress and public health. In India, catastrophic financial losses due to TB are severe, stressing the need for social safety net care.[4] The HIV pandemic proved to be a boon in disguise wherein concentrated efforts could be made and proved the potential of efforts and treatment in TB care. Though all these countries have been making efforts for TB control for more than 3–4 decades the decline of DSTB is not yet converted to benefits in MDR-TB management for various reasons. Identifying areas of either delay or failure in intervention and then targeted interventions are essential in regions with weak healthcare systems where MDR-TB is closely tied to socio-economic challenges.

DEFICIENCIES IN EVOLVING OR WEAK HEALTHCARE SYSTEMS

Evolving healthcare systems, while marked by ongoing progress, may appear weak due to persistent challenges such as limited resources and infrastructure, which can result in overcrowded facilities, long wait times, reduced care quality, and inadequate medical supplies. These evolving systems often struggle with a shortage of trained healthcare professionals and restricted access to diagnostic tools and treatment options, leading to delays in accurate diagnoses and timely interventions. Additionally, the absence of robust health information systems hinders effective data collection, monitoring of health trends, and strategic public health planning. However, it is important to note that most weak healthcare systems are in an evolving phase, gradually overcoming these barriers. There are very few healthcare systems that are inherently weak and stagnant, showing little to no progress over time. Addressing these challenges is crucial for enhancing effective disease management and improving health outcomes, particularly in the context of MDR-TB, as these evolving systems strive toward greater resilience and capability.

Challenges in Managing TB and MDR-TB in Resource-limited Settings in Weak Healthcare Systems: A Complex Interplay of Factors

The challenges encompass diagnostic barriers, treatment complications, and broader socioeconomic and structural issues. These intricately interconnected factors are depicted comprehensively in **Flowchart 1**.

Diagnostic challenges: Managing TB and MDR-TB in resource-limited settings is critically hindered by the limited access to advanced diagnostics, such as polymerase chain reaction (PCR)-based nucleic acid amplification tests (NAATs) like GeneXpert and TrueNat. This scarcity delays the detection of TB and drug resistance, particularly rifampicin (RIF) resistance, and worsening disease progression and transmission. While national programs, including India's Programmatic Management of Drug-Resistant Tuberculosis (PMDT), have swiftly expanded universal drug susceptibility testing (UDST) facilities and adopted bedaquiline-based regimens, at places the development as well as acceptance of rapid diagnostic capacity by healthcare worker (HCW) has lagged behind, compromising treatment efficacy. The absence of rapid tools to identify resistance to second-line drugs like bedaquiline threatens to escalate drug resistance, a situation that could be catastrophic in these settings.[5] Reliance on slower diagnostics like culture alone or not adapting to already available rapid diagnostics of drug-resistant tuberculosis (DRTB) not only delays treatment but also significantly increases morbidity and mortality.

Treatment challenges: Although drugs exist to formulate an effective MDR-TB regimen, they are costly, more toxic, and less efficacious than first-line therapies, adversely affecting treatment outcomes. The prolonged treatment duration, often up to 2 years, along with a higher incidence of adverse drug reactions (ADRs), presents significant challenges. Noncompliance, provider errors in dosing or regimen adjustments, and drug shortages in weak healthcare systems further complicate management and worsen drug resistance, increasing the risk of treatment failure.

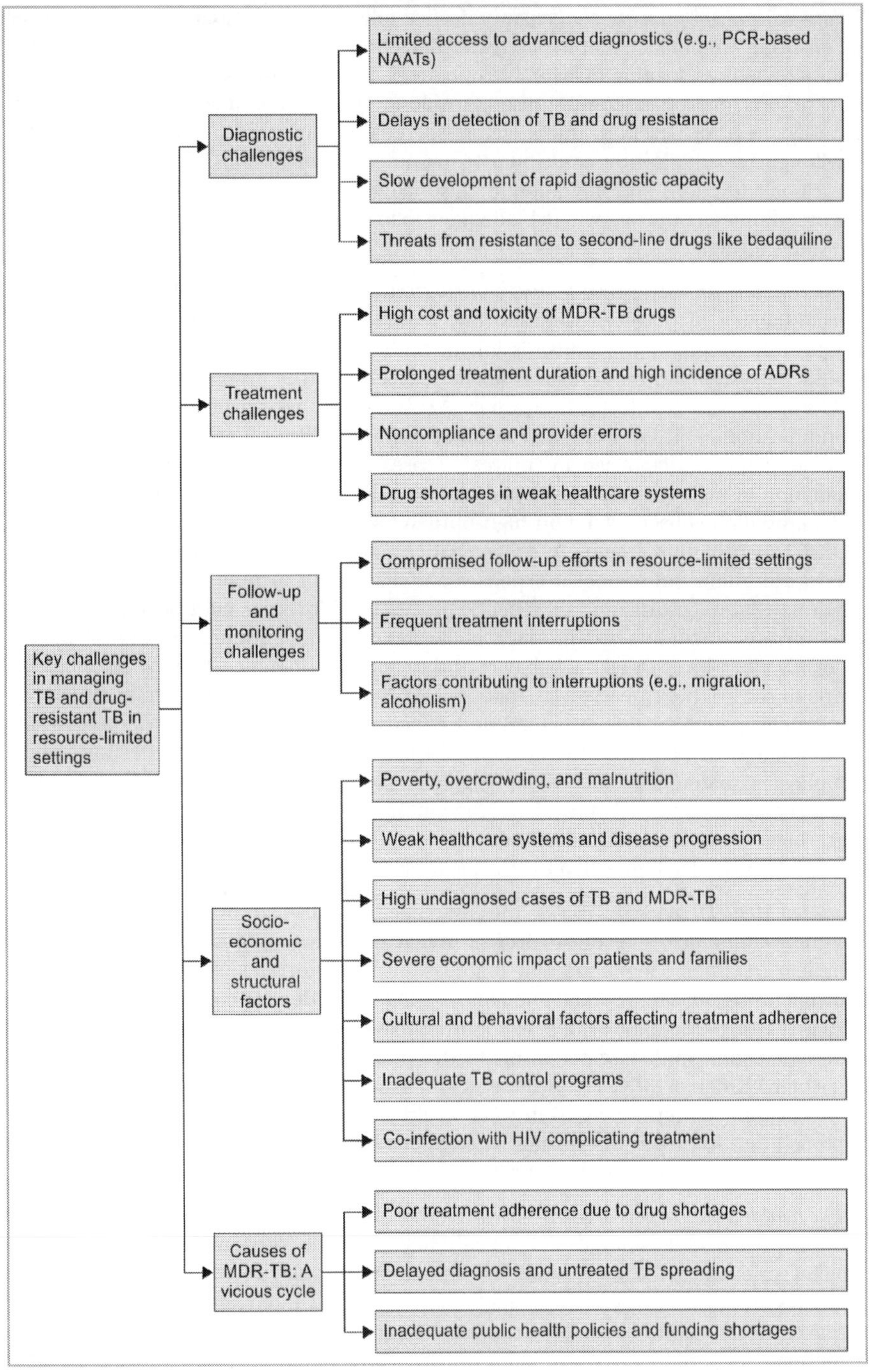

FLOWCHART 1: Key challenges in managing tuberculosis (TB) and drug-resistant TB in resource-limited settings.

(ADR: adverse drug reactions; HIV: human immunodeficiency virus; MDR-TB: multidrug-resistant tuberculosis; NAAT: nucleic acid amplification test; PCR: polymerase chain reaction)

Follow-up and monitoring challenges: Effective follow-up and monitoring are essential for ensuring treatment compliance, early detection of complications, and preventing treatment failures, leading to favorable outcomes. However, in resource-limited settings, these efforts are often compromised, resulting in frequent treatment interruptions and the spread of DRTB. In India, factors such as migration, alcoholism, and patient's unwillingness significantly contribute to treatment interruptions.[6] Similar challenges of various addictions and migration are also likely to be present in other high-burden, resource-limited countries, where inadequate follow-up is also linked to resource scarcity and staff shortages.

Socioeconomic and structural factors contributing to MDR-TB: In high-burden countries, the confluence of poverty, overcrowding, malnutrition, and compromised immunity significantly amplifies the transmission of both DSTB and MDR-TB. The fragility of healthcare systems in these regions further exacerbates the propagation of the disease and its progression in infected individuals. A substantial disparity persists between global TB notifications and the estimated incidence of MDR-TB, primarily attributable to the large number of undiagnosed and untreated cases. Notably, approximately 35% of the TB population in high-burden countries remains undiagnosed, a stark contrast to the 20% undiagnosed rate observed in non-high-burden regions.[7] The economic repercussions of MDR-TB are profound, frequently driving patients and their families into extreme poverty due to exorbitant out-of-pocket expenses and significant income loss incurred during the prolonged diagnostic and therapeutic processes.[4] Moreover, cultural and behavioral determinants, including stigma, lack of awareness, and entrenched cultural beliefs, adversely affect health-seeking behavior and treatment adherence, thereby complicating efforts to control the spread of TB. Inadequate TB control programs, often hampered by insufficient resources, infrastructure, and effective monitoring, further perpetuate the dissemination of MDR-TB. The challenge is compounded by HIV coinfection, which complicates treatment protocols and heightens the risk of MDR-TB, particularly in high-burden countries where HIV prevalence remains high despite recent declines. This scenario exacerbates the economic burden and leads to a significant loss in disability-adjusted life years (DALYs) and a diminished work capacity among the younger population.

Causes of MDR-TB: A vicious cycle—The emergence of MDR-TB is primarily driven by poor treatment adherence, often due to drug shortages and interrupted supplies, which prevent complete treatment. Inadequate or inaccessible laboratory resources delay diagnosis, allowing untreated TB to spread and contributing to the development of MDR-TB. These challenges are particularly evident in countries like India, where diagnostic and treatment efforts are significantly hampered. Ineffective public health policies, funding shortages, and a high burden of MDR-TB further exacerbate inadequate TB management.

Addressing TB and MDR-TB in weak healthcare systems requires a comprehensive approach that improves diagnostics, strengthens follow-up systems, and addresses the socioeconomic and structural factors contributing to the disease burden.

Public health implications of MDR-TB and strategies for control in weak healthcare systems: MDR-TB presents a substantial public health challenge, both within national borders and on a global scale, due to the high mobility of populations through migration and travel, which facilitates the spread of the disease. Inadequate screening and treatment protocols in one region can lead to outbreaks in others, exacerbating the issue. MDR-TB often emerges from incomplete or improper TB treatment, which fosters the development of drug-resistant strains, complicating efforts to control and treat the disease. The reactivation of MDR-TB further perpetuates resistance, escalating morbidity and mortality rates. A pressing concern is the irrational use of newer drugs like bedaquiline, which, while essential for treating drug-resistant TB, is now available in the private sector in countries like India, where studies have highlighted poor prescription patterns.[8] Inadequate follow-up and misuse of bedaquiline, particularly in the private sector, heighten the risk of resistance, which is difficult to diagnose and treat in resource-limited settings.[5] The economic impact of failing to meet the end-TB mortality target by 2030 could be severe, particularly in sub-Saharan Africa, where 15 countries face the potential for a gross domestic product (GDP) reduction exceeding 10%. This underscores the urgency for increased financing from affected countries, donors, and the private sector, as the economic benefits of controlling MDR-TB are substantial.[9] However, implementing effective control measures in high-burden countries remains challenging due to resource limitations, diagnostic delays, inconsistent drug supplies, and a shortage of trained healthcare professionals, especially in rural areas. Low public awareness, stigma, weak policies, and insufficient funding further hinder efforts, making a multisectoral approach, including health system strengthening and community engagement, essential for effective control.

STRATEGIES TO COMBAT MULTIDRUG-RESISTANT TUBERCULOSIS IN WEAK HEALTHCARE SYSTEMS

Addressing MDR-TB in regions with weak healthcare systems requires a multifaceted approach **(Flowchart 2)**.

- *Strengthening healthcare infrastructure*: Investing in healthcare infrastructure is essential to effectively combat TB. This involves constructing and upgrading medical facilities, securing a consistent supply of essential equipment and medications, and enhancing the overall capacity to manage TB cases. Establishing dedicated respiratory medicine departments in medical colleges is vital for providing specialized care. Additionally, it is imperative to strengthen capacity-building efforts to ensure the timely delivery of rapid diagnostic reports to both doctors and patients, supported by robust systems for efficient sample transportation to laboratories.
- *Improving diagnostic and treatment capabilities*: Enhancing diagnostic and treatment capabilities is crucial for managing TB, particularly drug-resistant forms. This includes rapid expansion of access to advanced tools like GeneXpert machines, ensuring the availability of effective second-line drugs, and training HCWs in the latest treatment protocols. Regulating the use of drugs like bedaquiline and ensuring rigorous patient's follow-up are vital to prevent further drug resistance. Rapid deployment of validated, cost-effective diagnostics for DRTB is essential. Additionally, integrating IT-enabled platforms in national programs, utilizing technology for patient awareness and counseling, and employing artificial intelligence (AI)-equipped drug-vending machines with local language interfaces are innovative solutions that should be adopted at the programmatic level for effective diagnosis and management.
- *Targeting latent drug-resistant TB infections*: Testing and treating individuals with latent DRTB, particularly household contacts of MDR-TB patients, is crucial. Latent MDR-TB cases can be classified into contacts of known MDR-TB patients and those of undiagnosed or unknown cases. Current guidelines primarily focus on the former group, while the latter remains challenging to diagnose and guide for treatment regimens for these contacts which should align with the drug-resistance profile of the index TB case.[10] If a country has data of baseline drug resistance patterns in community done at intervals of at least a decade it can further guide in deciding regimens.
- *Incorporating surgical and rehabilitation options*: Treatment programs should incorporate surgical interventions when appropriate, particularly for localized TB cases, to enhance patient's outcomes. Additionally, integrating pulmonary rehabilitation into posttreatment care is crucial for optimizing recovery. Establishing partnerships with both surgical centers and pulmonary rehabilitation centers, along

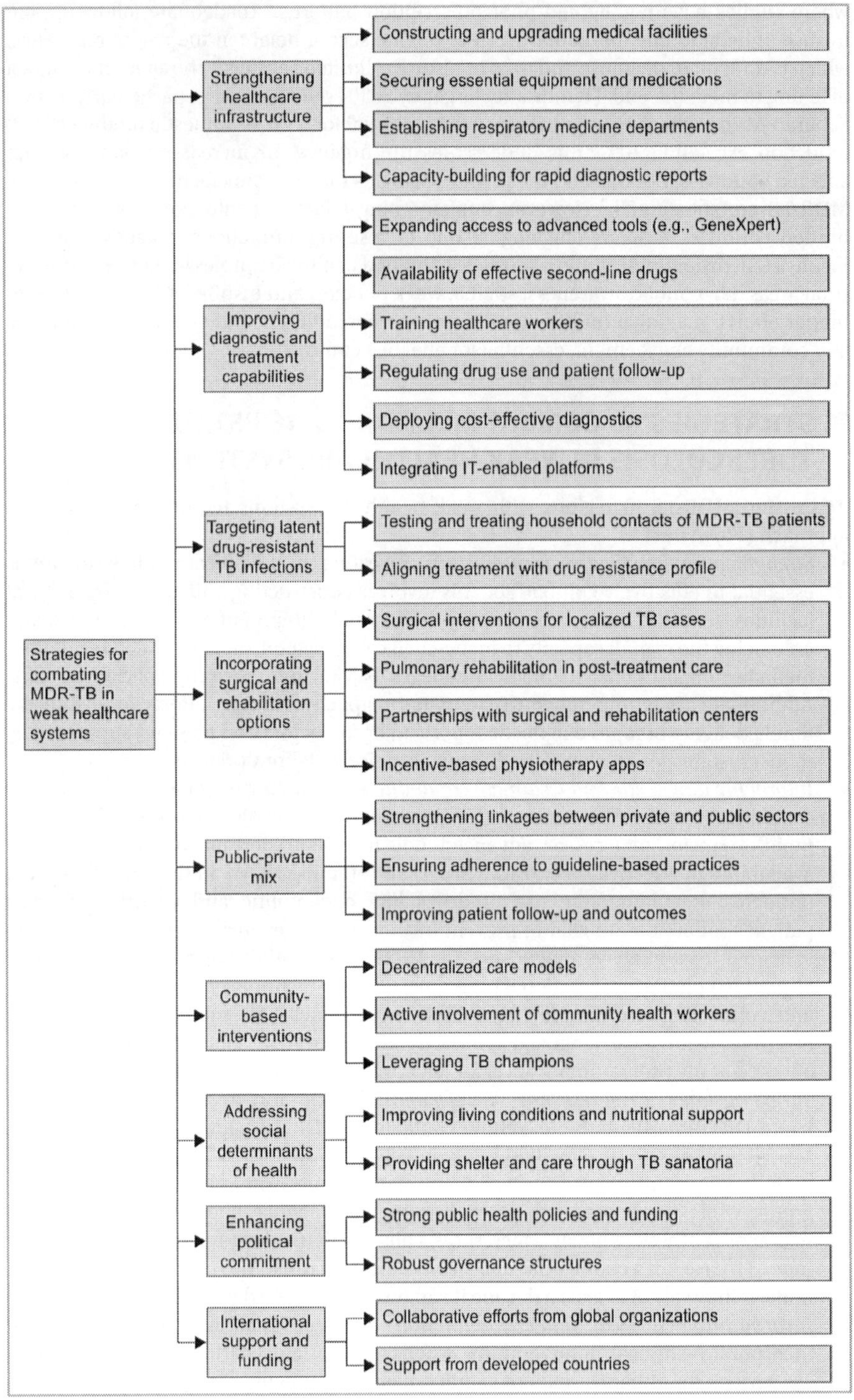

FLOWCHART 2: Strategies for combating multidrug-resistant tuberculosis (MDR-TB) in weak healthcare systems.

with utilizing incentive-based physiotherapy apps, can significantly enhance the effectiveness of these efforts.

- *Public-private mix*: In all countries with weak healthcare systems, initial care for TB often occurs in the private sector, where diagnostic and treatment practices are frequently suboptimal and disorganized, exacerbating the challenge of TB control.[8,11] Given that TB is a notifiable disease in most countries, it is crucial to move beyond mere notification and establish mechanisms to correct any faulty management of reported cases.[11] Strengthening the linkages between the private and public sectors for the diagnosis and treatment of DRTB will not only reduce the economic burden on patients but also ensure adherence to guideline-based diagnostic and treatment practices, while improving patient's follow-up and treatment outcomes.
- *Community-based interventions*: Decentralized care models and the active involvement of community health workers are vital for improving treatment adherence and providing essential patient support. These community-based interventions ensure continuous care within local settings and help to build trust between healthcare providers and patients. Additionally, leveraging DRTB patients who have achieved successful treatment outcomes as TB champions can further strengthen these initiatives and promote effective disease management within communities. Especially in counseling or supporting to get over ADR and continuing treatment.
- *Addressing social determinants of health*: Implementing policies and programs that improve living conditions, provide nutritional support, and enhance access to healthcare can significantly impact TB control efforts. For particularly vulnerable subgroups, such as those lacking social or economic support, reopening TB sanatoria could provide essential shelter and care throughout their treatment. It is noteworthy that the Madras trial, which recommended against sanatorium-based treatment, excluded DRTB patients from its study; hence, its findings may not be directly applicable to MDR-TB cases for various reasons.[12]
- *Enhancing political commitment*: Strong political commitment is pivotal in the fight against MDR-TB. Effective public health policies, adequate funding, and robust governance structures are essential for the successful implementation and sustainability of TB control programs.
- *International support and funding*: Collaborative efforts from global health organizations, governments, and nonprofits can bridge gaps in funding and expertise. International support is vital for bolstering local capacities to manage MDR-TB effectively. Developed countries should support countries with weak healthcare systems.

The multifaceted challenges posed by MDR-TB necessitate a comprehensive and coordinated approach. Addressing medical, social, and political dimensions is essential to effectively control and eventually eliminate the disease, particularly in regions burdened with weak healthcare systems.

RECENT ADVANCES AND RESEARCH

Latest advancements in MDR-TB treatment and management: Recent advancements in the treatment of MDR-TB have culminated in the development of the all-oral 6-month BPaLM regimen, which consists of bedaquiline, pretomanid, linezolid, and moxifloxacin. This regimen has demonstrated a substantial improvement in treatment success rates, achieving an 89% success rate compared to the 52% associated with older regimens.[13] The World Health Organization (WHO) now recommends the BPaLM regimen as the standard of care for MDR-TB cases. This shorter regimen offers significant advantages, particularly in resource-limited settings, by alleviating the treatment burden on patients, enhancing adherence, and reducing the risk of loss to follow-up. However, it is essential to ensure a reliable baseline drug-sensitivity profile for all drugs in the regimen, as undiagnosed baseline resistance could lead to poor outcomes in these shorter MDR-TB regimens.[5] Furthermore, meticulous post-treatment completion follow-up monitoring is indispensable to ensure a sustained and relapse-free cure. Therefore, ongoing research in this domain is still imperative to optimize and safeguard the efficacy of this promising therapeutic approach.

Innovations in diagnostic technologies: Rapid molecular tests like Xpert *Mycobacterium tuberculosis* (MTB)/RIF enable quick detection of TB and drug resistance within hours.[14] There is a critical need for similar rapid molecular diagnostic tests detecting resistance to both first- and second-line drugs, essential for identifying MDR-TB, pre-XDR-TB, and XDR-TB.[5] this would help to avoid delays, counseling, and better adherence right from the time of first contact with the healthcare delivery system.

Vaccine development: New TB vaccines are urgently needed. The M72/AS01E candidate shows promise in preventing active TB in those with latent infection.[15] Recombinant Bacillus Calmette–Guérin (BCG) revaccination in adults also holds potential. Ongoing trials are evaluating their efficacy and safety.

CONCLUSION

Multidrug-resistant tuberculosis remains a significant obstacle to global TB elimination, particularly in regions with fragile healthcare systems. The persistence of MDR-TB is fueled by socioeconomic inequities, inadequate infrastructure, and gaps in diagnostics and treatment. While advancements in diagnostic tools and therapies exist, their limited accessibility in resource-poor settings diminishes their potential impact. The economic burden on patients, exacerbated by prolonged treatment and high out-of-pocket costs, highlights the need for a holistic and patient-centered approach. A comprehensive strategy that strengthens healthcare systems, enhances diagnostic and therapeutic capacities, and ensures equitable resource distribution is crucial. Strong public health policies, unwavering political commitment, and global collaboration are essential to overcoming these challenges. As we aim to end the TB epidemic, intensified efforts are required to address MDR-TB in high-burden, resource-limited areas, recognizing it as both a public health crisis and a moral imperative. Encouragingly, treatment for MDR-TB has proven feasible and successful even in low-resource settings, with promising results from pilot programs introducing rapid diagnostics and newer drugs. It is imperative that the same dedication shown in controlled studies is applied in real-world conditions to generalize these findings and improve community outcomes.

REFERENCES

1. Munje R, Deshmukh R, Tumane K. Multidrug-resistant TB among previously treated TB cases: A retrospective study in Nagpur, India. Indian J Tuberc. 2015;62(4):207-10.
2. World Health Organization (2023). Global tuberculosis report 2023. [online] Available from https://iris.who.int/ [Last accessed Sept., 2024].
3. Lv H, Zhang X, Zhang X, Bai J, You S, Li X, et al. Global prevalence and burden of multidrug-resistant tuberculosis from 1990 to 2019. BMC Infect Dis. 2024;24(1):1-9.
4. Chatterjee S, Das P, Stallworthy G, Bhambure G, Munje R, Vassall A. Catastrophic costs for tuberculosis patients in India: Impact of methodological choices. PLoS Global Public Health. 2024;4(4):e0003078.
5. Mishra GP, Mulani J. Implications of bedaquiline-resistant tuberculosis. Lancet Infect Dis. 2022;22(2):166.

6. Mishra GP, Gandhi SA, Ghorpade SV. Study of Various Causes of Treatment Interruption Among Tuberculosis Patients. Indian J Basic Applied Med Res. 2016;6(1):382-6.
7. Kim J, Keshavjee S, Atun R. Health systems performance in managing tuberculosis: analysis of tuberculosis care cascades among high-burden and non-high-burden countries. J Glob Health. 2019;9(1):010423.
8. Mishra G, Mulani J. Tuberculosis prescription practices in private and public sector in India. Natl J Integr Res Med. 2013;4(2):71-8.
9. Silva S, Arinaminpathy N, Atun R, Goosby E, Reid MJ. Economic Impact of TB Mortality in 120 Countries and What It Will Cost If We Don't Achieve the End TB Targets: A Full-Income Analysis. SSRN Electr J. 2020.
10. Mishra G, Mulani J. Latent Multi-drug Resistant Tuberculosis: An Unaddressed Problem. Arch Pulmonol Respir Care. 2020;6(1):084-6.
11. Mishra GP. Public-private mix in tuberculosis. Lancet Infect Dis. 2012;12(12):908-9.
12. Dawson JJ, Devadatta S, Fox W, Radhakrishna S, Ramakrishnan CV, Somasundaram PR, et al. A 5-year study of patients with pulmonary tuberculosis in a concurrent comparison of home and sanatorium treatment for one year with isoniazid plus PAS. Bull World Health Organ. 1966;34(4):533.
13. World Health Organization (WHO). (2022). WHO Consolidated Guidelines on Tuberculosis. Module 4: Treatment—Drug-Resistant Tuberculosis Treatment, 2022 Update. [online] Available from https://www.who.int/publications/i/item/9789240063129 [Last accessed Sept, 2024].
14. World Health Organization (Organization). (2021). Consolidated Guidelines on Tuberculosis Treatment. Module 3: Diagnosis. Rapid Diagnostics for Tuberculosis Detection, 2021 Update. [online] Available from https://www.who.int/tb/publications/2019/consolidated-guidelines-drug-resistant-TB-treatment/en/ [Last accessed Sept, 2024].
15. Tait DR, Hatherill M, Van Der Meeren O, Ginsberg AM, Van Brakel E, Salaun B, et al. Final Analysis of a Trial of M72/AS01E Vaccine to Prevent Tuberculosis. N Engl J Med. 2019;381(25):2429-39.

CHAPTER

2

How Multidrug-resistant Tuberculosis Poses a Major Challenge to Global TB Control Efforts?

R Sridhar, N Meenakshi

Abstract

According to Global Tuberculosis (TB) report in 2024, 87% of new cases occurred in 30 high-TB burden countries and two out of five patients with drug-resistant TB accessed treatment in 2022. The consumption expenditure incurred by multidrug-resistant tuberculosis (MDR-TB) patients were many more, when compared to drug-sensitive tuberculosis (DSTB). There is an urgent need for the effective implementation of Universal Health Coverage in low- and middle-income countries with a well-knit social protection scheme and rapid scale up of rapid molecular diagnostic test [WHO-recommended rapid diagnostic (WRD) test], and newer regimens such as bedaquiline, pretomanid, and linezolid (BPaL)/bedaquiline, pretomanid linezolid, and moxifloxacin (BPaLM) to increase the drug-resistant TB (DRTB) cases diagnosed, to improve the cure rate, and to decrease the economic burden of treating DRTB in these countries.

Keywords: Drug-resistant TB, rapid molecular test, universal health coverage, BPaL/BPaLM regimens

INTRODUCTION

According to Global Tuberculosis (TB) Report, in 2022, 87% of new TB cases occurred in 30 high-TB burden countries. Only two out of five people with drug-resistant TB (DRTB) accessed treatment in 2022. Globally, about 50% of TB patient and their households face total costs (direct and indirect) that are catastrophic. Under the above-mentioned circumstances rapid molecular diagnostic tests for the diagnosis of DRTB and shorter multidrug-resistant (MDR)/extensively drug-resistant tuberculosis (XDRTB) treatment regimens are the need of the hour to bring down the level of infectious DRTB patients.

Three countries accounted for 42% of the estimated global number of people who developed MDR/rifampicin-resistant tuberculosis (RRTB) in 2022—India (27%), Philippines (7.5%), and Russian Federation (7.5%).

A World Health Organization (WHO)-recommended rapid diagnosis test (WRD) was used as the initial test for 47% of the 7.5 million people newly diagnosed with TB in 2022. Higher level of coverage was in the European region 77%, Western Pacific Region 65%, and lower was in the South-East Asian Region 39%. As per the global target set in 2023 coverage of "Rapid Diagnostic Testing for TB" should be reached to 100% by 2027.

UNIVERSAL HEALTH COVERAGE[1]

The WHO is developing a post-2015 Global Strategy, which highlights the need for all countries to progress toward Universal Health Coverage to ensure universal access to needed health services without financial hardship in paying for them, as well as *Social Protection Mechanisms* for income replacement and social support in the event of illness. Social protection involves scheme to cover costs beyond direct medical cost, including compensation of lost income. Examples of social protection schemes include sickness insurance, disability grants, other conditional or unconditional cash transfers, food assistance, travel vouchers, and other support packages.[2]

FINANCIAL BURDEN FOR LOW- AND MIDDLE-INCOME COUNTRIES

As per the systematic review done by Tadayuki Tanimura et al.,[3] covering 49 studies revealed on average cost incurred before TB treatment was initiated and represented 50% of the total cost **(Fig. 1)**. Indirect costs dominated both before and during treatment, and direct costs were relatively more important before than during treatment.

Total cost for MDR-TB was higher when compared with drug-sensitive tuberculosis (DSTB)—total costs as percentage of reported individual income for MDR-TB patients and DSTB patients were 223% versus 31% in Ecuador, 76% versus 24% in Cambodia and 34% versus 27% in Brazil.

Commonly reported coping mechanisms included taking a loan, selling household items, using savings, and transfers from relatives.

How to reduce the burden of multidrug-resistant tuberculosis treatment costs?

Cost of treatment of DRTB patients is a key healthcare challenge for most low- and middle-income countries. Cost-saving and cost-effective DRTB treatment options are critically needed to reduce the economic pressure in these countries.

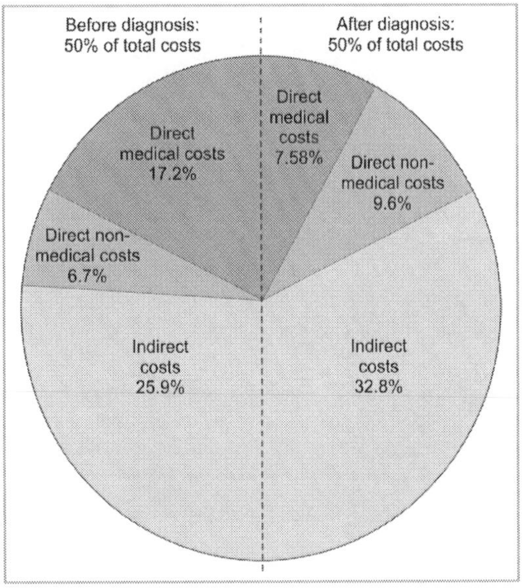

FIG. 1: Breakdown of direct and indirect costs before and during treatment (eight studies) percentages are proportion of respective subcomponent cost out of the total cost.

TB Alliance and the Swiss Tropical and Public Health Institute have developed SLASH-TB (Savings from Leveraging and Adopting Shorter and Highly Effective TB Treatments).[4] The tool calculates the costs and cost-effectiveness when a country continues with the standard regimens compared using bedaquiline, pretomanid, and linezolid (BPaL) and bedaquiline, pretomanid, linezolid, and moxifloxacin (BPaLM).[5] Applied the tool for four countries Pakistan, the Philippines, South Africa, and Ukraine.

Table 1 gives the cost comparison for these four countries.[5]

TABLE 1: Cost comparison for SSOR, SLOR, BPaL, and BPaLM.

					Savings when using BPaL/M instead of SSOR and SLOR	
Regimen outcome	**SSOR (USD)**	**SLOR (USD)**	**BPaL (USD)**	**BPaLM (USD)**	**Annual**	**Per patient**
Pakistan						
Estimated number of patients on treatment in 2022, *n*	2,839	982	1,201	2,620		
Total cost	3,598,662	3,142,085	1,195,782	2,694,750	2,850,215	746
Per patient cost	1,268	3,200	996	1,029	42%	
Cost per successful treatment with SSOR/SLOR versus BPaL/BPaLM	2,271		1,112			
Philippines						
Estimated number of patients on treatment in 2022, *n*	5,154	2,501	161	7,494		
Total cost	9,115,023	6,507,564	246,336	11,714,494	3,661,758	478
Cost per successful treatment with SSOR/SLOR versus BPaL/BPaLM	2,698		1,685			
South Africa						
Estimated number of patients on treatment in 2022, *n*	4,965	2,820	730	6,665		
Total cost	6,237,855	9,449,067	950,968	8,839,013	5,896,940	757
Per patient cost	1,256	3,351	1,303	1,328	38%	
Cost per successful treatment with SSOR/SLOR versus BPaL/BPaLM	3,268		1,437			
Ukraine						
Estimated number of patients on treatment in 2022, *n*	2,581	2,709	1,642	3,648		

Continued

Continued

Regimen outcome	SSOR (USD)	SLOR (USD)	BPaL (USD)	BPaLM (USD)	Savings when using BPaL/M instead of SSOR and SLOR	
					Annual	Per patient
Per patient cost	3,394	6,920	2,545	2,573	51%	
Cost per successful treatment with SSOR/ SLOR versus BPaL/ BPaLM	7,969		2,739			

(BPaL: bedaquiline, pretomanid, and linezolid; BPaLM: bedaquiline, pretomanid, linezolid, and moxifloxacin; SLOR: standard long oral regimen; SSOR: standard short oral regimen)

TABLE 2: Budget impact analysis: Savings when switching from SSOR and SLOR to BPaL/ BPaLM.

	Pakistan		Philippines		South Africa		Ukraine	
	5-year span	10-year span	5-year span	10-year span	5-year span	10-year span	5-year span	10-year span
Number of people treated	32,812	81,481	74,946	154,216	48,069	97,119	30,551	71,512
Total savings	14,002,655	37,678,985	23,153,108	53,301,425	34,430,535	69,563,734	61,606,894	152,921,201
Provider cost saving	13,457,879	36,211,235	19,408,472	44,797,456	30,152,151	60,919,652	46,114,424	114,373,593
Patient cost saving	544,776	1,467,751	3,744,636	8,503,969	4,278,384	8,644,082	15,492,470	38,547,608
Savings per patient	427	462	309	346	716	716	2,017	2,138
Total savings, %	44	48	15	17	36	40	60	65%

(BPaL: bedaquiline, pretomanid, and linezolid; BPaLM: bedaquiline, pretomanid, linezolid, and moxifloxacin; SLOR: standard long oral regimen; SSOR: standard short oral regimen)

INCREMENTAL EFFECTIVES

In the four analyzed countries, the treatment success rate for standard short oral regimen (SSOR) ranged between 67 and 81%.

- *Standard long oral regimen (SLOR)*: 53–73%
- *BPAL/BPALM*: 90%

Using BPaL/BPaLM instead of SSOR and SLOR not only results in considerable cost savings but leads to an increased number of patients annually with successful treatment outcomes.

SAVINGS (TABLE 2)[5]

Over 5 years, depending on each country's DRTB burden and the speed of switch from current to new TB regimens, the savings are 44%, 15%, 36%, and 60% for Pakistan, Philippines, South Africa, and Ukraine, respectively.

CONCLUSION

There is an urgent need for adopting "Universal Health Coverage" for all the low- and middle-income countries in order to effectively address DSTB and DRTB. Availability of rapid molecular diagnostic test and shorter regimens like BPaL/BPaLM for DRTB will reduce the economic burden of the countries and, in turn, will achieve better cure rates, reduction in the pool of infectious cases and lesser transmission in the society resulting in long-term gain for these countries. Social protection schemes are the need of the hour to cut down both direct and indirect cost of this diagnostic and treatment of DRTB, reducing the catastrophic costs incurred by patients and their family members.

REFERENCES

1. World Health Organization. (2010). The world health report: Health System Financing: The path to universal Coverage 2010, Geneva. [online] Available from https://iris.who.int/handle/10665/44371 [Last accessed Sept., 2024].
2. International Labour Office (ILO) and the World Health Organization (WHO). (2009). A joint crisis initiative of the UN Chief executive board for co-ordination on the social protection floor Geneva: The Social Protection Floor 2009. [online] Available from chrome-extension://efaidnbmnnnibpcajpcglclefindmkaj/https://www.un.org/en/ga/second/64/socialprotection.pdf [Last accessed Sept., 2024].
3. Tanimura T, Jaramillo E, Weil D, Raviglione M, Lonnorth K. Financial burden for tuberculosis patients in low- and middle-income countries: a systematic review. Eur Respir J. 2014;43:1763-75.
4. Institute for Health Metrics and evaluation. (2020). Global Burden of disease collaborative network, Global Burden of Disease Study 2019 (GBD 2019 results – Seattle, WA USA). [online] Available from https://ghdx.healthdata.org/gbd-2019. [Last accessed Sept., 2024].
5. Auer C, Gupta A, Malbacius C, Ghafoor A, Kock Y, Medvedieva O, et al. Savings from the introduction of BPaL and BPaLM regimens at the country level. IJTLD Open. 2024;1(7):314-9.

CHAPTER

3

Hotspots of Drug-resistant Tuberculosis as Key Drivers of Epidemic Intelligence for Public Health Action

Shikha Dhawan

Abstract

India accounts for the largest global drug-resistant tuberculosis (DRTB) burden. Population-based estimation of DRTB hotspots can guide effective prevention and control strategies. A mix of conventional and modern methods is essential for mapping DRTB hotspots to provide valuable information on drug-resistance patterns and transmission dynamics of resistant strains to guide public health action and policy decisions to allocate resources and services.

Keywords: Epidemic intelligence, hotspots, drug-resistant tuberculosis, National Tuberculosis Elimination Program, Universal Drug Susceptibility Testing, heatmaps

INTRODUCTION

Epidemiological indicator of effective implementation of the National TB Elimination Program (NTEP), Government of India, is the primary and acquired resistance to the anti-TB drugs. As TB-causing bacteria are airborne, primary resistance develops through transmission from a drug-resistant tuberculosis (DRTB) affected patient while emergence of secondary or acquired resistance is multifactorial due to the health system and patient-related factors. Hence, reliable estimates of DRTB are crucial for NTEP to upscale and strategize DRTB management. Thwarting TB and DRTB transmission can be achieved by relentless TB infection control measures, augmenting screening efforts by mapping hotspots and protecting the most vulnerable from becoming victims to this scourge. Strengthening laboratory capacity for quality assured diagnostic, treatment, and care are also crucial to hammer the nail for management of all forms of TB. The need of the hour is to strengthen epidemic intelligence for public health interventions catering to local geographies and demographics.

DRUG-RESISTANT TB SCENARIO IN INDIA

The NTEP outlines drug-resistant patterns based on drug susceptibility as multi-drug resistant (MDR), mono rifampicin resistant (RR), pre-extensively drug-resistant (XDR) with resistance to rifampicin (MDR/RR) plus any fluoroquinolone (FQ), XDR with resistance to rifampicin (MDR/RR), plus any FQ with bedaquiline and/or linezolid and isoniazid (INH)-resistant.[1] As per the India TB report (2023), the estimated incidence of

MDR/RR TB in the country was 119,000 (2021). In 2022, the MDR/RR cases increased by 32% with total 63,801 diagnosed cases comprising 12,002 pre-XDR, 85 XDR and 15,953 INH mono-/poly-DRTB. Of these 91% were initiated on treatment and from the 2021 cohort, 82% were successfully treated.[1]

NATIONAL ANTI-TB DRUG RESISTANCE SURVEY

The National Anti-TB Drug Resistance Survey (2014–2016) deployed drug susceptibility testing of 5,280 samples from 120 tuberculosis units (TU) across the country. The survey demonstrated the prevalence of DRTB to be 6.19% [confidence interval (CI) 5.54–6.90%] among all cases of TB with new cases being 2.84% (CI 2.27–3.50%) while previously treated were 11.60% (CI 10.21–13.15%).[2] Add on resistance to any FQ and any second-line injectable drug was 21.82% (CI 17.33–26.87%) and 3.58% (CI 1.8–6.32%), respectively.[2] Alarming high-isoniazid resistance 11.06% (CI 9.97–12.22%) and 25.09% (CI 23.1–27.11%) was reported in new and previously treated cases.[2] Resistance to any first- or second-line anti-TB drug was 28.0% (CI 26.77–29.29%) that encompassed 22.54% (CI 21.10–24.10%) from new cases and 36.82% (CI 34.64–39.04%) from previously treated cases while prevalence of XDR-TB was 1.3% (CI 0.36–3.30%).[2] An interesting finding was the absence of mono-RR in new TB cases and was always associated with INH resistance.[2] The study findings exemplified the need to strengthen our fight against DRTB and make key changes in the manner DRTB is managed in the country.

WHY ARE WE FAILING TO MANAGE DRUG-RESISTANT TUBERCULOSIS?

India stands at the top with regard to the highest (27%) global MDR/RR TB burden followed by the Philippines (7.5%) and the Russian Federation (7.5%).[3] Crackdown on DRTB requires microbiological confirmation of TB causing bacteria along with its drug-susceptibility profiles deciphered through culture methods, molecular tests, or sequencing methods. With the launch of Universal Drug Susceptibility Testing (UDST), NTEP has made major strides in upfront diagnosis of DRTB by combining (CBNAAT/TrueNat), line probe assay (LPA) (first- and second-line), and liquid culture and drug-susceptibility testing (C&DST) in a logically integrated DRTB diagnostic and treatment algorithm. Yet, the country is plagued to bridge the diagnostic and treatment delays for DRTB that fuel primary transmission. We are also struggling to manage socioeconomic determinants of TB and DRTB like poverty, low literacy, overcrowding, and malnutrition in addition to health systems gaps in infrastructure and facilities.

Drug-resistant tuberculosis diagnostic services are still limited at peripheral laboratories. Regular need for specimen transport to centralized laboratories for extended drug-susceptibility testing leads to patient's loss, diagnostic delays, impediment in treatment initiation, and patients' shopping for health in the unregulated private sector with huge out of pocket expenditures. Poor DRTB treatment outcomes are due to inherent limitations in missed drug mutations by the available diagnostic arsenal compounded with diagnostic capacity gaps, nonadherence to toxic drugs, inadequate treatment, mono-isoniazid resistance, over-the-counter (OTC) misuse of FQs, delay in regimen modification for nonresponders, individualized treatment management, rudimentary infection prevention measures interlinked with patient and the providing health system fueled lacunas. Though, the NTEP has rolled out shorter and oral DRTB regimens, the country is yet to reap its benefits as beneficiaries' enrollment is limited due to the rampant background drug resistance to FQs, adherence challenges and adverse drug reactions to toxic drugs.

IS HOTSPOT MAPPING THE ANSWER TO EFFECTIVELY MANAGE DRUG-RESISTANT TUBERCULOSIS IN INDIA?

Being a vast country, the burden of DRTB is heterogenous across India. Populous metros and multiple geographies in India with easy access to DRTB diagnostic facilities and fulfillment of UDST report local clusters of hotspots of DRTB.[4,5] However, there is an urgent need for epidemiologically relevant geographical surveillance to identify hotspots of DRTB and guide epidemic intelligence. Cluster-based analysis would be useful to decipher if geographically bundled DRTB cases grouping around high population densities are a chance phenomenon or are statistically insignificant spatial clusters of low values.[4] Spatial correlations over time may also be used to study whether the patterns are clustered, dispersed, or random to reflect availability and access to diagnostic tests for DRTB in the given geography. The benefits of hotspot mapping include improved surveillance to identify geographical information systems (GISs) tagged clusters of DRTB cases for better targeted interventions and public health action such as intensified case finding, contact tracing, drug susceptibility testing, linkage to treatment and care and guiding resource allocation and equity in improving resilience for DRTB management.

Choropleth thematic maps are used to visualize the distribution of DRTB cases over large geographic areas. These maps use varying colors or shades to represent different variables in data sets to provide visual representation of spatial patterns within the framework of regional boundaries. Heatmaps are another effective way for visualizing hotspots of DRTB cases. They display the density and distribution of individual data points in more details based on latitude and longitude or the address of the reported case. These maps can be used to identify clusters of high DRTB incidence that can be shown to have correlation with diverse local variables like access to quality-assured diagnosis, treatment facilities, urban versus rural areas, population density, socioeconomic factors, education, gender, family size, family income, past history of TB, indoor pollution, alcohol use, smoking, diabetes, hypertension, etc. Data over multiple years can also be analyzed for temporal trends in incidence of DRTB over time. Hotspots thus plotted can be used to direct resources and interventions where they are most needed by informing public health policies and strategies for prevention and control.

Sequencing-based hotspot mapping linked to GIS tagged clusters is another approach to enrich knowledge on understanding transmission dynamics of DRTB strains. It strengthens molecular epidemiology to guide strategies for individualized treatment regimens based on accurate resistance prediction thereby fostering a healthy provider and beneficiary relationship with better treatment outcomes. Though sequencing-based DRTB hotspot mapping is cost intensive and other challenges include need for specialized trained manpower and data analysis acumen, it is a powerful tool as it detects novel mutations missed by other diagnostics. Investments in sequencing techniques and molecular epidemiology will bolster public health action and control strategies. It will also shed light on transmission dynamics and save lives through appropriate drug regimen, strengthen prevention measures and augment treatment outcomes. This has been elaborated by a year-wise hotspot analysis study that showed new hotspots arising in the proximity of the old hotspots suggesting community-based primary transmission mandating better risk determination, intensified surveillance, and management of DRTB.[4]

Studying hotspots is also essential as the DRTB clusters may be limited to specific regions requiring local interventions but will drive the overall prevalence of a state as seen in case of Sahariya tribes in Madhya Pradesh and Mumbai, Maharashtra. The Sahariya tribes of Madhya Pradesh have higher DRTB prevalence in new TB cases (9.9%), a situation exacerbated by lack of access to quality-assured public diagnostic facilities, illiteracy, poverty, malnutrition, and unregulated private sector.[6] Mumbai is a well-established hotspot of primary DRTB (7.72%) due to higher prevalence of human immunodeficiency virus (HIV)/acquired immunodeficiency syndrome (AIDS), unregulated private sector, previously treated cases, poverty, malnutrition, and population living in unventilated overcrowded slums.[2,7] Undiagnosed DRTB cases are fueling community-wide primary transmission in Mumbai thumping the need for localized intensified active case finding by engaging community-based civil organizations, treatment supporters, and molecular epidemiology to sequence the transmitting-resistant strains. Localized interventions guided by hotspot mapping thus have the potential to either revitalize better adherence to first-line anti-TB drugs in case of secondary DRTB transmission or to revamp the prevention and control aspects of programmatic management of drug-resistant TB (PMDT) in case of primary DRTB transmission.

CONCLUSION

Recognizing transmission dynamics and DRTB hotspots in community settings using conventional and modern approaches are crucial. A better understanding of hotspots leveraged from patterns of drug resistance and strains is essential for guided interventions in high-burden areas to foster success in DRTB management. Multipronged interventions encompassing government leadership, infection prevention strategies, ramping diagnostic infrastructure, resistance-guided individualized treatment and curtailing primary transmission are instrumental to make progress against DRTB and ultimately to achieve India's TB elimination goals.

REFERENCES

1. Central TB Division, DGHS, MOHFW. (2023). India TB Report 2023, National TB Elimination Program, Annual Status Report. [online] Available from tbcindia.mohfw.gov.in/wp-content/uploads/2023/05/5646719104TB_AR_2023_04-04-2023_LRP_final.pdf. [Last accessed Sept, 2024].
2. Ministry of Health and Family Welfare , Government of India. (2023). First National anti-TB Drug resistance Survey India (NDRS) (2014–2016). [online] Available from https://tbcindia.mohfw.gov.in/wp-content/uploads/2023/05/4187947827National-Anti-TB-Drug-Resistance-Survey.pdf [Last accessed Sept, 2024].
3. World Health Organization. (2023). Global Tuberculosis Report 2023. [online] Available from https://iris.who.int/bitstream/handle/10665/373828/9789240083851-eng.pdf?sequence=1 [Last accessed Sept, 2024].
4. Ladha N, Bhardwaj P, Chauhan NK, Naveen KHS, Nag VL, Giribabu D. Determinants, risk factors and spatial analysis of multidrug resistant pulmonary tuberculosis in Jodhpur, India. Monaldi Arch Chest Dis. 2022;92(4).
5. Dorjee K, Sadutshang TD, Rana RS, Topgyal S, Phunkyi D, Choetso T, et al. High prevalence of rifampin-resistant tuberculosis in mountainous districts of India. Indian J Tuberc. 2020;67(1):59-64.
6. Prakash R, Kumar D, Gupta VK, Jain S, Chauhan DS, Tiwari PK, et al. Status of multidrug resistant tuberculosis (MDR-TB) among the Sahariya tribe of North Central India. J Infect Public Health. 2016;9:289-97.
7. FirstPost. (2023). TB trends in Mumbai: Past, present and future. [online] Available from https://www.firstpost.com/health/tb-trends-in-mumbai-past-present-and-future-13139522.html, 2023. [Last accessed Sept., 2024].

CHAPTER

4

Antibiotic Resistance Factors in Multidrug-resistant Tuberculosis

Karthikasri K, Shobana S

Abstract

This review investigates the factors influencing antibiotic resistance in multidrug-resistant tuberculosis (MDR-TB). The primary focus of this review is on genetic mutations that provide resistance to both first-line and second-line anti-TB medications. It also examines the impacts of efflux pump mechanisms, cell wall changes, and metabolic adjustments on developing resistance to antibiotics. The review also discusses how persistence, dormancy, and compensatory mutations boost resistance and assist in bacterial survival. Additionally, it explores how horizontal gene transfer, epigenetic elements, and the formation of biofilms affect drug resistance. These multiple resistance mechanisms highlight the challenges in managing and controlling TB infections, especially MDR-TB. Understanding the factors of antibiotic resistance is essential for creating new diagnostic tools, treatment strategies, and targeted medications. Dealing with MDR-TB requires a comprehensive strategy involving advances in drug development, enhanced diagnostics, and specialized treatment methods due to the complexity of drug resistance in *Mycobacterium tuberculois* (*M. tuberculosis*). As the bacteria continues to adapt and develop new forms of resistance, ongoing research and surveillance of the evolution of MDR-TB are important in addressing the challenges of controlling and treating TB. This review helps in the understanding of resistance mechanisms as it is necessary for healthcare professionals and researchers to possess a comprehensive knowledge to address the worldwide problem of drug-resistant TB effectively.

Keywords: Drug-resistant tuberculosis, genetic mutations, efflux pumps, metabolic adaptations, persistence, and dormancy

INTRODUCTION

Multidrug-resistant strains of tuberculosis are the main reason why TB continues to remain a health challenge across the globe. The evolution of complex drug resistance mechanisms in *Mycobacterium tuberculosis* arises from various genetic and physiological mechanisms including the mutations in specific genes conferring resistance to first-line and second-line anti-TB drugs, efflux pump mechanisms, cell wall modifications, and metabolic adaptations. The treatment of *M. tuberculosis* remains difficult due to its ability to persist and remain dormant, which makes the bacteria survive even in the presence of antibiotics. Additionally, compensatory mutations help multidrug-resistant tuberculosis (MDR-TB) strains to keep their virulence and transmission ability. Even though horizontal gene transfer (HGT) is less frequent in *M. tuberculosis* than in other bacteria, it helps in the acquisition of resistance genes. Epigenetic factors and biofilm formation enhance the bacteria's resistance to antibiotics, highlighting the complex nature of drug resistance in TB.

GENETIC MUTATIONS CONFERRING RESISTANCE TO FIRST-LINE ANTITUBERCULOSIS DRUGS

The key to the development and spread of drug-resistant TB are the mutations in the genes that resist the first line of anti-TB drugs. Isoniazid resistance generally occurs due to mutations in the *katG* gene and *inhA* promoter region, whereas rifampicin resistance is primarily caused by mutations in the *rpoB* gene, specifically within the 81 base pair rifampicin-resistance-determining region (RRDR).[1] Ethambutol resistance is caused by mutations in the *embB* gene at the codon 306, whereas pyrazinamide resistance is caused by a variety of mutations in the *pncA* gene. Streptomycin resistance is caused by mutations in the *rpsL* and *rrs* genes. Combinations of these mutations, plus additional genetic changes, result in MDR-TB and extensively drug-resistant TB (XDR-TB). Understanding these changes is critical for developing rapid molecular diagnostic tests and guiding effective treatment plans.

RESISTANCE MECHANISMS AGAINST SECOND-LINE TUBERCULOSIS DRUGS

Challenges in treating drug-resistant tuberculosis also arise due to new resistance mechanisms against second-line TB drugs. Genetic mutations and physiological adaptations are the mechanisms through which *M. tuberculosis* resists the effects of the antibiotics. Mutations in the *gyrB* gene as well as overexpression of efflux pumps contribute to resistance against fluoroquinolones. Mutations in the *tlyA* gene and *eis* promoter region causes resistance against injectable agents. Mutations in *atpE* and *Rv0678* genes cause bedaquiline resistance, while delamanid resistance involves alterations in *fgd1, ddn,* and *fbi* genes. Linezolid resistance results from mutations in *rplC* and *23S* rRNA.

Clofazimine and bedaquiline share cross-resistance mechanisms and pretomanid resistance is like that of delamanid. Cycloserine and para-amino salicylic acid resistances are caused by mutations in *alr* and *folC* genes, respectively.[2] Processes such as higher efflux pump function and changes in cell wall permeability can provide resistance to various type of drugs. Comprehending these distinct resistance mechanisms is essential for developing new diagnostic tools and implementing better drug treatments.

EFFLUX PUMP MECHANISMS IN MULTIDRUG-RESISTANT TUBERCULOSIS STRAINS

Efflux pump mechanisms are significantly involved in the survival of MDR-TB strains during antibiotic treatment. Efflux pumps in *M. tuberculosis* are protein complexes found in the cell membrane that function by reducing intracellular drug levels to sublethal amounts. In MDR-TB strains, many efflux pump systems play a key role in conferring resistance. The most significant include the MmpL (mycobacterial membrane protein large) family, particularly *MmpL5*, which is known to be resistant against bedaquiline and clofazimine.

Overexpression of genes encoding these pumps, which is commonly caused by mutations in the regulatory genes like *Rv0678*, resulting in increased drug efflux. *Rv1258c* which encodes for the Tap efflux pump contributes to resistance against rifampicin and several other antibiotics,[3] which encodes for the P55 pump is involved in resistance against drugs such as rifampicin, clofazimine, and bedaquiline. To develop a high level of resistance, these efflux pump mechanisms frequently interact with other resistance mechanisms, such as target mutations and the complexity of these efflux systems in *M. tuberculosis* possesses a greater challenge for the drug development and treatment strategies.

ROLE OF MYCOBACTERIAL CELL WALL MODIFICATIONS IN DRUG RESISTANCE

The mycobacterial cell wall has a unique structure with a high amount of lipids and complexity, which serves as a built-in protection against numerous antibiotics and the mutations in the cell wall enhanced resistant to drugs. Alterations in the composition and structure of mycolic acid are important because they affect the cell wall permeability and fluidity. Gene mutations such as *kasA* and *inhA* related to mycolic acid biosynthesis not only provide resistance to drugs such as isoniazid but also aids in the reduction of cell wall permeability.

In addition, changes in arabinogalactan and peptidoglycan layers might affect the penetration of drugs such as ethambutol. Some resistant bacteria produce extracellular polymeric substances (EPSs), which creates an additional physical barrier to drug penetration. Modifications in cell wall proteins and porins contribute to the resistance by limiting the influx of antibiotics. Importantly, these cell wall modifications frequently interact with other resistance mechanisms, such as efflux pumps and drug-modifying enzymes, to form a multifaceted defense against antibiotics.

ANTIBIOTIC TOLERANCE PROMOTED DUE TO METABOLIC ADAPTATIONS

In TB infections, dormancy and/or persistence are the metabolic adaptations which enable the bacteria to enter a state of decreased metabolic activity. These modifications make the bacteria less susceptible to antibiotics that target actively dividing cells. One of the primary adaptations involves the transitioning to alternative energy sources and metabolic pathways. During TB infection, bacteria make use of lipids as their main carbon source which also leads to higher antibiotic tolerance. To order to withstand host immune responses and exposure to antibiotics, the bacteria activate the stress response pathways, such as the dormancy survival regulon (DosR).

The modulation of central carbon metabolism is one other important adaptation. The tricarboxylic acid (TCA) cycle can affect the production of reactive oxygen species and the bactericidal activity of some antibiotics. The bacteria can also enter a state of replicative quiescence, making them less susceptible to drugs that target cell division mechanisms. Moreover, *M. tuberculosis* can create small colony variants with altered metabolism, thereby increasing their resistance to antibiotics. The synthesis of specialized metabolites like mycothiol helps to defend against oxidative stress caused by both host defenses and certain antibiotics.

PERSISTENCE AND DORMANCY LINKS TO ANTIBIOTIC RESISTANCE

The key factors contributing to the antibiotic resistance are the persistence and dormancy, which make the TB treatment and control more challenging. The bacteria enter a state of metabolic dormancy or reduced growth, allowing them to survive in environments with antibiotics and developing high tolerance to most antibiotics that target actively growing cells. This tolerance is caused by physiological adaptations rather than genetic changes, resulting in a subpopulation of persister cells capable of withstanding drug treatment. The activation of stress response pathways is the key to this process, particularly the DosR, which regulates multiple genes involved in metabolic slowdown.[4]

Persisters exhibit altered cell wall composition and decreased permeability, which improves their drug tolerance. These dormant bacteria can become active under suitable conditions, potentially resulting in the relapse of the infection. The bacteria acquire genetic mutations during its switch between active and dormant states which confer resistance when exposed to sublethal antibiotic concentrations. Persistence and its associated evolution of genetically encoded resistance highlights the challenge in eliminating TB infections. Additionally, the use of prolonged and multiple-drug treatment strategies is required due to the presence of various bacterial subgroups with diverse metabolic processes in an organism.

COMPENSATORY MUTATIONS ENHANCING THE RESISTANCE

In the MDR-TB strains, compensatory mutations improve the resistance to a greater extent. These genetic mutations enable the MDR-TB strains to maintain their virulence and their ability to transmit while also maintaining their resistance characteristics. An example could be mutations in *rpoA* and *rpoC* genes, which encode for RNA polymerase subunits, can counterbalance the negative effects caused by *rpoB* mutations in strains resistant to rifampicin.[5] In isoniazid-resistant strains, mutations in the *ahpC* promoter region compensates for the decrease in catalase-peroxidase activity due to *katG* mutations. Compensatory genetic mutations in the *rpsL* or *gidB* genes help in restoring the functionality of the ribosomes in strains resistant to streptomycin. These adaptive alterations not only help to stabilize the MDR-TB strains but also improve their growth rates and their survival ability in stressful conditions. Notable compensatory mutations can amplify resistance to the original drug or confer resistance to alternative antibiotics.

HORIZONTAL GENE TRANSFER AND ACQUISITION OF RESISTANCE

In *M. tuberculosis*, HGT is a less common phenomenon than in other bacterial pathogens, but this plays a notable role in the acquisition of drug resistance and genetic diversity. Due to its intracellular nature and lack of plasmids, *M. tuberculosis* has been considered to have limited potential for genetic exchange. Nevertheless, recent studies have shown that HGT does take place in *M. tuberculosis*, mainly via conjugation, transduction, and, to a lesser extent, transformation. Conjugation allows for the movement of large portions of genomic DNA between mycobacterial cells, which may also include the genes for drug resistance. Through the integration of prophages, phage-mediated transduction can introduce new genetic elements which confer resistance. Though rare, it has been experimentally demonstrated that even transformations have the possibility of resistance gene acquisition from lysed bacteria in mixed infections.

The transfer of genomic islands related to virulence or resistance has been noted, demonstrating the bacteria's ability to adapt. Although HGT events are not as common in *M. tuberculosis* as they are in other bacteria, their occurrence highlights the ability of rapid evolution of drug resistance. This phenomenon emphasizes the significance of continuous surveillance of resistance patterns and the need for strategies to control the dissemination of new resistance mechanisms among TB populations.

EPIGENETIC FACTORS CONTRIBUTING TO ANTIBIOTIC RESISTANCE

Heritable changes in gene expression without DNA sequence alterations are referred to as epigenetic factors. Several mechanisms of epigenetics influence the resistance in *M. tuberculosis*. Alterations in the DNA methylation patterns can affect gene expression. For instance, the methylation of the *iniBAC* promoter region leads to increased expression of these genes responsible for resistance against isoniazid. Modifying histone-like proteins such as *Lsr2* can alter the chromatin structure and accessibility of genes, which can influence the expression of multiple genes, including the genes related to drug efflux mechanisms.

Under stress conditions, small regulatory RNAs like *MTS1338* may impact antibiotic tolerance through the regulation of cell wall lipid composition. Antibiotics or host immune factors may result in stress-induced epigenetic changes that cause adaptive responses, such as the increased expression of efflux pumps like *Rv1258c* when exposed to rifampicin. These factors are involved in regulating persistence and dormancy, as demonstrated by the epigenetic regulation of the *dosR* regulon, which is crucial for antibiotic tolerance in dormant cells. Some of these epigenetic modifications may be inherited across bacterial generations, and may potentially create stable antibiotic-tolerant subpopulations, as seen in the heritable phenotypic heterogeneity of mycobacterial populations.

IMPACT OF BIOFILM FORMATION ON DRUG RESISTANCE

Bacterial communities surrounded within the extracellular matrix produced by themselves impact drug resistance through different mechanisms. The matrix acts as a physical barrier, preventing the entry of antibiotics, particularly hydrophilic drugs, into the cells. Cells within the biofilm show variation in metabolism, with some becoming dormant or growing slowly, which hinders the effectiveness of antibiotics targeting actively growing cells. Quorum-sensing facilitates coordinated resistance mechanisms and controls the resistance gene expression. Certain biofilms produce enzymes that break down or modify antibiotics, while the hypoxic microenvironment in thick biofilms affects antibiotic activity and alters bacterial metabolism. Moreover, biofilms shield bacteria from the immune system of the host, ultimately aiding in antibiotic resistance through prolonged survival.

CONCLUSION

The complex nature of drug-resistant mechanisms in *M. tuberculosis* underscores the difficulty in managing and addressing TB infections. Comprehending these various resistance pathways is crucial for the development of new diagnostic tools, treatment approaches, and drug targets. A comprehensive approach is necessary to tackle MDR-TB due to the interactions between genetic mutations, physiological adaptations, and environmental factors. Ongoing research and monitoring are crucial to stay ahead of emerging resistance patterns as the bacteria keep evolving and adapting. In the end, dealing with the problem of MDR-TB involves a multi-faceted strategy incorporating new drug research, enhanced testing, and specific treatment plans for the resistance mechanisms involved.

REFERENCES

1. Libiseller-Egger J, Phelan J, Campino S, Mohareb F, Clark TG. Robust detection of point mutations involved in multidrug-resistant *Mycobacterium tuberculosis* in the presence of co-occurrent resistance markers. PLoS Comput Biol. 2020;16(12):e1008518.
2. Chizimu JY, Solo ES, Bwalya P, Kapalamula TF, Mwale KK, Squarre D, et al. Genomic Analysis of *Mycobacterium tuberculosis* Strains Resistant to Second-Line Anti-Tuberculosis Drugs in Lusaka, Zambia. Antibiotics. 2023;12(7):1126.
3. Farzaneh SS, Norouzi F, Fazeli H, Salehi M, Safari M, Esfahani BN. Novel mutation in efflux pump Rv1258c (Tap) gene in drug resistant clinical isolates of *Mycobacterium tuberculosis* in Iran. J Infect Dev Ctries. 2024;18(2):235-42.
4. Zeng S, Yang D, Rens C, Fontaine V. The *Mycobacterium bovis* BCG GroEL1 Contributes to Isoniazid Tolerance in a Dormant-Like State Model. Microorganisms. 2023;11(2):286.
5. Napier G, Campino S, Phelan JE, Clark TG. Large-scale genomic analysis of *Mycobacterium tuberculosis* reveals extent of target and compensatory mutations linked to multi-drug resistant tuberculosis. Sci Rep. 2023;13(1):623.

CHAPTER

5

Trends in Multidrug-resistant Tuberculosis

Nishi Aggarwal, Sanjay Rajpal, Kamal Chopra

Abstract

The increasing prevalence of multidrug-resistant tuberculosis (MDR-TB) presents a major global public health challenge, especially in countries such as India, China, and Russia, which carry a large portion of the TB burden. The rise of MDR-TB and XDR-TB, which increase the risk of death in TB patients, is major challenge. The present article reviews trends, challenges, and prevalence globally and in India, emphasizing the need for improved surveillance and diagnostic capacities.

Keywords: Tuberculosis, multidrug resistance, TB prevalence, TB incidence, XDR-TB

INTRODUCTION

Tuberculosis (TB) is a significant health challenge globally, with an estimated incidence of 10.6 million new cases, and there were 1.6 million deaths reported occurring in 2021 globally.[1]

Multidrug-resistant TB (MDR-TB), a severe form of drug-resistant TB, continues to present a threat to global TB control efforts. India has the highest MDR-TB (26%) burden.[2] MDR-TB is caused by bacilli, which is resistant to rifampicin and isoniazid, due to improper use of antibiotics during treatment the disease becomes more challenging to treat and increases the risk of transmission.[3] About 464,000 global cases of rifampicin-resistant TB, 78% of which were MDR-TB, were noticed globally in 2019,[4,5] and approximately 25% of deaths related to TB can be attributed to antimicrobial drug resistance.[6] There were an estimated 450,000 MDR-TB cases in 2021, representing a 3.1% increase from the previous year.[4]

The aim to cut global TB deaths by 95% by 2035 faces major hurdles, as highlighted in the World Health Organization (WHO) End-TB Strategy and the United Nations Sustainable Development Goals (2015). The rise of MDR-TB and extensively drug-resistant tuberculosis (XDR-TB), which increase the risk of death in TB patients, is hindering the achievement of this goal. To end the global TB epidemic, urgent action is needed. There is a lack of data resources to estimate the global incidence trends of MDR-TB and XDR-TB for the current situation, which is crucial for preventing and treating TB, thereby reducing TB-related deaths.[1]

Globally, countries have been expanding diagnostic capacity over recent years, detecting more patients with MDR-TB. Still, many cases have not been reported, especially in some Central Asian countries, like China, India, Russia, and Eastern Europe.[6]

There have been several studies which are published during 2016–2022 reported the prevalence of MDR-TB among new and previously treated patients in various sites in India, with the pooled prevalence of MDR-TB among new cases as 3.9% [95% confidence interval (CI) 2.2–6.1)] and 13.4% (95% CI 8.8–18.7) among previously treated cases.[7] A study published during 2001–2016,[7] including a systematic review of the prevalence of MDR-TB in India, showed a wide range of proportions and uncertainty that exists around the population-based estimates of MDR-TB.

Between 2014 and 2016, the first and the largest ever National Anti-TB Drug Resistance Survey (NDRS) that involved drug susceptibility testing for 13 anti-TB drugs was conducted in India.[8] The NDRS considered only TB cases registered with the Revised National TB Control Program—presently referred to as National Tuberculosis Elimination Program (NTEP) and thus lacked representation of patients exclusively treated in the private sector.

Additionally, the age-standardized rate (ASR) of MDR-TB was 5.63 [95% UI (uncertainty interval) = 3.12–9.73] per 100,000 among 450,600 cases (95% UI = 247,830–785,370), with a global incidence rate of 5.30% in 2019.[7] The distribution of cases from 2010 to 2019 was almost U-shaped. The average annual decrease in ASR was 1.36% (95% CI –2.19 to –0.52) during the same timeframe. Most regions and countries saw a decline in MDR-TB incidence trends, while the incidence of XDR-TB rose. The highest incidence rates for MDR-TB and XDR-TB were found in individuals aged 35–44 and 55–64 years, with the peak for both occurring in the 35–44 years age group. The peaks for MDR and XDR rates were consistent with the first peaks of the incidence rates of MDR-TB and XDR-TB, which was logical since high drug resistance leads to high incidence rate in drug-resistant TB. A reasonable explanation for the absence of second peaks for MDR and XDR rates is that the mortality rate of TB is high among the elderly.[9] Regions with a higher sociodemographic index (SDI) generally exhibited lower age-standardized rates of MDR-TB ($p < 0.001$, ρ^* –0.43)[7].

WHO report 2019 reports that out of the 21 geographical regions, 12 regions exhibited the age standardized rates of MDR-TB decreasing trends during 2010–2019, with the most significant decrease observed in East Asia followed by Central Asia and Eastern Europe.[7] **Table 1** show the incidence of MDR-TB and MDR rates in 2019 globally and in Asia.

India suffers from a significant burden of drug-resistance-TB, and its patterns and prevalence vary across time, region, and setting. India, which accounts for a high portion of the global TB burden, is currently at a critical juncture due to the growing prevalence of drug resistance TB. In India, the prevalence of "Adverse Drug Reaction" was 24.9% among new and 58.4% among previously treated TB cases. The prevalence of MDR was 3.5% among new and 26.7% among previously treated TB patients. Among the primary, the highest resistance was for isoniazid, followed by streptomycin. The trend of resistance was increasing among new and decreasing among previously treated. The prevalence of MDR was 5.1% among pediatric and 18.8% among HIV-TB co-infected patients. At the same time the prevalence among presumptive MDR was 23.3%.[7] The rates for MDR, single-drug resistant, and XDR were 3.5%, 24.9%, and 0.06% in new cases, while they were 26.7%, 58.4%, and 1.3% in previously treated cases, respectively. It is crucial to implement universal drug susceptibility testing across all districts and maintain continuous drug resistance-TB surveillance to ensure the success of these health programs. Regular monitoring of vital indicators is necessary to track progress toward the goal of eradicating TB and achieving a TB-free India.[8]

As of 2024, the incidence and prevalence of MDR-TB in India are significant public health concerns. According to the latest reports, the incidence rate of MDR-TB in India is approximately 8.5 per 100,000 population. The prevalence rate of MDR/RR-TB (rifampicin-resistant TB) is about 316 per 100,000 population. Additionally, MDR-TB occurs in 3.5% of

*The ρ value represents the strength of the correlation in Pearson's coefficient.

TABLE 1: The incidence of MDR-TB, ASR, and MDR rate of TB in Asian region in 2019.[7]

Characteristics	MDR-TB incidence No. × 10^3 (95% UI)	ASR per 100,000 No. (95% UI)	MDR rate (%)
Global	450.6 (247.83–85.37)	5.63 (3.12–0.73)	5.30
Asia Pacific	0.58 (0.14–1.84)	0.2 (0.05–0.64)	1.22
Central Asia	10.68 (7.03–14.94)	11.42 (7.55–6.05)	20.51
East Asia	31.26 (7.07–95.81)	1.81 (0.41–5.52)	4.10
South Asia	257.75 (72.44–595.41)	14.87 (4.18–3.94)	6.76
Southeast Asia	25.34 (14.88–41.38)	3.78 (2.23–6.16)	2.28

(ASR: age-standardized rate; MDR-TB: multidrug-resistant tuberculosis; UI: uncertainty interval)

new TB patients and 13% among previously treated patients.[7] India has made considerable progress in reducing TB cases with a 16% decline in new TB cases and an 18% reduction in mortality since 2015.[4] This progress should instill hope, but it is essential to remember that MDR-TB remains a challenging issue due to its resistance to standard treatments.[7]

A study by Stephanie Law and colleagues, published in "The Lancet Public Health," utilizes a dynamic model to forecast the progression of the TB epidemic in India over the next 20 years, focusing mainly on MDR-TB. The study highlights that India's private sector significantly contributes to antibiotic resistance. Key findings include a projected increase in MDR-TB cases from 3.9 to 14.1 per 100,000 people between 2012 and 2032. If current practices persist, the percentage of MDR-TB cases from primary transmission could rise from 15 to 85%. Correcting treatment errors or shifting more cases to the public sector will not significantly impact MDR-TB incidence, emphasizing that the epidemic is driven mainly by transmission.

The study highlights that India needs better national estimates for drug resistance; the current baseline figures for MDR-TB incidence and transmission are lower than other models, potentially exaggerating future increases. The model also needs calibration with past trends of MDR-TB in India, which may be more stable than the study projects. Due to lack of the data on MDR-TB incidence, this model could produce overly pessimistic projections of India's future epidemic.[10] India's National Tuberculosis Elimination Program needs to focus on these parameters to combat the current situation of MDR-TB. National estimates will be gathered by conducting surveys on drug-resistance TB from the public as well as private sectors to assess the situation.

Ultimately, the precise scale of these projections is less important than acknowledging that the past stability of India's MDR-TB epidemic does not guarantee that it will remain steady. As MDR-TB shifts from being primarily acquired during treatment to being predominantly transmitted, there is still a risk of a significant increase in cases—an outcome that could be avoided with a well-designed public health intervention.

CONCLUSION

Tuberculosis, particularly MDR-TB, poses a critical global health challenge, with countries like India bearing a significant portion of the burden. The growing prevalence of drug-resistant forms of TB, driven by improper antibiotic use and inadequate healthcare infrastructure, highlights the need for urgent action. While global efforts, such as the WHO End-TB Strategy, aim to reduce TB deaths by 2035 drastically, MDR-TB remains a formidable obstacle. Despite advances in diagnosis and treatment, including India's progress in reducing TB cases and mortality, the rise of MDR-TB, especially in previously treated patients, continues to hinder these efforts. The projected increase in MDR-TB incidence, particularly driven by transmission, underscores the need for robust public health interventions, improved drug resistance surveillance, and universal drug susceptibility testing. By addressing these challenges, there is hope for overcoming the epidemic and achieving a TB-free future.

REFERENCES

1. Lohiya A, Suliankatchi R, Rath ARS, Jacob O, Chinnakali P, Goel AD, et al. Prevalence and patterns of drug-resistant pulmonary tuberculosis in India—A systematic review and meta-analysis. J Glob Antimicrob Resist. 2020;22:308-16.
2. World Health Organization. (2022). Global Tuberculosis Report 2022. Geneva: World Health Organization; 2022. [online] Available from https://www.who.int/teams/ global-tuberculosis-programme/TB-reports/global-tuberculosis report-2022 [Last accessed Sept., 2022].
3. World Health Organization. (2023). Global Tuberculosis Report 2023. License: CC BY-NC-SA 3.0 IGO. Geneva: World Health Organization; 2023.
4. Bagchi S. WHO's Global Tuberculosis Report 2022. Lancet Microbe. 2023;4:e20.
5. World Health Organization. (2020). Global Tuberculosis report 2020. [online] Available from https://www.who.int/publications-detail-redirect/9789240013131 [Last accessed Sept, 2024].
6. Hengliang Lv, Zhang X, Zhang X, Bai J, You S, Li X, et al. Global prevalence and burden of multidrug-resistant tuberculosis from 1990 to 2019. BMC Infect Dis. 2024;24:243.
7. Bu Q, Qiang R, Fang L, Peng X, Zhang H, Cheng H. Global trends in the incidence rates of MDR and XDR tuberculosis: Findings from the global burden of disease study 2019. Front Pharmacol. 2023;14:1156249.
8. Ministry of Health and Family Welfare and World Health Organization. (2017). First National anti-TB Drug Resistance Survey India (NDRS) (2014–2016). [online] Available from https://tbcindia.Gov.in/showfile.php?Lid=3315 [Last accessed Sept., 2024].
9. Dhamnetiya D, Patel P, Jha RP, Shri N, Singh M, Bhattacharyya K. Trends in incidence and mortality of tuberculosis in India over past three decades: A join point and age-period-cohort analysis. BMC Pulm Med. 2021;21(1):375.
10. Fojo AT, Dowdy DW. Multidrug-resistant tuberculosis in India: looking back, thinking ahead. The Lancet Public Health. 2017;2(1):e8-e9.

CHAPTER

6 Barriers in the Development of Specific Drug Susceptibility Testing

Zeeshan Sidiq

Abstract

Drug-susceptibility testing (DST) is crucial for the effective treatment of infectious diseases, yet it encounters several substantial obstacles. Traditional testing methods are often time-consuming, and the complexity of pathogen biology presents additional challenges, especially as new resistance mechanisms continue to emerge rapidly. The economic landscape also poses difficulties, with high costs and scarce resources, particularly in low-income regions, making widespread implementation difficult. The regulatory approval process adds another layer of complexity, varying widely from one region to another, while the lack of standardization can lead to inconsistent outcomes. Furthermore, integrating DST into clinical practice is complicated by challenges in interpreting results, as well as by inadequate infrastructure and training. Overcoming these barriers require technological advancements, cost reduction, improved standardization, and enhanced training efforts, alongside collaborative work between scientific and regulatory communities.

Keywords: Drug susceptibility testing, technical limitations, pathogen biology, resistance mechanisms, economic challenges, regulatory issues, standardization, clinical integration

INTRODUCTION

Accurate and reliable drug-susceptibility testing (DST) is a key component in the management of infectious diseases as it ensures that the chosen treatment is effective against the pathogen. Despite its critical role, the development and implementation of specific-drug susceptibility testing face numerous challenges. This chapter looks into the barriers obstructing the development of DST with a focus on the technical limitations, economic challenges, regulatory hurdles, and problems related to clinical integration.

Technical Limitations

Drug-susceptibility testing faces a number of technical limitations that affect its efficiency. These challenges can be broadly categorized into following key areas:

- *Complexity of traditional methods:* Traditional methods such as broth microdilution or agar diffusion are time-consuming and may not provide results quickly enough to guide treatment decisions effectively.

- *Complexity of pathogen biology:* Different pathogens, particularly those with complex life cycles or genetic variability, present challenges in developing universally applicable testing methods. For example, multidrug-resistant tuberculosis (MDR-TB) and drug-resistant malaria strains require very specific tests due to unique mutations in the genes and the resistance mechanisms. MDR-TB requires testing for specific mutations in genes like *rpoB*, *katG*, and *inhA*, while drug-resistant malaria involves identifying mutations in genes like *pfcrt* and *pfmdr1*.[1]
- *Emergence of novel resistance mechanisms:* The rapid evolution of resistance mechanisms necessitates constant updates to testing methodologies. For example, the emergence of drug-resistant tuberculosis (DR-TB) and carbapenem-resistant *Enterobacteriaceae* (CRE) has resulted in a need for advanced molecular assays capable of detecting novel resistance genes.[2]

While recent advancements, like molecular assays and next-generation sequencing (NGS), have sped up testing, they introduce their own set of challenges. For example, molecular assays such as the GeneXpert *Mycobacterium tuberculosis* (MTB)/rifampicin (RIF) provide rapid results but may miss certain resistance mutations. In contrast, sequencing technologies offer more comprehensive data but require advanced equipment and expertise.[3]

Economic Challenges

Drug susceptibility testing is highly affected by economic difficulties in terms of both development and availability.

- *High costs of development and implementation:* The development of new tests for detecting the susceptibility of microbes requires a substantial amount of funds for research and development, technology, and validation procedures. To give an example, the cost of implementing NGS for susceptibility testing for pathogens like drug resistant *Mycobacterium tuberculosis* is still too high for many healthcare settings.[4]
- *Limited resources in low-resource settings:* In many low- and middle-income countries, the financial burden caused by advanced susceptibility testing technologies is a barrier to their adoption. This is particularly critical for managing diseases such as tuberculosis and human immunodeficiency virus (HIV)/acquired immunodeficiency syndrome (AIDS), which are highly prevalent in these regions.[5]

Efforts to reduce the cost by technological innovations, such as point-of-care tests and low-cost sequencing platforms are ongoing and might be the way to the future.

Regulatory Issues

The regulatory approval process for new DST methods is complex and varies across regions. Ensuring these new tests meet rigorous standards for accuracy and reliability while also addressing the urgent need for rapid diagnostics is a delicate balance.[3] To accelerate the availability of new DST technologies, it is crucial to streamline regulatory processes while maintaining high standards for test quality. This requires collaboration among regulatory bodies, researchers, and manufacturers to ensure innovations are both effective and timely.

Standardization Issues

The lack of standardized techniques for susceptibility testing can result in an inconsistent and variable outcome. The standardization of methodologies among laboratories is crucial to achieve reliable and consistent outcomes.[6]

Clinical Integration

Incorporating susceptibility testing into a clinical workflow is difficult for many reasons.

- Interpretation of susceptibility test results does require clinical expertise since it involves deducing the microbiological and treatment response context. Potential misinterpretation of results can result in treatment decisions. One example is presence of resistance genes that do not always reflect phenotypic resistance.[7]
- *Infrastructure and training*: Suitable infrastructure, as well-trained staff is essential for implementing DST. Also, in a wide range of circumstances, an absence of these capacities limits regular use of broad testing strategies.

It is important to improve education for clinicians and laboratory personnel, so that better training programs are established and more resources are available.

CONCLUSION

Specific-drug susceptibility testing presents a number of obstacles for development and implementation such as technical limitations, economic labyrinth as well as regulatory hurdles and standardizations requirements that can complicate matters further together with clinical integration. The means to overcome those challenges is a multipronged approach that includes technological advancements, cost mitigation activities, standardization efforts and improving training, and infrastructure. Further research and open dialogue across scientific domains along with international cooperation will be key in addressing these challenges so that susceptibility testing can appropriately inform treatment decisions leading to better patient's outcomes.

REFERENCES

1. Zhang Y, Yew WW. Drug resistance mechanisms in Mycobacterium tuberculosis. J Antimicrob Chemother. 2023;78(1):1-11.
2. Nordmann P, Poirel L. The challenges of detecting and combating carbapenem-resistant bacteria. Nat Rev Microbiol. 2023;21(6):339-53.
3. Aarons R, Brown T, Jones M. Advances in molecular diagnostics for drug resistance detection. J Clin Microbiol. 2017;55(4):789-98.
4. Gordon NC, Wareham DW. High-throughput sequencing in antibiotic resistance research. Clin Microbiol Rev. 2024;37(2):e00012-23.
5. Kang Y, Lee SH. Cost-effective strategies for implementing next-generation sequencing in clinical settings. J Clin Microbiol. 2023;61(4):e02345-22.
6. Foster K, McCauley K. Navigating regulatory landscapes for new susceptibility tests. Regulat Toxicol Pharmacol. 2023;101:1-8.
7. Jones TS, Patel S. Standardization of drug susceptibility testing: Current challenges and future directions. J Clin Pathol. 2024;77(2):123-30.

Section 2: Diagnostic

CHAPTER

7

Decoding Resistance: Role of Mutations in Tuberculosis Treatment Failure

Salil Bhargava, Jaya Lalwani, Nagraj Perumal

Abstract

Tuberculosis (TB), a persistent global health burden, continues to pose a significant challenge due to the emergence of drug-resistant strains. Despite the availability of various anti-tubercular drugs, treatment regimens often require prolonged durations, even in drug-sensitive cases. The emergence of drug-resistant strains further complicates treatment, necessitating extended therapy, increasing the risk of adverse effects, relapse, and the development of more severe forms of TB, such as extensively drug-resistant TB (XDR-TB). Genetic mutations within the *Mycobacterium tuberculosis* (MTB) genome play a pivotal role in conferring drug resistance. These mutations can alter the structure or function of target proteins, rendering them ineffective against anti-TB drugs. This phenomenon, observed with both older and newer antibiotics, presents significant challenges in designing effective treatment plans. Advances in next-generation sequencing (NGS) offer promising potential for more accurate and rapid drug susceptibility testing, facilitating more targeted therapeutic approaches compared to the traditional drug susceptibility testing methods. By elucidating the complex interplay between genetic mutations and drug resistance, this chapter aims to contribute to the development of innovative strategies to combat TB and improve patient outcomes.

Keywords: Multidrug-resistant TB (MDR-TB), extensively drug-resistant TB (XDR-TB), resistance mechanisms, genetic mutations, treatment failure

INTRODUCTION

Mycobacterium tuberculosis (MTB), the causative agent of tuberculosis (TB), remains a significant global public health threat, claiming millions of lives annually. Despite advancements in recent years, challenges like drug-resistant TB (DR-TB) and the COVID-19 pandemic pose a formidable challenge to disease control efforts. Treating TB is inherently complex, requiring a multidrug regimen due to MTB's intricate defense mechanisms. However, a major hurdle arises when treatment fails despite adherence to seemingly appropriate therapy. This treatment failure often stems from the emergence of MTB strains harboring mutations in genes critical for drug action. These mutations essentially create a shield, rendering the bacteria resistant to the drugs used in standard regimens. This resistance translates to significantly extended treatment durations, the use of more toxic medications with increased side effects, and ultimately, reduced treatment adherence and treatment success rates. Understanding the precise mechanisms by which these mutational changes confer resistance is crucial for developing effective strategies to combat this evolving pathogen. This chapter delves into the intricate world of mutational adaptations in MTB and their role in treatment failure. We will explore the specific mutations associated with resistance to various TB drugs, the impact of these mutations on treatment outcomes, and the complex challenges they pose for effective TB control.[1]

MULTIFACETED DETERMINANTS OF TREATMENT FAILURE

Treatment failure is a critical concept in TB management. It is defined as a scenario where a patient's TB infection remains viable, as evidenced by a positive smear or culture test for MTB, after completing a prescribed course of treatment. Several established factors that can influence treatment outcomes include adherence to lengthy regimens, potential sex and age disparities, diagnostic delays, and the presence other concomitant diseases like HIV coinfection. Although previous exposure to TB medications, particularly if treatment was incomplete or inappropriate, adverse drug effects in an individual and drug interactions can significantly increase the risk of resistance development and subsequent treatment failure, drug resistance is undoubtedly the primary determinant of treatment failure. Drug resistance arises when mutations occur in the genes of MTB that encode targets for anti-TB drugs. These mutations can alter the structure or function of the target protein, rendering the drug ineffective. The development of drug resistance significantly complicates treatment. Multidrug-resistant tuberculosis (MDR-TB) arises when MTB exhibits resistance to the two most potent first-line drugs, isoniazid (INH) and rifampicin. Extensively drug-resistant tuberculosis (XDR-TB) presents an even greater challenge, as this subset of MDR-TB displays additional resistance to a fluoroquinolone antibiotic and at least one of the second-line injectable anti-TB drugs. Distinguishing between treatment failure due to drug resistance from other factors like poor adherence or reinfection is crucial for guiding appropriate management strategies.[2]

MUTATION VARIANTS AND TREATMENT OUTCOMES

Mycobacterium tuberculosis exhibits substantial genomic heterogeneity, posing a significant challenge to effective TB treatment. This variation encompasses mutations beyond those directly targeting genes associated with known anti-TB drugs. Notably, non-synonymous mutations, altering the amino acid sequence of encoded proteins, can significantly influence treatment outcomes. Examples include single nucleotide polymorphisms (SNPs) resulting in single amino acid substitutions and insertions/deletions (InDels) disrupting protein function. InDels in efflux pump genes, for instance, could decrease drug accumulation within the bacteria, making them less susceptible to the drug's effects. Furthermore, a broader spectrum of mutation variants can influence drug tolerance. These encompass feature ablation (complete gene deletion), frameshift mutations (insertion or deletion of nucleotides that disrupts the reading frame), in-frame insertions/deletions (maintaining the reading frame but potentially altering protein function), missense mutations (single amino acid substitutions), and various other types **(Table 1)**. These mutational variants associated with structural or functional related genes of MTB could lead to drug tolerance, thereby increasing the risk of developing resistance and relapsing after treatment. However, the silent/synonymous mutations may also occur in the DNA sequence but they do not lead to change in the amino acid sequence of the

TABLE 1: Mutation variants observed in candidate resistance genes.

Drug	Candidate resistance genes	Mutation variants
AMK	*bacA, ccsA, eis, rrs, Rv2477c, whiB6, whiB7*	Feature ablation, frameshift, inframe deletion, inframe insertion, initiator codon, loss of function, missense, noncoding transcript exon, start lost, stop gained, stop lost, stop retained, synonymous, upstream gene
BDQ	*atpE, lpqB, mmpL5, mmpS5, mtrA, mtrB, pepQ, Rv0678, Rv1979c*	
CAP	*bacA, ccsA, rrl, rrs, Rv2680, Rv2681, tlyA, whiB6*	
CFZ	*fbiA, fbiB, fbiC, fgd1, mmpL5, mmpS5, pepQ, Rv0678, Rv1979c, Rv2983*	
DLM	*ddn, fbiA, fbiB, fbiC, fgd1, ndh, Rv2983*	
EMB	*aftB, embA, embB, embC, embR, glpk, Rv2477c, Rv2752c, ubiA*	
ETO	*ethA, ethR, inhA, mshA, ndh, Rv0565c, Rv3083*	
INH	*ahpC, dnaA, glpK, hadA, inhA, katG, mshA, ndh, Rv0010c, Rv1129c, Rv1258c, Rv2752c*	
KAN	*bacA, ccsA, eis, rrs, Rv2477c, whiB6, whiB7*	
LFX	*glpK, gyrA, gyrB, Rv2477c, Rv2752c*	
LZD	*rplC, rrl, tsnR*	
MFX	*glpK, gyrA, gyrB, Rv1129c, Rv2477c, Rv2752c*	
PZA	*clpC1, panD, pncA, PPE35, rpsA, Rv1258c, Rv3236c, sigE*	
RIF	*glpK, lpqB, mtrA, mtrB, nusG, rpoA, rpoB, rpoC, Rv1129c, Rv2477c, Rv2752c*	
STM	*bacA, gid, glpK, rpsL, rrs, Rv1258c, Rv2477c, whiB7*	

(AMK: amikacin; BDQ: bedaquiline; CAP: capreomycin; CFZ: clofazimine; DLM: delamanid; EMB: ethambutol; ETO: ethionamide; INH: isoniazid; KAN: kanamycin; LFX: levofloxacin; LZD: linezolid; MFX: moxifloxacin; PZA: pyrazinamide; RIF: rifampicin; STM: streptomycin)

protein and, therefore, they typically have no impact on drug susceptibility. Overall, the presence of diverse mutation variants in MTB populations contributes to the emergence of drug tolerance and necessitates further research to improve TB diagnostics and treatment strategies.[3-6]

OVERVIEW OF MUTATION CATALOGS

To combat the growing challenge of DR-TB, two crucial resources have emerged—the World Health Organization (WHO) Mutation Catalogue and the Indian Mutation Catalogue. Released in 2021 with a second edition in 2023, the WHO Catalogue provides a global reference for interpreting mutations associated with resistance to 13 anti-TB drugs. This vital resource analyses a vast collection of isolates worldwide. In 2022, India followed suit with the introduction of the first country-specific catalog for MTB, and version 2 in 2024 offering insights into over 10,673 mutations prevalent in circulating strains within the nation. These catalogs serve a critical role in deciphering genotypic data for clinicians, informing effective treatment decisions for patients with TB. Additionally, they guide researchers in developing novel molecular drug susceptibility tests, including targeted next-generation sequencing (NGS), paving the way for more efficient and accurate TB diagnostics.[3-6]

FIRST-LINE ANTI-TUBERCULAR DRUG RESISTANCE AND ASSOCIATED MUTATIONS

The cornerstone of effective TB treatment lies in a combination of four first-line antibiotics—INH, rifampin (RIF), pyrazinamide (PZA), and ethambutol (EMB). When properly administered, this regimen effectively eliminates MTB, rendering patients noninfectious and preventing further transmission. However, the emergence of drug resistance poses a significant challenge. This section explores the mechanisms behind resistance to each of these first-line drugs and the associated mutations within the bacterial genes.

Rifampicin is the most effective and first-line drug for TB treatment. Resistance to rifampicin primarily develops due to point mutations in RIF resistance-determining region (RRDR) an 81-bp region (codons 426–452) of the *rpoB* gene that encodes the β-subunit of the RNA polymerase. Mutations in the *rpoB* gene at codons 430, 435, 445, and 452 are commonly associated with rifampicin resistance. However, rare mutations outside the RRDR have also been shown to cause resistance. Notably, these mutations often involve single-nucleotide changes leading to amino acid substitutions, in-frame deletions, or insertions within the *rpoB* gene. The Version 2.0 Indian catalog reported 63 mutations in the *rpoB* gene and 25 mutations in the *rpoC* gene, suggesting a potential role for this gene in rifampicin resistance. Furthermore, several other candidate genes are likely involved in this complex resistance mechanism.

Resistance to the other most important anti-tubercular drug, INH, is a complex phenomenon associated with mutations in multiple genes, primarily *katG* and *inhA*. INH, a prodrug, requires activation by the bacterial enzyme KatG. It then inhibits mycolic acid synthesis, a critical component of the mycobacterial cell wall encoded by the *inhA* gene. Point mutations within these genes are predominantly associated with INH resistance. The most common mutations linked to resistance include promoter mutations upstream of the fabG1-inhA (C15T and T8C) and furA-katG (S315T, S315N, and W328L) operons. Mutations in the inhA promoter region can lead to its overexpression, causing relative INH resistance. Notably, inhA mutations may also confer cross-resistance to ethionamide (ETO). While mutations in katG were assumed to result in a loss-of-function (LoF) phenotype and consequently, high-level INH resistance, but it has now been shown that other nonsynonymous mutations in katG or its upstream regulatory region can also contribute to INH resistance.

Pyrazinamide resistance in MTB primarily arises from mutations in the *pncA* gene, which encodes the enzyme pyrazinamidase responsible for converting the prodrug PZA to its active metabolite, pyrazinoic acid. Pyrazinoic acid disrupts critical cellular processes like energy production (pncA), trans-translation (rpsA), and pantothenate/coenzyme A (panD) which are essential for the pathogen's survival. Mutations in the *pncA* gene and its promoter, particularly nonsense mutations and InDels within the coding region (e.g., A11G and A11C), are likely to cause LoF mutations which may lead to high-level PZA resistance. Additionally, mutations in the *rpsA* gene, such as the single point mutation (R212R), have also been reported to confer PZA resistance.

Ethambutol disrupts MTB cell wall synthesis by targeting arabinosyl transferase, an enzyme encoded within the *embCAB* operon. This operon is essential for the biosynthesis of arabinogalactan, a crucial component of the mycobacterial cell wall. Mutations within the *embCAB* operon, particularly within the *embB* gene, are primarily associated with EMB resistance. These mutations encompass nonsynonymous substitutions in the *embB* coding sequence, its promoter region, and even an intergenic mutation located upstream of *embA*. Notably, mutations in the *ubiA* gene have also been implicated in EMB resistance.[3-6]

AMINOGLYCOSIDES RESISTANCE AND ASSOCIATED MUTATIONS

Aminoglycosides, including amikacin (AMK), capreomycin (CAP), and kanamycin (KAN), serve as second-line therapeutic options for MDR-TB. However, resistance to any of these injectable antibiotics defines XDR-TB. Their mechanism of action involves binding to the 16S rRNA within the 30S ribosomal subunit, thereby inhibiting protein synthesis in mycobacteria. Point mutations in specific genes are the predominant mechanism underlying aminoglycoside resistance. AMK resistance is frequently associated with mutations in the *rrs* (ribosomal RNA small subunit) and *eis* genes, or the promoter region of the *whiB7* gene. Specific mutations in *rrs* gene (e.g., A1401G, G1484T, C1402T) and a mutation in the *eis* gene promoter (C14T) serve as well-characterized genotypic predictors of AMK resistance. Likewise, mutations in genes such as *rpsL* (K43R, K88M, K88R) and *rrs* (A514C, C517T) are functionally well-understood determinants of streptomycin (STM) resistance. It is noteworthy that KAN and CAP are no longer recommended for standard TB treatment regimens due to the emergence of resistance. Resistance to these drugs, along with STM, is believed to arise from unlinked chromosomal mutations.[3-6]

FLUOROQUINOLONES RESISTANCE AND ASSOCIATED MUTATIONS

Fluoroquinolones, including levofloxacin (LFX), ofloxacin (OFX), and moxifloxacin (MFX), have become increasingly important antibiotics for treating MDR-TB. Their mechanism of action involves targeting DNA gyrase, an enzyme essential for MTB DNA replication. DNA gyrase is a complex enzyme composed of two A and two B subunits encoded by the *gyrA* and *gyrB* genes, respectively. The development of fluoroquinolone resistance in MTB is primarily attributed to mutations within specific regions of these genes, designated as the quinolone resistance-determining region (QRDR). The QRDR encompasses conserved sequences within gyrA and gyrB where mutations can hinder fluoroquinolone binding and reduce the drug's effectiveness. The most frequently observed mutation associated with fluoroquinolone resistance is D94V in the *gyrA* gene. This mutation is often linked to high-level resistance against LFX and MFX. Additionally, the G88A mutation in *gyrA* is specifically associated with OFX resistance.[3-6]

ETHIONAMIDE AND PROTHIONAMIDE RESISTANCE AND ASSOCIATED MUTATIONS

Ethionamide and prothionamide (PTO) have gained prominence as part of the WHO's recommended Group C drugs for treating TB resistant to rifampicin (RR-TB) and MDR-TB. Both drugs share structural similarities with INH and act as prodrugs, requiring activation by the enzyme EthA, a NADPH-dependent flavin adenine dinucleotide-containing monooxygenase. The activated form of ETO mirrors the action of INH, forming an ETO-NAD adduct that inhibits InhA, a vital enzyme for mycolic acid biosynthesis in MTB. Development of resistance to ETO is primarily associated with mutations within the *ethA* gene. These mutations can significantly impair EthA function, rendering the bacteria incapable of activating the drug. Common resistance mechanisms include premature stop codons and InDels within the ethA coding sequence. These mutations disrupt the gene's reading frame or prematurely terminate protein translation, resulting in a nonfunctional EthA enzyme and subsequent ETO resistance.[3-6]

RESISTANCE AND ASSOCIATED MUTATIONS IN NEWER ANTI-TUBERCULAR AGENTS

The emergence of DR-TB has driven the development and use of newer antitubercular agents like bedaquiline (BDQ), delamanid (DLM), linezolid (LZD), clofazimine (CFZ), and carbapenems. While these drugs offer hope for treating MDR-TB and RR-TB, the specter of resistance looms large. Mutations within specific genes, including *Rv0678, atpE,* and *pepQ,* have been implicated in resistance to BDQ and/or CFZ. Furthermore, BDQ-CFZ cross-resistance can develop through several mechanisms: pre-existing resistance in the infecting strain, the presence of heteroresistant bacterial subpopulations harboring resistance mutations, and de novo resistance evolution during treatment. Similarly, DLM resistance is associated with a specific mutation in the *ddn* gene and potential LoF mutations in five other genes (*fbiA, fbiB, fbiC, fgd1,* and *Rv2983*). Mutations in two key genes, *rplC* and *rrl,* specifically at codons 154 (C154R) and 2814 (G2814T), have been identified as potential mechanisms for LZD resistance. This underscores the fact that mutational drug resistance in MTB remains a therapeutic and diagnostic challenge not only in the yesteryears anti-tubercular drugs but also the newer therapeutic options being explored.[3-6]

CHALLENGES AND WAY FORWARD

Effective TB management hinges on accurate drug susceptibility testing and devising the treatment regimens based upon the findings of phenotypic and genotypic drug resistance data available from these drug susceptibility tests. However, current methods present distinct limitations. While genotypic drug susceptibility testing (gDST) offers rapid turnaround times, it may not detect all resistance mechanisms. Conversely, phenotypic drug susceptibility testing (pDST), the gold standard, can be time-consuming and laborious. NGS holds immense promise for comprehensive strain characterization and resistance detection. However, its widespread application in resource-constrained settings is hindered by high costs, infrastructure requirements for data processing and analysis, and the need for expertise in interpreting complex genetic data. Standardization of NGS protocols for TB diagnostics is also ongoing. Looking ahead, overcoming these diagnostic hurdles is crucial. Research into novel technologies like advanced molecular assays, microfluidics-based platforms, and machine learning algorithms offers promise for improving diagnostic sensitivity, specificity, and turnaround times.

In addition to these benchside dilemmas, there are many bedside issues in translation of this information into clinical application for patient management. This requires better and in depth understanding of the anti-tubercular drugs, their resistance mechanisms, and development of strategies and regimens to overcome the resistance. The need of the hour may be tailor made well thought out regimens in the patients exhibiting drug resistance based on the scientific evidence and the individual strain mutations and resistance profile. Data about the resistance mutations also needs to be collected and documented on a routine basis from the local circulating stains for developing robust scientific evidence.

CONCLUSION

The emergence and spread of DR-TB strains pose a formidable challenge to global TB control efforts. Understanding the intricate link between mutations in the MTB genome and their impact on drug resistance is crucial for developing effective treatment strategies. By addressing the limitations of current diagnostic methods, exploring the potential of

NGS and alternative technologies, and investing in research on novel treatment options, we can move closer to achieving faster, more accurate, and comprehensive TB diagnostics. Ultimately, this will contribute to better patient outcomes and more effective TB control strategies.

REFERENCES

1. World Health Organization. Global tuberculosis report 2023. Geneva: World Health Organization; 2022.
2. Mushtaq F, Raza SM, Ahmad A, Aslam H, Adeel A, Saleem S, et al. Antimicrobial drug resistant features of *Mycobacterium tuberculosis* associated with treatment failure. PLoS One. 2023;18(10): e0293194.
3. World Health Organization. Catalogue of mutations in *Mycobacterium tuberculosis* complex and their association with drug resistance. Geneva: World Health Organization; 2021.
4. World Health Organization. Catalogue of mutations in *Mycobacterium tuberculosis* complex and their association with drug resistance, second edition. Geneva: World Health Organization; 2023.
5. ICMR, NIRT. (2022). Indian catalogue of *Mycobacterium tuberculosis* mutations and their association with drug resistance. 2022. [online] Available from https://www.nirt.res.in/pdf/2022%20India%20Mutations%20Catalogue_CDC%20Cleared.pdf [Last accessed September, 2024].
6. ICMR, NIRT. (2024). Indian Catalogue of *Mycobacterium tuberculosis* mutations and their association with drug resistance, Version 2.0, 2024. [online] Available from https://nirt.res.in/pdf/mutation_catalogue_v2.pdf [Last accessed September, 2024].

CHAPTER

8

Early Detection Tools of Pulmonary Tuberculosis Affecting Treatment Outcome

Ritu Singhal

Abstract

Prompt and accurate diagnosis of tuberculosis (TB) and drug-resistant TB (DR-TB) is essential for early start of appropriate anti-TB treatment, thereby ensuring favorable outcome for the patient. Early treatment initiation is also crucial for rendering patient noninfectious and curtailing spread of TB. Presently, there are many accurate and rapid molecular diagnostic tests available for detection of TB and DR-TB approved by the World Health Organization (WHO) which provide early information about drug susceptibility to important antibiotics used for the treatment of TB and thus influence better treatment outcome. While antigen detection is crucial in human immunodeficiency virus (HIV) patients, microscopy continues to play a role in monitoring treatment response in patients.

Keywords: Diagnosis, drug susceptibility, molecular test

INTRODUCTION

Prompt diagnosis of tuberculosis (TB) is essential to the early start of drug-sensitive anti-TB treatment, thereby rendering patients noninfectious and curtailing the spread of TB. Also crucial is accurate determination of drug-resistant TB (DR-TB), which is central to designing proper treatment regimen for DR-TB patients and reducing spread of DR-TB. Last decade has seen emergence of many accurate and rapid molecular diagnostic tests for detection of TB and DR-TB, while extensive research into developing both nucleic acid and antigen-based tests for application in resource-poor and peripheral settings is ongoing. Presently, early diagnosis of TB is based on microscopic and nucleic acid-based methods mainly and also antigen detection. Most nucleic acid-based methods additionally provide early information about drug susceptibility to important antibiotics used for the treatment of TB.[1,2]

DIRECT MICROSCOPY

Direct microscopy has traditionally been done using Ziehl–Neelsen (ZN) staining for detecting presence or absence of acid-fast bacilli (AFB). It is one of the most inexpensive methods available with results on same day and is of high specificity (83.4–99%). Its accuracy is highly dependent on the technical operator, thus resulting in a broad range of sensitivities of 25–81.6% and lesser in pediatric age group and human immunodeficiency virus (HIV). Since 2012, there has been an introduction of light-emitting diode (LED) fluorescence microscopy as an improvement on ZN microscopy. Microscopy remains an integral part of TB detection and monitoring response to treatment, measuring infectiousness, and predicting the likelihood of relapse in patients.[3]

NUCLEIC ACID AMPLIFICATION TESTS

The World Health Organization (WHO) has recommended the use of many nucleic acid amplification tests (NAATs) for TB detection instead of smear microscopy, due to better sensitivity, particularly in patients with paucibacillary disease and HIV. Also, most can detect TB drug resistance and associated mycobacterial gene mutations, allowing clinicians to design effective TB treatments. Besides, these are high throughput tests. These assays rely on polymerase chain reaction (PCR) amplification of targeted genetic region of the *Mycobacterium tuberculosis* (MTB) complex and simultaneously provide results of drug-susceptibility testing (DST) for crucial antibiotics. Rapid diagnosis of accurate DST prompts early initiation of correct treatment and therefore favorable treatment outcome. Real-time PCR methods are simplest and hence, presently are most widely used molecular tests endorsed by the WHO. Various types of molecular assays approved by the WHO are summarized in **Table 1**.[2,4,5]

Line Probe Assays

Line probe assays (LPAs) are deoxyribonucleic acid (DNA) strip-based tests which can detect the MTB DNA and DST to antibiotics by binding DNA amplification products to probes that target specific parts of the MTB genome, resistance-associated mutations,

TABLE 1: Various types of molecular assays for approved by WHO.

Type of assay	Level of complexity	Assays name and manufacturer
Real-time PCR	Low	• Xpert MTB/RIF and Xpert MTB/RIF Ultra assays (Cepheid, Sunnyvale, USA), Truenat MTB, MTB Plus, and MTBRIF Dx tests (Molbio Diagnostics, Goa, India) • Xpert® MTB/XDR (Cepheid)
	Moderate	• Abbott RealTime® MTB and Abbott RealTime MTB RIF/INH (Abbott) • BD MAX™ MDR-TB (Becton Dickinson) • cobas® MTB and cobas MTB-RIF/INH (Roche) • FluoroType® MTBDR and FluoroType® MTB (Hain Lifescience/Bruker)
Hybridization-based assays	High	• GenoType® MTBDR*plus* v1 and v2; GenoType MTBDR*sl*, (Hain Lifescience/Bruker), • GENOSCHOLAR™ NTM + MDRTB II; Genoscholar PZA-TB II (Nipro)
Target NGS assays	High	• Deeplex® Myc-TB test (Genoscreen) • AmPORE-TB® test (Oxford Nanopore Diagnostics) • TBseq® test (Hangzhou ShengTing Medical Technology Co)

(NGS: next-generation sequencing; PCR: polymerase chain reaction; WHO: World Health Organization)

or corresponding wild-type DNA sequences. Commercial LPAs for detecting MTB and resistance to rifampicin (RIF) and isoniazid (INH) in sputum smear-positive specimens (direct testing) and in cultured isolates of MTB (indirect testing) were approved in 2008. LPAs are technically complex tests, designed for referral laboratory setting. The results can be obtained in 2–3 working days.

Genotype MTBDRplus or first-line LPA detects susceptibility to RIF by means of *rpoB* gene at a sensitivity of over 95%, while INH susceptibility is detected by *katG* and *inhA* genes which provide susceptibility to high-dose and low-dose INH, respectively, at sensitivity of 78.5%. Mutation in *inhA* promoter genes additionally tell resistance to ethionamide (ETH). Genotype MTBDR*sl* 2.0 assay or second-line LPA detects resistance to fluoroquinolones (FQ) using mutations in FQ (*gyrA* and *gyrB*) and SLID (*rrs* and *eis*). Reported sensitivity is around 90% for FQ and 87% for SLID. For FQ, the test provides information on high/low level of resistance as the presence of mutant 3B, 3C, and 3D in *gyrA* gene are associated with high-level FQ resistance. Test tells about low-level kana resistance. Specificity of detection of resistance is above 95–100% for each antibiotic.

Rifampicin/INH forms part of drug-sensitive regimen and FQ is an important component of most drug-resistant treatment regimens. LPAs provide prompt recognition and level of resistance, which is crucial for treatment modification so that patients can be started on appropriate regimen. This decreases opportunity of drug resistance to develop nor are patients exposed to burdensome, longer drug regimens with higher potential for toxicity unnecessarily.[2,4,5]

Xpert/Xpert Ultra/Omni/Xpert Extensively Drug Resistant

Cepheid has introduced cartridge-based NAAT which detects the presence of TB DNA, as well as common mutations associated with RIF resistance within 1.5–2 hours. In Xpert MTB/RIF sample processing, PCR amplification and detection are integrated into self-enclosed automated in single Xpert MTB/RIF cartridge, fairly simple to use. Assay's sample reagent, used to liquefy sputum, is tuberculocidal and therefore can be used in the peripheral-level laboratories with minimum biosafety. However, machine and its operation are expensive and require uninterrupted electrical power supply, room temperature, and yearly calibration. The test has sensitivity comparable to culture in diagnosing pulmonary TB in adults is however lower in pediatric and HIV population. Xpert ultra was introduced in 2017 with objective of increasing sensitivity of Xpert to 16 bacilli/mL by having a larger chamber for DNA amplification, two multicopy amplification namely, *IS6110* and *IS1081*.

These modifications have increased ultra's overall sensitivity from 85 to 88%. Specificity of Xpert is very high at 98% but slightly lower for Xpert ultra at 95% since it detects dead bacilli in patients with recently cured TB. Lower specificity however is a cause of concern in regions with high numbers of HIV-TB coinfections or recurrent TB cases.

The latest WHO recommendation suggests use of Xpert MTB/RIF and Xpert Ultra as an initial test for detection of TB and RIF resistance in all adults with signs and symptoms of pulmonary TB in sputum. In children, this is expanded to gastric aspirate, nasopharyngeal aspirate, and stool.

GeneXpert Omni (Omni; Cepheid) is a battery-operated, handheld device modification of regular Xpert, a cost-effective method for using as point of care.

Xpert MTB/XDR assay as low-complexity, automated NAAT for the detection of resistance to INH, FLQ, ETH, and SLID by detecting 16 clinically relevant mutations, intended for use as a reflex test in specimens determined to be MTB positive, they offer rapid DST in intermediate and peripheral laboratories. Results are available in under 90 minutes, leading to faster time to results than LPAs and culture-based DST. Sensitivity is around 91% for INH, 90% for FQ, and 85% for SLIDS in preliminary trials.[2,4,5]

Truenat

In 2020, three real-time PCR-based molecular assays, Truenat MTB, MTB Plus, and MTB-RIF Dx assays from Truenat™ (Molbio Diagnostics, Goa, India), had been approved by the WHO for initial diagnosis of TB and subsequent detection of RIF resistance in adults and children with signs and symptoms of pulmonary TB. Truenat MTB and Truenat MTB plus detect MTB and are used as initial diagnostic tests for TB, whereas Truenat MTB-RIF Dx identifies resistance to RIF and is used as a reflex test in those with positive results on MTB platform. These three tests are run on the portable, automated, battery-operated devices with minimal user input and provide results in an hour or two. Therefore, these tests are being used at the same health system level as Xpert MTB/RIF.[2,4,5]

Moderate Complexity Test

Moderate complexity tests are commercially available semiautomated/automated real-time PCR-based molecular tests available for detection of MTB and RIF and INH resistance. These tests are faster, less complex to perform than phenotypic DST and LPA, and are largely automated with high throughput. Four moderate-complexity tests approved by the WHO in 2020–2021 include Abbott Real-Ti*me* MTB, BD MAX™ MDR-TB, *Bruker-Hain Diagnostics*, and *Roche Diagnostics* (Roche) as detailed in **Table 2**. These tests have very low limit of detection, ranging from 6 to 60 colony-forming units (CFU)/mL. They offer potential for rapid provision of accurate results and testing efficiency, where high volumes of tests are required daily. The tests have been recommended for use on respiratory samples for people with signs and symptoms of pulmonary TB for detection of pulmonary TB and RIF and INH resistance rather than culture and phenotypic DST. Application of this technology will give advantage of detecting both RIF and INH resistance upfront on clinical samples in presumptive pulmonary TB patients.[2]

Targeted Next-generation Sequencing

Targeted next-generation sequencing (tNGS) rapid molecular assays are based on amplification of larger regions of selected genes with NGS technology in order to identify most mutations across multiple genes. Presently, the WHO-approved tNGS offer great potential in appropriate treatment, as these cover extensive list of anti-TB drugs and provide drug-susceptibility results to newer and repurposed anti-TB drugs being used in recent newer DR-TB regimens.[2,6]

TABLE 2: WHO endorsed moderate complexity tests.

Parameters	Abbott Real-Time MTB	Becton Dickinson (BD)	Bruker–Hain Diagnostics	Roche Diagnostics (Roche)
Tests	• RealTi*me* MTB test • RealTi*me* MTB RIF/INH	BD MAX™ MDR-TB for both MTB and RIF and INH detection	• FluoroType® MTB, which detects *Mtb* • FluoroType MTBDR for RIF and INH detection	• cobas® MTB assay to detect *Mtb* • cobas® MTB-RIF/INH assay for RIF and INH detection
Targets	Multicopy: IS*6110* genetic element and the *pab* gene	Multicopy: IS*6110* and IS*1081*	Multicopy: rpoB	6 single-copy targets: 16S rRNA, *esxJ, esxK, esxM, esxP, esxW*

(INH: isoniazid; MTB: *Mycobacterium tuberculosis*; RIF: rifampicin)

LIPOARABINOMANNAN

Lipoarabinomannan assay (LAM) is an inexpensive biomarker-based antigen detection test which detects lipopolysaccharide present in mycobacterial cell walls. Presently, Alere Determine TB LAM Ag, Abbott, San Diego, USA is the only WHO-approved, commercially available urinary LAM test. It has utility in resource-limited settings and/or nonavailability of sputum sample. However, it has poor sensitivity, 42% in HIV, and failure to differentiate between mycobacterial species and can cross-react with other fungal diseases.

The WHO recommends lateral-flow LAM (LF-LAM) to assist in the diagnosis of active pulmonary TB in HIV-positive adults, adolescents, and children with signs and symptoms and those with advanced HIV disease.[2,7]

CONCLUSION

To conclude, last decade has seen emergence of plethora of molecular tests for detection of TB and DR-TB approved by WHO, thus facilitating correct anti-TB treatment and better treatment outcome. However, microscopy is a rapid test that continues to play role in monitoring treatment response.

REFERENCES

1. World Health Organization (WHO). (2023). WHO standard: Universal access to rapid tuberculosis diagnostics. [online] Available from https://www.who.int/publications/i/item/9789240071315 [Last accessed September, 2024].
2. World Health Organization (WHO). (2024). WHO consolidated guidelines on tuberculosis: module 3: diagnosis: rapid diagnostics for tuberculosis detection, 3rd edition. [online] Available from https://www.who.int/publications/i/item/9789240089488 [Last accessed September, 2024].
3. Central TB Division, Ministry of Health and Family Welfare (MoHFW), Government of India. (2020). Training Modules (1-4) For Programme Managers & Medical officers. [online] Available from https://tbcindia-wp.azurewebsites.net/wp-content/uploads/2023/05/NTEPTrainingModules1to4.pdf [Last accessed September, 2024].
4. Ministry of Health and Family Welfare (MoHFW), Government of India. (2021). Guidelines for programmatic management of drug resistant tuberculosis in India. [online] Available from https://tbcindia.mohfw.gov.in/wp-content/uploads/2023/05/8368587497Guidelines-for-PMDT-in-India-1.pdf [Last accessed September, 2024].
5. Emily MacLean, Mikashmi Kohli, Stefan F Weber, Anita Suresh, Samuel G Schumacher, Claudia M Denkinger, et al. Advances in Molecular Diagnosis of Tuberculosis. J Clin Microbiol. 2020;58(10):e01582-19.
6. World Health Organization. Use of targeted next-generation sequencing to detect drug-resistant tuberculosis. Rapid communication, World Health Organization 2023, 978-92-4-007637-2 (electronic version).
7. Cara M Gill, Lorraine Dolan, Laura M Piggott, Anne Marie McLaughlin. New developments in tuberculosis diagnosis and treatment. Breathe 2022;18:210149.

CHAPTER

9

How One Can Lead to Extensively Drug-resistant Tuberculosis?

Sangeeta Sharma

Abstract

Mismanagement of tuberculosis leads to augmentation and worsening of drug-resistance resulting in emergence of extensively drug-resistant (XDR) strains. Main risk factors are wrong regimen given at wrong dosages with poor compliance and presence of uncontrolled comorbidities in a patient. Lack of implementation of preventive strategies for high-risk groups results in transmission. Redressal warrants timely physician, patient, and provider centric interventions.

Keywords: Extensively drug-resistant TB, XDR-TB, risk factors

INTRODUCTION

Extensively drug-resistant tuberculosis (XDR-TB) remains a major public health problem negating the effectiveness of strategies under the TB control programs. Reliable epidemiological and surveillance data on the global trends of actual disease burden is essential to determine the effectiveness TB treatment and prevention strategies directed to achieve the milestones and targets of the WHO's End TB Strategy and the UN Sustainable Development Goals. Globally in 2022, out of 10.6 million people who developed TB, 410,000 had multidrug-resistant TB (MDR-TB), and the estimated proportion of MDR/rifampicin-resistant (RR)-TB cases with pre-XDR-TB (i.e., resistance to any fluoroquinolone) and XDR-TB, i.e., resistance to other Group A drugs along with fluoroquinolone) was 18% [95% confidence interval (CI) 16–20%]. The number of people diagnosed and started on treatment was much lower—175,650 people in 2022, equivalent to about two in five of those in need and still below the prepandemic level of 181,533 people in 2019. An estimated 160,000 deaths attributed largely to lack of access to effective TB treatment. India contributed to 27% of this global burden although reliable country data on XDR-TB is not available. This is a cause of further concern as the burden may be even higher than estimated due to underreporting and underdiagnosis.[1]

TEXT

Factors such as spontaneous genetic mutations occurring in the *Mycobacterium tuberculosis* (MTB) at predictable rates confer resistance to first-line drug (FLD) and second-line drug (SLD) anti-TB drugs, coupled with inherent genetic susceptibility of the host are factors beyond human control for acquiring primary XDR-TB. But there are many more important preventable TB risk determinants which can lead to emergence of XDR-TB in a patient.[2,3] The most powerful predictor for the presence of XDR-TB in a patient is past history of inadequate irregular drug-sensitive or drug-resistant TB treatment, generally resulting in sequential selection of mutant strains with each course of irregular antitubercular therapy (ATT). Thus, mismanagement of TB with resultant worsening of drug-resistance (DR) pattern leads to augmentation of secondary DR and emergence of XDR strains.[2,3]

Implementation of protocol-based programmatic management guidelines for drug-resistant tuberculosis (PMDT) and streamlined services ensuring universal health coverage (UHC) so that preventive and treatment facilities are readily available and accessible to all those who actually need them.[4] This is a significant challenge and disruptions, if frequent, can lead to amplification of resistance increasing the risk of XDR-TB, its prevalence, transmission, further worsening of resistance and mortality.[2-4] Redressal warrants timely physician, patient, and provider centric interventions.[1,4]

Physician centric interventions target continuum of care starting from early accurate diagnosis, initiation of appropriate treatment regimen in right dosages, ensuring compliance, and timely follow-ups for a successful final outcome.[4]

Implementation of universal drug-sensitivity testing (DST) and availability of reliable DST results for patients with treatment failure and MDR-TB patients cannot be undermined and are of utmost importance while the physician builds upon the second-line treatment regimen prescription.[4] Further, diagnosis is particularly difficult in highly vulnerable DR-TB populations such as children, human immunodeficiency virus (HIV), homeless, and prisoners. Limited skilled staff with expertise and training in the differential presentation of TB in children and people living with HIV (PLHIV) can result in diagnostic delays.[2,3] Access to diagnosis of XDR-TB can be challenging with limited availability of DST to new and repurposed antituberculosis drugs (ATDs) bedaquiline, linezolid, clofazimine, delamanid, and pretomanid.[5] Genotypic testing [drug-resistance testing (DRT)] based on molecular markers of bedaquiline and linezolid resistance is not yet fully understood, therefore phenotypic testing (DST) on culture isolates is currently the only reliable test available. Resistance-conferring genetic mutations are scattered without a defined hotspot region, meaning that the development of a rapid molecular test might not be feasible for bedaquiline in the near future. This is a significant gap in the expansion of DST for monitoring of the emergence of further resistance when all RR/MDR/Pre-XDR/XDR regimens being used at present are bedaquiline based.[5] By performing whole-genome sequencing (WGS) or next-generation sequencing (NGS) of serial strains, low-frequency resistance mutations and heterogeneous resistance with high sensitivity can be detected. Emphasis should therefore be to recommend conducting reliable drug susceptibility tests, including WGS or TGS at the beginning of treatment and repeating the DST when the sputum conversion is delayed in all DR-TB patients.[6]

Linking of correct laboratory results to individual patients and their clinical data in a timely manner is pertinent for these to be meaningful and actionable. Further nowadays, results of most diagnostic tests, molecular assays and liquid culture DST (MGIT) including their rapid analysis, are available in a digital format which can be communicated with help information technology connectivity to the desired physician, a transition from paper-based recording and reporting systems to case-based digital surveillance systems. However, its implementation is hindered by the absence of unique patient identification codes, multiple samples being tested from the same patient bearing different codes, recurrent referrals to different health facilities for testing of the same patient and connectivity issues. This results in decreased notification rates at most centers even in expected patients.[7]

Physician's prescription errors include failure to identify preexisting resistance profile, disease severity and charting of drugs used by the patient in the past, selection of ineffective drug combinations incorporating several less active drug classes, incorrect inappropriate regimen required for a particular resistance pattern, the addition of a single drug to a failing regimen, inadequate drugs dosages as per body weight, and dosing intervals, incomplete treatment duration of anti-TB drugs are all treatment factors that predispose a MDR-TB patient to the emergence of further resistance and XDR-TB.[2,3,7]

Long and toxic MDR-TB treatment regimens can result in poor adherence in some, with the patient missing drug doses during their present or past ATT courses. This piles up as augmentation of resistance, adding up with development of compounding resistance to drugs with each course. Nonadherence to prescribed treatment is often underestimated by physicians and is difficult to predict. Habitual defaulters may have associated factors such as psychiatric illness, emotional and physical stress, alcoholism, drug addiction, homelessness, and poverty.[2,3,7] Multisectoral action is needed to address these TB risk determinants.[4]

There is some evidence emerging linking comorbidities such as HIV/acquired immunodeficiency syndrome (AIDS), hepatitis, malnutrition, other chronic conditions, smoking, socioeconomic factors like poverty, and overcrowding with XDR-TB.[2,3] Diabetes mellitus (DM) and malnutrition are well-known risk factors for TB in the past. But recently, some studies have shown significant association of these with treatment failure and emergence of XDR-TB. There is a higher chance of inadequate immune response of the host, persistence of TB bacilli with higher mycobacterial loads, hence a higher chance of random bacillary mutation and the emergence of MDR and XDR-TB strains. This necessitates stringent control of comorbidities alongside longer TB treatment, on a case to case basis. Further, uncontrolled DM and malnutrition have recently been linked to variations in the drug bioavailability or blood pharmacokinetic (PK) levels resulting in increased odds of unfavorable treatment outcome, particularly death.[7] The global convergence of the accelerating type 2 DM pandemic, emergence of XDR mutants has become a serious challenge to clinicians worldwide.[4]

Another important contributing factor are the logistic difficulties governed by centralized services. Poor political commitment and administrative control can result in frequent stock-outs or shortages of drugs and diagnostics due to limited procurement, poor quality control, distribution, and supply chain management. Shortage of drugs can be a common reason forcing patients to stop treatment, especially in resource-limited settings because of the patient's inability to support expensive reserve drugs. Limited training of human resources at all levels can mar the availability of expertise and skilled workers resulting in deficits in the optimal continuum of care and preventive facilities.[4,7]

Tuberculosis control programs implemented in the past had poor infrastructure, using conventional diagnostics, empirical treatment strategies based upon local susceptibility patterns, poor follow-ups, all having partly contributed to the building up of DR over the years.[2,3,7]

CONCLUSION

The ultimate multipronged strategy to control XDR-TB is a comprehensive targeted approach incorporating all the good preventive and treatment practices, based upon sustained political commitment; a rational case-finding with quality assured, accurate diagnosis through rapid molecular methods, and liquid culture DST; appropriate treatment regimen ensuring compliance; uninterrupted supply of quality-assured diagnostics and ATDs; standardized recording and reporting system; and preventive therapy for high-risk groups.

REFERENCES

1. WHO. Global tuberculosis report 2023. Geneva: World Health Organization; 2023.
2. Saifullah A, Mallhi TH, Khan YH, Iqbal MS, Alotaibi NH, Alzarea AI, et al. Evaluation of risk factors associated with the development of MDR- and XDR-TB in a tertiary care hospital: a retrospective cohort study. PeerJ. 2021;9:e10826.
3. Sinulingga HE, Sinaga BY, Siagian P, Ashar T. Profile and risk factors of pre-XDR-TB and XDR-TB patients in a national reference hospital for Sumatra region of Indonesia. Narra J. 2023;3(3):e407.
4. WHO. WHO consolidated guidelines on tuberculosis. Module 4: treatment-drug-resistant tuberculosis treatment, 2022 update. Geneva: World Health Organization; 2022.
5. Kadura S, King N, Nakhoul M, Zhu H, Theron G, Köser CU, et al. Systematic review of mutations associated with resistance to the new and repurposed Mycobacterium tuberculosis drugs bedaquiline, clofazimine, linezolid, delamanid and pretomanid. J Antimicrob Chemother. 2020;75:2031-43.
6. Chen X, He G, Lin S, Wang S, Sun F, Chen J, et al. Analysis of Serial Multidrug-Resistant Tuberculosis Strains Causing Treatment Failure and Within-Host Evolution by Whole-Genome Sequencing. mSphere. 2020;5(6):e00884-20.
7. Pedersen OS, Butova T, Kapustnyk V, Miasoiedov V, Kuzhko M, Hryshchuk L, et al. Treatment outcomes and risk factors for an unsuccessful outcome among patients with highly drug-resistant tuberculosis in Ukraine. Clin Microbiol Infect. 2024;30(3):360-7.

CHAPTER 10

Strain Typing Methods in the Identification of Drug Resistance in *Mycobacterium Tuberculosis*

Priya Rajendran, Sivakumar Shanmugam, Banurekha V Velayutham

Abstract

Tuberculosis (TB), caused by the bacterium *Mycobacterium tuberculosis* (MTB), remains one of the serious health problems worldwide. The different strains of MTB have been associated with drug resistance, transmission, and outbreaks. Hence many studies focused on the identification of the strains belonging to different lineages using various molecular typing methods. Insertion sequence IS6110-based restriction fragment length polymorphism (RFLP) analysis was considered as the gold standard for the molecular typing of MTB. However, newer methods such as spacer oligonucleotide typing (spoligotyping); mycobacterial interspersed repetitive units-variable number tandem repeats, (MIRU-VNTR); and the recently developed whole genome sequencing (WGS) demonstrated higher resolution and discriminatory power. With the provision of considerable data and unprecedent accuracy, WGS paves a revolutionary path in drug resistant MTB strain identification, transmission dynamics, and outbreak investigations.

Keywords: Drug resistance, lineages, molecular typing, WGS

INTRODUCTION

Tuberculosis (TB) disease, caused by *Mycobacterium tuberculosis* (MTB), is a serious threat with high disease burden reported worldwide. In addition, multidrug-resistant (MDR)-TB, that is resistant to at least two first-line drugs isoniazid (INH) and rifampicin (RIF), and extremely drug-resistant XDR (TB), a MDR-TB that is resistant to a fluoroquinolone, and bedaquiline and/or linezolid have poses a greater threat.[1] The drug resistance is mediated through, single nucleotide polymorphism/insertion/deletion (mutation) of nucleotides from the gene conferring resistance. These mutations arise due to drug pressure leading to resistance toward the anti-TB drugs. However, all mutations in a gene do not necessarily lead to phenotypic resistance and are graded based on their ability to increase the minimal inhibitory concentration (MIC) of the drug toward MTB. Such mutations are characterized and catalogued by the World Health Organization (WHO) for the lineages reported worldwide and by Indian Council of Medical Research (ICMR)-National Institute for Research in Tuberculosis (NIRT) for the lineages prevalent in India.

A total of nine lineages have been identified so far with MTB *sensu stricto*, including lineages 1 (East African Indian/EAI), 2 (Est Asian/Beijing), 3 (Central Asian Strain/CAS),

4 (Euro American), 7, and 8, and MTB var. africanum, including lineages 5, 6, and 9. There is a major difference seen in disease severity, transmission pattern and drug resistance based on the lineage distribution in MTB. For example, compared to lineage 7, lineages 3, 4, and 5 are more virulent while lineages 2 and 3 are prone to gaining genetic determinants of drug resistance.[2] Hence, in addition to diagnosis of MTB and its drug resistance, strain identification to lineage level is important for the disease control, since it has a major impact on development of MDR/XDR-TB, treatment outcome, and epidemiological outbreaks. Commonly used MTB strain typing methods are, insertion sequence IS*6110*-based RFLP analysis, spacer oligonucleotide typing (spoligotyping), mycobacterial interspersed repetitive units-variable number tandem repeats (MIRU-VNTR) and whole genome sequencing (WGS). We have described here the evolution of different typing methods and current progress made in strain identification of MTB.

IS6110-BASED RESTRICTION FRAGMENT LENGTH POLYMORPHISM

The insertion sequence IS6110 of MTBC is usually present in multiple copies ranging from 0 to 25 based on the frequency of transposition and the genomic region of transposition. The difference in this copy number and its location in the genome is responsible for its high polymorphism and influences IS6110 as molecular marker for MTB strain identification. The method in brief involves polymerase chain reaction (PCR) amplification followed by digestion using restriction enzyme *PvuII*, gel electrophoresis, and southern blot hybridization **(Fig. 1)**. Being a commonly used and standardized method, the fingerprints generated from various studies are digitalized and catalogued to compare by a computer program developed exclusively for the fingerprint analysis. This method serves as an useful tool for identification of transmission events, investigation of outbreaks, and differentiation between reactivation and reinfection.[3] Despite its high discriminatory

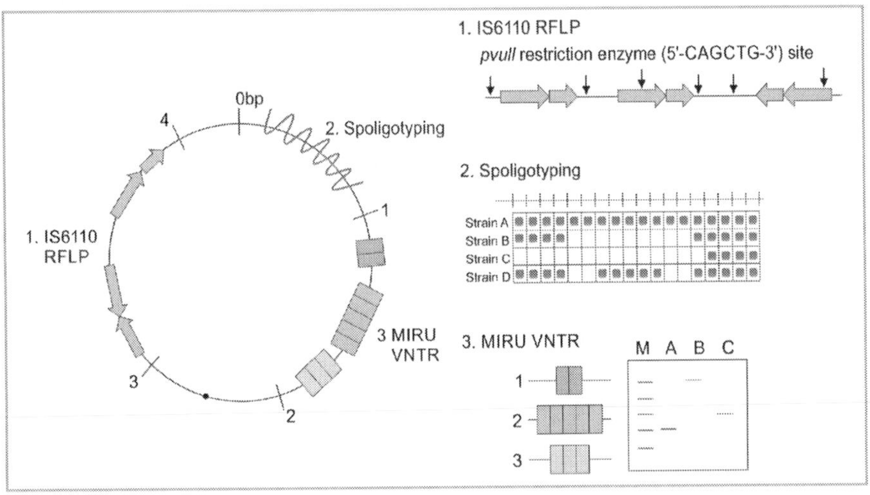

FIG. 1: Molecular genotyping methods found in the *Mycobacterium* genome [modified from Chae et al. (2018)]. 1—IS 6110 RFLP carried out on specific transposase gene carrying restriction enzyme (*PvuII*). 2—Spoligotyping of direct repeat of 36-bp length interspersed by unique spacers [spoligotypes patterns represented by black (presence of spacers) and white (absence of spacers) boxes]. 3—Variable number tandem repeats (VNTR) of mycobacterial interspersed repetitive units (MIRU) are also employed as unique markers.

power, reproducibility, and stability of the patterns obtained, IS6110 RFLP is not used in recent studies owing to its technical limitations. The need for high-quality DNA, expensive computer software and personnel with great technical expertise reduced its utility in MTB molecular epidemiology studies.

MYCOBACTERIAL INTERSPERSED REPETITIVE UNIT-VARIABLE NUMBER TANDEM REPEAT

The MIRU is a minisatellite-like structure found in MTB genome composed of 40–60 base pair unit repetitive sequence that is used in strain identification by variation in its number. MIRU-VNTR is being preferred in many countries over spoligotyping and IS6110 RFLP in recent years. The major advantage behind this preference is the quick process with high accuracy and need for small amount of DNA. The principle involved behind this method is analysis of variable tandem repeat loci that are amplified using specific primers complementary to the flanking regions **(Fig. 1)**. The tandem repeat units generated are changed into numerical code to get digital format results. The digits thus obtained represent the number of copies at a particular locus and digitalization of the technique has led to the development of a free software tool named VNTR plus. This webtool can be used for strain similarity search, constructing phylogenetic trees, and geographic information mapping and this in turn will help in transmission studies, and to study association of drug resistance. Although MIRU-VNTR has higher resolution compared to IS6110 RFLP, 12- and 15-MIRU-VNTR still has lower discriminatory power. Hence, use of 24-MIRU-VNTR is preferred in recent years but with the limitation of complex process involved and mandate of high-end system for analysis.

SPOLIGOTYPING

Spoligotyping is a hybridization assay based on the amplification of spacers comprising 43 short sequences. Based on the variation in spacers for different strains, the spot patterns obtained in hybridization process will vary for the samples tested **(Fig. 1)**. These spots are translated into numerical code of 15 digits (octal code), leading to generation of >3,800 spoligotypes. The lineage association with drug resistance has been documented by spoligotyping studies worldwide. For example, MDR-TB isolates from Northern and Central India, China, Korea, and Taiwan seemed to have significantly higher frequencies of association with Beijing strains. Reports from other studies have documented the association of Beijing strains with streptomycin (Poland), ethambutol, and linezolid resistance (China).[4] Possibility of generating spoligotypes data from WGS data is being explored in various studies and the prediction of spoligotypes is done usually by SpolPred software. However, with increase in generation of MTB WGS data in recent times, a new software termed Spolpred2 have been developed that can be integrated with the TB-Profiler tool, a pipeline used for detection of MTB resistance and strain type from WGS data.[5] Although, spoligotyping seems to be useful in epidemiological studies, the agreement at the lineage relationship particularly at the level of sub lineage was low. This limitation could be tackled by using this SpolPred2 tool, since dual method of strain typing is involved. In such instances, understanding the association of lineage with drug resistance becomes easier and more studies in future using this approach are needed.

WHOLE GENOME SEQUENCING

With the provision of considerable data and unprecedent accuracy, WGS paves a revolutionary path in the clinical management of drug-resistant TB, since it can identify even small insertions and deletions (indels). The high sensitivity and specificity of WGS have been demonstrated by a systematic review for the first-line drugs INH and RIF.[6] However, significantly high variation in other first- and second-line drugs indicates that identification of MTB drug resistance may be more intricate than anticipated. This limitation could be attributed to complicated genetic mechanisms involved in conferring resistance, or resistance being driven by nonspecific mechanisms such as efflux pumps which requires attention when WGS is used to make clinical decisions. Another major hindrance of using WGS in clinical setting is relying on culture for DNA extraction and sequencing which is still time consuming for patient management. Although, direct WGS from samples has been shown to be successful in few studies, the discordance between phenotypic and genotypic results needs to be resolved with larger datasets before completely switching to direct WGS.

While there are various technical limitations in implementing WGS, a significant progress has been made in terms of data analysis and standardization tool development. Several online database tools, such as ReSeqTB, TBPortal, TBprofiler, and GenTB served in interpreting and linking genetic drug resistance result to phenotypic data thus allowing periodic surveillance of drug resistance at global level. Using such tools, the association of drug resistance at lineage level could be documented. For example, when a phylogenetic analysis was performed on a dataset of 5310 WGS MTB sequences isolated from five different continents, global spread of both Beijing and non-Beijing strain with at least 32 different MDR-TB clades were documented.[7] While studies on resistance conferring determinants are linked to lineages 2 and 4 globally, Indian studies have documented that lineage 1, being predominant in South India and 3 in North India are more commonly involved with drug resistance.[8]

CONCLUSION

In summary, while other typing methods are getting outdated, WGS is likely to be the sole reliable method in epidemiological and evolutionary studies along with drug-resistance testing in future. With the reduction in cost of sequencing, improved sequencing technologies and development of analytic tool, implementing WGS in TB laboratories will increase. However, the major challenges pointed out in various studies worldwide namely failure to demonstrate the impact on treatment outcome; relying on culture for DNA isolation; discrepancies between genotypic and phenotypic resistance results; and lack of a well-established IT infrastructure need to be addressed for better performance and data interpretation of WGS.

REFERENCES

1. Dheda K, Mirzayev F, Cirillo DM, Udwadia Z, Dooley KE, Chang KC, et al. Multidrug-resistant tuberculosis. Nat Rev Dis Primers. 2024;10(1):22.
2. Shanmugam SK, Kumar N, Sembulingam T, Ramalingam SB, Selvaraj A, Rajendhiran U, et al. Mycobacterium tuberculosis Lineages Associated with Mutations and Drug Resistance in Isolates from India. Microbiol Spectr. 2022;10(3):e0159421.
3. Park YK, Bai GH, Kim SJ. Restriction fragment length polymorphism analysis of Mycobacterium tuberculosis isolated from countries in the western pacific region. J Clin Microbiol. 2000;38(1):191-7.
4. Panwalkar N, Chauhan DS, Desikan P. Spoligotype defined lineages of Mycobacterium tuberculosis and drug resistance: Merely a casual correlation? Indian J Med Microbiol. 2017;35(1):27-32.
5. Napier G, Couvin D, Refregier G, Guyeux C, Meehan CJ, Sola C, et al. Comparison of in silico predicted Mycobacterium tuberculosis spoligotypes and lineages from whole genome sequencing data. Sci Rep. 2023;13(1):11368.
6. Papaventsis D, Casali N, Kontsevaya I, Drobniewski F, Cirillo DM, Nikolayevskyy V. Whole genome sequencing of Mycobacterium tuberculosis for detection of drug resistance: a systematic review. Clin Microbiol Infect. 2017;23(2):61-8.

7. Cohen KA, Manson AL, Abeel T, Desjardins CA, Chapman SB, Hoffner S, et al. Extensive global movement of multidrug-resistantM. tuberculosis strains revealed by whole-genome analysis. Thorax. 2019;74(9):882-9.
8. Poonawala H, Kumar N, Peacock SJ. A review of published spoligotype data indicates the diversity of Mycobacterium tuberculosis from India is under-represented in global databases. Infect Genet Evol. 2020;78:104072.

CHAPTER

11

Pattern and Characteristics of Mutation in Drug Resistant Clinical Isolates of Extrapulmonary Tuberculosis

Ramakant Dixit, Ankur Gupta

Abstract

Genomic alterations in the specific genes of *Mycobacterium tuberculosis* determine the resistance to drugs. The genetic changes that confer resistance to major antimycobacterial drugs differ geographically and are influenced by many factors. MTBDRplus assay is a rapid and reliable molecular-based testing assay to detect gene mutations responsible for drug resistance in tuberculosis isolates both from pulmonary and extrapulmonary sites. There is limited literature on pattern and characteristics of mutation in tuberculosis isolate from extrapulmonary tuberculosis sites. Therefore, it is important to identify resistance mutation patten not only to guide effective antituberculosis treatment but also for epidemiological purpose.

Keywords: Genetic mutations, drug resistance, extrapulmonary tuberculosis

INTRODUCTION

Genome-wide analysis of multidrug resistance (MDR) and extensively drug-resistant *Mycobacterium tuberculosis* (XDR MTB) reveals that drug resistance arises due to mutations in the gene and/or the promoter region.[1] Accurate and rapid detection of MDR-tuberculosis (TB) is critical for decreasing the transmission of TB and reducing the amplification of drug resistance. Acquisition of drug resistance in MTB does not occur as a result of horizontal transfer of resistance-determining genes or region, but results from mutations (caused by substitutions or deletions or insertions of nucleotide sequences) in specific resistance-determining regions of the gene targets or their promoters or activating enzymes of anti-TB chemotherapeutic agents.[2] However, based on the knowledge of reported mutations of the anti-TB drug resistance genes, rapid molecular diagnostic line probe assay (LPA) has been developed for the detection of drug resistance in MTB. In 2008, Genotype MTBDRplus LPA has been recommended for rapid detection of drug resistance of MTB by World Health Organization (WHO). Many studies have shown that the specificity and sensitivity of genotype MTBDRplus assay for rifampicin (RIF) and isoniazid (INH) resistance are found to be comparable to conventional phenotypic drug susceptibility testing (DST).[2] A meta-analysis study carried out in 2008 found that the genotype MTBDRplus assay has a sensitivity of 98% for detecting RIF resistance and 89% for detecting INH resistance, and specificity of 99% for both RIF and INH.[3] Similarly, mutations in several genetic loci have been implicated in development of resistance to second-line anti-TB drugs.

Globally, many reports have been published on detection and diagnosis that are based on rapid advanced molecular assays. However, owing to the geographical diversity of MTB clinical isolates across the world, there is a possibility of varying efficacy of molecular genotyping methods, which may have diagnostic implications. In addition, the mutations responsible for resistance could differ with region and thus provide an insight into the epidemiology of the disease. In **Table 1,** the magnitude of drug-resistant (DR) MTB isolates and pattern of drug resistance mutations is not well known. As far as monoresistance is concerned, resistance to INH (7.2%) exceeds other first-line anti-TB drugs [6.85% for streptomycin (SM), 1.6% for ethambutol, and 4.6% for RIF].[4]

Phenotypic methods of DST are widely used in developed countries, whereas in developing countries genotypic methods are used to avoid culture and biosafety constraints. Genotypic methods show only the screen for mutations in resistance genes, while phenotypic methods detect resistance accompanied by risk factors associated with the problem. There is a scarcity of data on the drug-specific resistance patterns of extrapulmonary tuberculosis (EPTB), particularly in countries with high TB burdens, as a result of the lack of extrapulmonary specimens and DST capabilities. Unlike pulmonary TB, systematic drug resistance surveillance in EPTB is not carried out, and consequently there are no reliable estimates of the level of drug resistance in EPTB.[5]

In a study from selected health facilities in Addis Ababa, Ethiopia,[6] all RIF resistant isolates from EPTB sites had rpoB mutations at codon 530–533, which showed the absence of the wild-type band (WT8) with the appearance of MUT and an amino acid mutation at the S531L position 2. All INH resistance mutation patterns were in katG and among them 11.4% were missing from the WT at codon 315, 6.8% had an amino acid mutation at the S315T1 position, and 2.3% isolate had one at the S315T2 position.

Of the 151 extrapulmonary isolates is another study from Ethopia,[7] the sensitivity and specificity of MTBDRplus in detecting INH resistance were 90.9% and 100%, respectively.

TABLE 1: Mutations implicated in resistance of tubercle bacilli to different drugs.

Drug	Resistance genes	Gene function	Mechanism
Rifampicin	*rpoB*	RNA polymerase	Target modification
Isoniazid	*katG*	Catalase-peroxidase enzyme	Decreased drug activation
	inhA	NADH-dependent enoyl-acyl carrier protein	Target amplification or modification
Pyrazinamide	*pncA*	Pyrazinamidase	Decreased drug activation
Ethambutol	*embCAB operon*	Arabinosyltransferase	Target modification
Levofloxacin Moxifloxacin	*gyrA gyrB*	DNA gyrase A DNA gyrase B	Target modification
Linezolid	*Rrl*	23S rRNA	Target modification
Cycloserine	*Ald*	L-alanine dehydrogenase	Substrate shunting
Amikacin, capreomycin, and kanamycin	*Rrs*	16S rRNA	Target modification
Streptomycin	*rpsL*	12S ribosomal protein	Target modification
Kanamycin	*Eis*	Aminoglycoside acetyltransferase	Inactivating mutation

While for RIF, it was 100% and 99.3% for sensitivity and specificity, respectively. The katG S315Tl was the most common mutation observed in 85.7% of the INH-resistant isolates. In the case of RIF, the most common mutation (61.9%) was observed at position rpoB S531L. Two percent of MTB isolates had discordant results between the genotypic MTBDRplus test and the phenotypic DST. Discordant results between phenotypic and genotypic DST may be due to the fact that not all mutations conferring resistance to anti-TB drugs are included in the LPA assay. Mutations in the gyrA promoter region were strongly associated with levofloxacin and moxifloxacin resistance. A mutation in the gyrA codon was found in 14.3% of fluoroquinolone (FQ)-resistant isolates. This mutation confers resistance to levofloxacin and is associated with low-level resistance to moxifloxacin. The gyrA mutations were predominantly found to occur in codons 92–96. The predominant *rrs* gene mutation was A1401G (7.1%). This is a common mutation to be associated with high-level resistance to amikacin, capreomycin, and kanamycin.

In a study from China,[8] 111 DR-EPTB isolates included pre-XDR-TB (53.2%), MDR-TB (29.7%), and poly–DR-TB (12.6%). The resistant drugs were INH followed by RIF and SM. The genotypes of 111 strains were lineage 2 and lineage 4. KatG_p.Ser315Thr was main gene mutation for resistance to INH; rpsL_p.Lys43Arg for SM, rpoB_p.Ser450Leu for RIF, embB_p.Met306Val for ethambutol, gyrA_p.Asp94Gly for FQs, and pncA_p.Thr76Pro for pyrazinamide (PZA). The residence was a significant risk factor for cluster transmission by patients and phenotypic DR types of strains for lineage 2 transmission.

A cross-sectional study analyzed 218 fine-needle aspirate (FNA) samples from tuberculosis lymph nodes (TBLN) patients and among the 50 culture-positive isolates, 14% had drug resistance caused by a gene mutation. Out of these, 8% isolates were mono-resistant to INH drug, which is caused by a gene mutation in katG in the region of interrogated at codon 315 in the amino acid sequence of S315T1, and 6% isolates were resistant to both RIF and INH drugs. The mutation was observed for katG (at codon 315 with a change in the sequence of amino acid S315T) and rpoB [at codon 530–533 with a change in the sequence of amino acid *S531L* (*S450L*)] genes. The most prevalent spoligotypes were orphan and SIT53 strains. The orphan and SIT53 (T) strains were the most common in the study area, and a DR strain caused by a common gene mutation could indicate the transmission of clonal-resistant strains in the community. Four isolates tested resistant to the INH drug of the *katG* gene only with gene deletion in *katG/WT* and gene insertion in MUT1 (S315T1 change in amino acid sequences) conferring INH resistance. No inhA drug resistance-associated gene mutation was observed in this study. In the case of RIF, study identified a mutation in the region interrogated at codon530–533 with a change in the amino acid sequence of S531L insertion. The 50 isolates were further characterized by RD9 deletion-based polymerase chain reaction (PCR) followed by spoligotyping and no *Mycobacterium bovis* was found suggesting that bovine TB may play a minor role in humans.[9]

A study from Iran[10] demonstrated sequence alterations in codon 513 of the 81 bp region of the *rpoB* gene as the most common mutation occurred in 75.6% of molecularly confirmed RIF-resistant strains from different extrapulmonary sites. In addition, simultaneous mutation at codons 512 and 513 was demonstrated in 34.3% of the isolates. However, our findings lead to the conclusion that based on molecular identification and drug susceptibility results, we can demonstrate mutations and correlate the genetic events within the isolates to their resistance. The rate of rpoB mutations in this study was high stressing on further studies to clarify the epidemiology of resistant MTB. Sequence analysis of the 81 bp region of the *rpoB* gene demonstrated mutations in 61.2% sequenced samples. Several point mutations including deletion mutations at codons 510, 512, 513, and 515, with 45% and 51% of the mutations in codons 512 and 513, respectively were seen, along with 26% replacement mutations at codons 509, 513, 514, 518, 520, 524, and 531. The most common alteration was Gln → His, at codon 513, presented in 75.6% isolates.

Another study from 60 TBLN isolates, 8.3% were identified MDR-TB cases and one isolate was INH mono-resistant. Most of the RIF-resistant isolates showed mutation in codon S531L and all isolates mutated in the *katG* gene conferring INH-resistant strains had mutations in codon of S315T1. Five and six resistance-associated mutation isolates were found in *rpoB* and *katG* genes, respectively and five isolates (8.3%) were MDR-TB. There were no isolates that showed the mutation in the inhA promoter region gene. Of five RIF resistant isolates, missing WT along with known mutations could be detected in all resistant isolates. Of these, 80% of them showed mutations in codon S531L and one isolate was in codon H526Y mutation.[11]

A study from north India on DR-EPTB, phenotypic DST and gene sequencing revealed 100% concordance for gryA, gryB, and rss. The most common single mutation in gryA was D 94 A (aspartic acid-alanine, 8.2%). Other mutations included D 94 Y (aspartic acid-tyrosine, 4.1%) and A 90 V (alanine-valine, 2%) isolates. In gryB, a single mutation was observed at position 1496 (AAC-ACC) which led to an amino acid change, asparagine 499-threonine in 2% isolates. In rss, one isolated mutation was observed at position 1401 (CAC-CGC) in 4% isolates.[12]

In a study from Varanasi,[13] India, out of 14 MDR-TB strains from EPTB samples, 12 had mutations in rpoBS531L (MUT3 band) and 2 had mutations in *rpoB* MUT D516V (MUT1 band). KatG mutation was predominant in all INH-resistant strains. All 14 MDR-TB strains and one INH mono-resistant strain had mutations in *katG* S315T1 (MUT1 band). Combined KatG and inhA mutations were found in one MDR-TB strain. Genotype MTBDRplus assay showed a good concordance with conventional DST. Mutation in codon s531L was detected in 78.57% of RIF-resistant isolates. There was 100% association of mutation in codon s315T1 of katG with INH resistance and combined mutation in inhA and *katG* gene was observed in 7.4% which is within a range of previously reported studies.

The most common FQ resistance gene mutation among extra-pulmonary DR TB isolates was MUT3C (50%) followed by WT3 mutation (33.3%) in a study from western part of India.[14] Furthermore, WT3 mutation was significantly associated with EPTB. (*p* value 0.001). These finding were different from Northen Indian data[12] where MUT 3B was most common mutation in EPTB (8.2%). No second-line aminoglycoside mutations were observed among extrapulmonary DR-TB samples in this study.

Resistance to drugs is due to particular genomic mutations in the specific genes of MTB. Timely genetic characterization will allow identification of resistance mutations that will optimize an effective antibiotic treatment regimen. The global rise of MDR-TB has emphasized the need for rapid, molecular-based testing to detect drug resistance in TB. Genotype MTBDRplus assay is a rapid and potentially reliable assay for detection of gene mutations associated with drug resistance in EPTB patients.

Genetic mutations play a crucial role in conferring anti-TB drug resistance in MTB. The presence of those genetic changes conferring resistance to key antimycobacterial drugs differs geographically and is influenced by factors such as the prevalence of DR-TB strains, treatment regimens, and patient adherence to therapy. Thus, understanding the types and frequency of those genetic changes is critical for effective DR strain detection, guiding treatment strategies, and monitoring the emergence of new resistance patterns. Moreover, to better understand the epidemiology and transmission dynamics of MDR-TB, further molecular epidemiology studies are needed to establish what proportion of MDR-TB cases are due to particular strains and what proportion of MDR-TB cases are due to ongoing transmission.

CONCLUSION

Genetic mutations play a crucial role in conferring anti-TB drug resistance in MTB. The presence of those genetic changes conferring resistance to key anti-mycobacterial drugs differs geographically and is influenced by factors like the prevalence of DR-TB strains, treatment regimens, and patient adherence to therapy. Thus, understanding the types and frequency of those genetic changes is critical for effective drug-resistant strain detection, guiding treatment strategies, and monitoring the emergence of new resistance patterns. Moreover, to better understand the epidemiology and transmission dynamics of MDR-TB, further molecular epidemiology studies are needed to establish what proportion of MDR-TB cases are due to particular strains and what proportion of MDR-TB cases are due to ongoing transmission.

REFERENCES

1. Ghosh A, N S, Saha S. Survey of drug resistance associated gene mutations in *Mycobacterium tuberculosis, ESKAPE* and other bacterial species. Sci Rep. 2020;10(1): 8957.
2. Bai Y, Wang Y, Shao C, Hao Y, Jin Y. GenoType MTBDRplus Assay for Rapid Detection of Multidrug Resistance in *Mycobacterium tuberculosis*: A Meta-Analysis. PLoS One. 2016;11(3):e0150321.
3. World Health Organization. (2018). WHO treatment guidelines for isoniazid resistant tuberculosis: Supplement to the WHO treatment guidelines for drug resistant tuberculosis. [online] Available from https://www.who.int/publications/i/item/9789241550079 [Last accessed September, 2024].
4. Polu GP, Mohammad Shaik J, Kota NMK, Karumanchi D, Allam US. Analysis of drug resistance mutations in pulmonary *Mycobacterium tuberculosis* isolates in the Southern coastal region of Andhra Pradesh, India. Braz J Infect Dis. 2019;23(5):281-90.
5. Singh PK. Epidemiological perspective of drug resistant extrapulmonary tuberculosis. World J Clin Infect Dis. 2015;5:77.
6. Alehegn E, Gebreyohanns A, Berhane BW, Wright JA, Hundie GB, Geremew RA, et al. Phenotypic Drug Resistance Pattern and Mutation Characteristics of *Mycobacterium tuberculosis* from Different Body Fluids Among Extra Pulmonary Patients Presented in Selected Hospitals in Addis Ababa, Ethiopia. Infect Drug Resist. 2023;16:5511-22.
7. Diriba G, Kebede A, Tola HH, Alemu A, Yenew B, Moga S, et al. Utility of line probe assay in detecting drug resistance and the associated mutations in patients with extrapulmonary tuberculosis in Addis Ababa, Ethiopia. SAGE Open Med. 2022;10:20503121221098241.
8. Shi T, Shou F, He Y, Zhou K, Gao W, Nie X, et al. Whole genome sequencing of drug resistance *Mycobacterium tuberculosis* from extra-pulmonary sites. Life Sci Alliance. 2023;6(11):e202302076.
9. Assefa G, Desta K, Araya S, Girma S, Hailu E, Mihret A, et al. Drug Resistance in Tuberculous Lymphadenitis: Molecular Characterization. Tuberc Res Treat. 2023;2023:3291538.
10. Khosravi AD, Meghdadi H, Ghadiri AA, Alami A, Sina AH, Mirsaeidi M. rpoB gene mutations among *Mycobacterium tuberculosis* isolates from extrapulmonary sites. APMIS. 2018;126(3):241-7.
11. Zewdie O, Mihret A, Abebe T, Kebede A, Desta K, Worku A, et al. Genotyping and molecular detection of multidrug-resistant *Mycobacterium tuberculosis* among tuberculosis lymphadenitis cases in Addis Ababa, Ethiopia. New Microbes New Infect. 2017;21:36-41.
12. Sharma SK, Chaubey J, Singh BK, Sharma R, Mittal A, Sharma A. Drug resistance patterns among extra-pulmonary tuberculosis cases in a tertiary care centre in North India. Int J Tuberc Lung Dis. 2017;21(10):1112-7.
13. Kumari R, Tripathi R, Pandey AP, Banerjee T, Sinha P, Anupurba S. Rapid Screening of MDR-TB in Cases of Extra Pulmonary Tuberculosis Using Geno Type MTBDRplus. PLoS One. 2016;11(7):e0159651.
14. Dixit R, Mohan E, Gupta A, Patni T. Pattern and characteristics of mutations conferring resistance to second line drugs in *Mycobacterium tuberculosis* isolates of pulmonary and extrapulmonary TB samples. Indian J Tuberc. 2024;71 Suppl 1:S37-S43.

CHAPTER

12

Impact of Genome Sequencing on Multidrug-resistant Tuberculosis Diagnosis and Prevalence

Chaitali Nikam

Abstract

Tuberculosis (TB) remains a major global health challenge, with multidrug-resistant TB (MDR-TB) complicating control efforts due to resistance to key anti-TB drugs. Traditional diagnostic methods are often slow and may miss novel resistance mutations, necessitating more advanced approaches. This chapter explores the impact of genome sequencing on the diagnosis and prevalence of MDR-TB, focusing on its advantages over conventional methods and its role in enhancing public health strategies.

Genome sequencing technology, including next-generation sequencing (NGS), whole-genome sequencing (WGS), and targeted sequencing assays. Genome sequencing offers significant improvements in sensitivity and specificity compared to traditional methods. It enables the precise identification of known and novel mutations associated with MDR-TB, facilitates rapid diagnosis with results available in days, and provides comprehensive genomic data for better surveillance and epidemiological mapping. Sequencing also supports the identification of previously unknown resistance mechanisms and improves understanding of transmission dynamics. Genome sequencing significantly impacts the diagnosis and control of MDR-TB by providing detailed genetic information and enabling more effective public health interventions. Addressing the associated challenges will be crucial for maximizing its benefits in global TB control efforts.

Keywords: TB, WGS, MDR, public health, diagnosis

INTRODUCTION

Tuberculosis (TB) continues to be a major global health challenge, with multidrug-resistant (MDR) TB presenting a significant obstacle to effective TB control programs worldwide. Patients with drug-resistant TB (DR-TB) may develop MDR or extensively drug-resistant (XDR) strains due to various factors, such as delayed diagnosis, improper treatment, or poor adherence to medication.[1] MDR-TB is characterized by resistance to at least two of the most effective first-line TB drugs—isoniazid (INH) and rifampicin (RIF). This resistance complicates both treatment and control strategies. Therefore, timely and accurate diagnosis of MDR-TB is essential for effective management and containment efforts.

Genome sequencing allows for a comprehensive analysis of *Mycobacterium tuberculosis* (MTB) genomes, identifying specific mutations linked to drug resistance. This method surpasses traditional techniques by detecting both known resistance mutations and novel variations that may not be captured by conventional susceptibility tests. Sequencing can provide insights into resistance mechanisms, including mutations in genes such as *rpoB*, *katG*, and *inhA*, which are crucial for RIF and INH resistance.

Controlling the high rates of DR-TB heavily relies on prompt laboratory diagnostics. Traditional methods for testing drug susceptibility, which involve culturing TB bacteria in solid or liquid media, can take several weeks or even months to produce results. The slow growth rate of MTB hinders the swift identification of drug resistance, thereby exacerbating the global spread of MDR-TB and XDR-TB. Recently, more rapid molecular diagnostic techniques, such as Xpert MTB/RIF and GenoType MTBDRplus, have been introduced into clinical practice.[2] While these methods offer quicker and simpler diagnosis, their implementation in resource-limited regions is constrained by high costs and limited availability.

SEQUENCING TECHNOLOGY

Recent advancements in genome sequencing technology have the potential to transform the landscape of MDR-TB diagnosis and prevalence monitoring, offering new tools for both clinical and public health applications. Genome sequencing determines the complete DNA sequence of an organism's genome. Next-generation sequencing (NGS) technologies, including whole-genome sequencing (WGS) and targeted sequencing, have revolutionized microbiology by allowing rapid, high-throughput sequencing at reduced costs. Unlike traditional methods that focus on a few genetic markers, sequencing provides comprehensive genomic data, facilitating the identification of mutations across the entire genome.

The World Health Organization (WHO) has recently approved two advanced amplicon-based sequencing assays for detailed DR-TB profiling directly from sputum samples.[3] The next-generation rapid drug susceptibility testing (DST) method evaluates mutations in gene regions of MTB associated with resistance to RIF, INH, fluoroquinolones, and second-line injectable drugs.[4] Meanwhile, the Deeplex R-MycTB assay utilizes a 24-amplicon panel to identify mutations across 18 genes related to resistance against 15 anti-TB drugs, including newer and repurposed medications such as bedaquiline (BDQ), clofazimine (CFZ), and linezolid (LZD).[5] Identifying resistance to these newer drugs is crucial, as they are now considered essential components in the WHO-recommended short MDR-TB regimens and emerging short-course DR-TB treatment protocols.[6,7] Successful application of the Deeplex assay using the portable Oxford Nanopore Technology MinION sequencer has been already demonstrated.

CURRENT WORKFLOW

The current MTB WGS workflow includes sputum decontamination followed by culture/enrichment (if not targeted) usually in a liquid media system, DNA extraction from culture, library preparation, and sequencing methods.[3] Sequence analysis involves validating data and performing quality control before mapping against a reference genome to identify genomic variations.

Recent studies have compared the accuracy of Xpert, line probe assays (LPAs), and WGS against phenotypic DST for detecting resistance to 15 different drugs. The agreement rates reported were 49% for Xpert, 63% for LPAs, and 93% for WGS.[8] Despite its high accuracy, the implementation of WGS in low-income, high TB-burden regions is challenging due to the need for specialized facilities, complex procedures, and highly skilled personnel for data analysis **(Fig. 1)**.

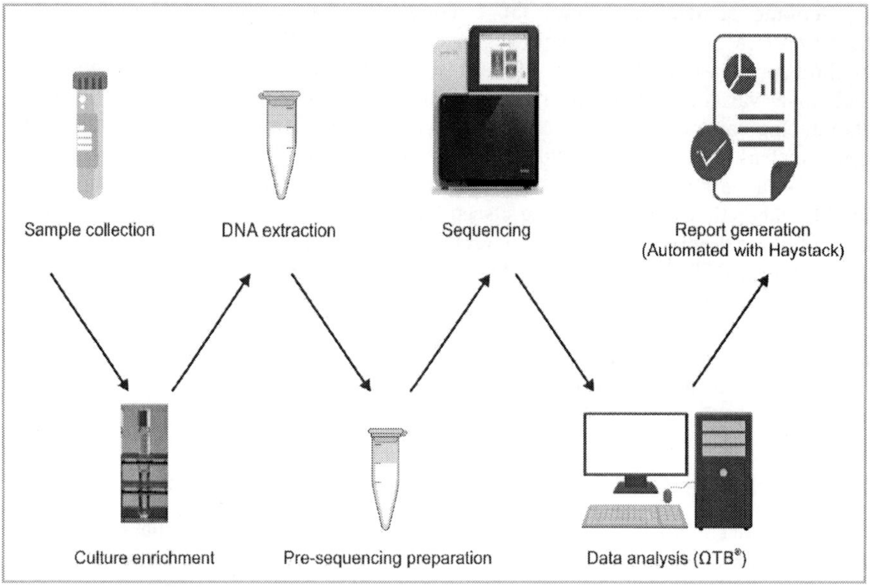

FIG. 1: Current flow of genome sequencing.

IMPACT ON DIAGNOSIS

Enhanced Sensitivity and Specificity

Genome sequencing provides a significant advantage over traditional diagnostic methods, such as culture-based techniques and molecular assays. Traditional methods often rely on detecting specific mutations associated with drug resistance, which may not identify all resistant strains. Sequencing, however, offers a comprehensive view of the genome, detecting a broad range of mutations linked to drug resistance along with coinfections and mixed infections.

Detection of Genetic Mutations

The MDR-TB is primarily caused by specific genetic mutations in the MTB genome. Sequencing can identify these mutations with high precision, including those in genes such as *rpoB*, *katG*, and *inhA*. By revealing these genetic markers, sequencing enables accurate identification of MDR-TB strains, leading to more effective treatment decisions.

Identification of Novel Resistance Mechanisms

Genome sequencing also aids in discovering novel resistance mechanisms that are not covered by conventional tests. This ability to identify previously unknown genetic variants associated with drug resistance expands our understanding of MDR-TB and informs the development of new diagnostic tools and treatments.

Rapid Turnaround Time

Traditional TB diagnostics, such as culture-based methods, can take weeks to yield results, which delays the initiation of appropriate treatment. In contrast, sequencing technologies can deliver results in a matter of days. This rapid turnaround is crucial in managing MDR-TB, especially in outbreak situations where timely intervention is necessary to prevent further spread.

IMPACT ON PREVALENCE

Improved Surveillance and Monitoring

Genome sequencing enhances surveillance by providing detailed genetic information on circulating TB strains. This data helps to track the spread of MDR-TB, identify outbreaks, and monitor trends in drug resistance. By mapping the genetic diversity of MDR-TB strains, public health officials can better understand the epidemiology of the disease including strain, lineages, etc.

Epidemiological Mapping

Sequencing data allows for precise geographic mapping of MDR-TB strains, identifying areas with high prevalence and pinpointing transmission hotspots. This information is crucial for directing resources and interventions to areas with the greatest need.

Understanding Transmission Dynamics

Sequencing technology enables a detailed analysis of transmission dynamics by tracking genetic variants of MTB. This tracking helps determine how MDR-TB strains spread within and between communities, informing targeted public health responses.

Public Health Interventions

Detailed genomic data supports the development of more targeted public health interventions. By understanding the genetic factors contributing to drug resistance and transmission, health authorities can design more effective strategies for controlling MDR-TB, including targeted screening, vaccination programs, and enhanced infection control measures.

LIMITATIONS

Despite its advantages, genome sequencing remains costly and may not be accessible in resource-limited settings. The high cost of sequencing technology and the need for specialized equipment and expertise can limit its widespread implementation.

The vast amount of data generated by sequencing can be challenging to interpret. Integrating genomic data into clinical practice requires sophisticated bioinformatics tools and expertise. Additionally, ensuring the accuracy and consistency of data interpretation across different laboratories is crucial for reliable results.

CONCLUSION

Genome sequencing has significantly impacted the diagnosis and management of MDR-TB, offering enhanced sensitivity, specificity, and rapid turnaround time. It has improved surveillance, monitoring, and understanding of MDR-TB prevalence and transmission dynamics. Despite challenges related to cost, data interpretation, and ethical concerns, the potential of sequencing technology to transform MDR-TB control efforts is immense. Continued investment in technological advancements and global collaborations will be key to harnessing the full potential of genome sequencing in the fight against MDR-TB.

REFERENCES

1. Kerubo G, Amukoye E, Niemann S, Kariuki S. Drug susceptibility profiles of pulmonary *Mycobacterium tuberculosis* isolates from patients in informal urban settlements in Nairobi, Kenya. BMC Infect Dis. 2016;l16:583.
2. Helb D, Jones M, Story E, Boehme C, Wallace E, Ho K, et al. Rapid detection of *Mycobacterium tuberculosis* and rifampin resistance by use of on-demand, near-patient technology. J Clin Microbiol. 2010;48:229-37.
3. The use of Next-generation Sequencing Technologies for the Detection of Mutations Associated with Drug Resistance in *Mycobacterium Tuberculosis* Complex: Technical Guide. Geneva: WHO
4. Colman RE, Mace A, Seifert M, Hetzel J, Mshaiel H, Suresh A, et al. Whole-genome and targeted sequencing of drug-resistant *Mycobacterium tuberculosis* on the iSeq100 and MiSeq: performance, ease-of-use, and cost evaluation. PLoS Med. 2019;16:e1002794.
5. Tagliani E, Hassan MO, Waberi Y, Filippo MR, De Falzon D, Dean A, et al. Culture and Next-generation sequencing-based drug susceptibility testing unveil high levels of drug-resistant-TB in Djibouti: results from the first national survey. Sci. Rep. 2017;7:17672.
6. Rapid Communication: Key Changes to the Treatment of Drug resistant Tuberculosis. Geneva: WHO; 2022.
7. WHO Consolidated Guidelines on Drug-resistant Tuberculosis Treatment. Geneva: WHO; 2019.
8. Heyckendorf J, Andres S, Köser CU, Olaru ID, Schön T, Sturegård E, et al. What Is Resistance? Impact of Phenotypic versus Molecular Drug Resistance Testing on Therapy for Multi- and Extensively Drug-Resistant Tuberculosis. Antimicrob Agents Chemother. 2018;62(2): e01550-17.

CHAPTER

13

Current Advances and Persistent Challenges in the Treatment of Pediatric Drug-resistant Tuberculosis

Nibedita Rath

Abstract

Tuberculosis (TB) remains a critical public health issue, with nearly 10 million new cases and millions of deaths annually. Children represent about 12% of these cases, yet a small fraction receive correct diagnosis and treatment. The emergence of drug-resistant TB (DR-TB) strains complicates control, with only 60% treatment success. Multidrug-resistant TB (MDR-TB) in children often goes undiagnosed due to lack of awareness and the targets for pediatric DR-TB treatment has only been met in just 15% goals. New drugs such as bedaquiline, delamanid, and pretomanid have been approved, but pediatric formulations are limited by a lack of clinical data. This chapter explores the development, efficacy, and safety of MDR-TB drugs in treating children with DR-TB.

Keywords: Pediatric TB, drug-resistant TB, MDR-TB

INTRODUCTION

Tuberculosis (TB) remains a significant global health issue, particularly affecting children. In 2022, approximately 1.25 million children and young adolescents contracted TB, with nearly half under the age of five making up 12% of the global 10.6 million cases. Tragically, around 214,000 of these young patients died, which translates to nearly 600 daily deaths from a preventable disease. Multidrug-resistant (MDR) and rifampicin-resistant (RR) TB are particularly severe, causing considerable mortality in children. Despite an estimated 30,000 annual cases of MDR-TB in children[1] < 5% are microbiologically confirmed, leading to poorer outcomes and higher mortality rates. Given the unique challenges of diagnosing and treating TB in children, it is essential to focus on improved early diagnosis and effective treatments to achieve the goal of zero TB deaths in children.

Treating MDR-TB is complex due to a limited selection of effective drugs, high pill burdens, extensive costs, lengthy treatments, and severe potential side effects. Drugs such as aminoglycosides, known to cause irreversible ototoxicity, hepatotoxicity, and neurological issues, complicate treatment further. After decades of stagnation in TB drug development, new medications such as bedaquiline, delamanid, and pretomanid have shown promise, particularly in adults. Significant progress has also been made in pediatric MDR-TB treatment, highlighting the need for continuous advancement in both diagnostics and therapeutics to combat this critical health challenge.

SAFETY AND EFFICACY OF BEDAQUILINE IN PEDIATRIC DRUG-RESISTANT TUBERCULOSIS

The use of bedaquiline to treat DR-TB in children has been somewhat restricted due to potential adverse effects. While ongoing clinical trials aim to thoroughly assess its safety and efficacy, information remains limited because children are often underrepresented in these trials. However, a compassionate use study involving children under the age of 15 indicated promising results, showing a higher rate of TB elimination after 6 months of bedaquiline treatment. Specifically, the study revealed that the drug could be highly efficacious in treating pediatric TB. A study found a 74.2% success rate among pediatric patients, with a mortality rate of 6.5% and a treatment failure rate of 2.9% connected to bedaquiline use.[2] Pediatric-focused clinical trials, such as the Janssen C211 and IMPAACT P1108, initiated in 2016 and 2017 respectively, are studying bedaquiline's efficacy in children across various age groups. Despite the limited data and small sample sizes, bedaquiline has been deemed safe for both adult's and children's cardiac health. The World Health Organization (WHO) recommends all-oral regimens for children under six, with dosages tailored according to age and weight. Though a pediatric-specific formulation is not yet available, the current version can be applied to treat MDR-TB in young patients.

SAFETY AND EFFICACY OF DELAMANID IN PEDIATRIC DRUG-RESISTANT TUBERCULOSIS

The WHO TB guidelines evaluate delamanid's role in long-term treatment plans for children with MDR/RR-TB. In one study, 116 out of 147 MDR-TB patients achieved negative cultures after 6 months of delamanid treatment, representing a success rate of 79%. Among pediatric patients, the success rate was slightly higher at 80%, with 20 out of 25 children showing negative cultures. Although 8% of the participants experienced QTc prolongation, no other severe adverse events were reported, suggesting that demand is both potent and safe for treating MDR-TB in both adults and children. The pharmacokinetic (PK) and safety of delamanid were also evaluated in children aged 0–17 years with MDR-TB through two clinical trials (NCT01856634 and NCT01859923).[3] The studies aimed to identify the appropriate dosage for different age groups and revealed that 89.2% of the participants exhibited a positive therapeutic response 24 months after the initial dose. The safety profile was found to be consistent across adults and children.

SAFETY AND EFFICACY OF PRETOMANID IN PEDIATRIC DRUG-RESISTANT TUBERCULOSIS

Pretomanid has received Food and Drug Administration (FDA) approval as part of innovative treatment regimens for MDR-TB. These regimens also include bedaquiline, pretomanid, linezolid (BPaL), and sometimes moxifloxacin BPaLM. However, there is limited research on pretomanid's effects in younger children. To address this, a phase I/II trial planned for 2023 aims to study the drug's PK following a single dose in this age group. The IMPAACT 2034 study is a phase I, multisite, open-label trial focusing on the PK, safety, tolerability, and acceptability of a single dose of pretomanid in infants, children, and teens under 18 years old. The study includes participants both with and without human immunodeficiency virus (HIV) who have confirmed or probable RR-TB. A common concern for the pediatric population is testicular atrophy and impaired fertility, which has been seen in rodents treated with pretomanid and similar nitroimidazoles like metronidazole. Nonetheless, a 2022 meta-analysis of four clinical trials found no evidence of reduced reproductive hormone levels in men treated with pretomanid-containing regimens, suggesting that therapeutic doses of pretomanid do not affect human fertility.[4]

SAFETY AND EFFICACY OF FLUOROQUINOLONES (MOXIFLOXACIN AND LEVOFLOXACIN) IN PEDIATRIC DRUG-RESISTANT TUBERCULOSIS

Fluoroquinolones, such as moxifloxacin and levofloxacin, play a vital role in treating drug-resistant (DR) TB. They work by inhibiting DNA gyrase, which leads to disrupted DNA synthesis and eventual cell death. Levofloxacin and moxifloxacin, being newer generation fluoroquinolones, are favored for TB treatment due to their increased effectiveness and reduced chances of resistance development. Of these two, levofloxacin is generally preferred when both options are available. This preference is due to its fewer known drug interactions, a better-understood safety profile in children, its more frequent use and supporting literature for TB and other conditions.[5] Additionally, moxifloxacin has a higher tendency to prolong QTc compared to levofloxacin.

SAFETY AND EFFICACY OF LINEZOLID IN PEDIATRIC DRUG-RESISTANT TUBERCULOSIS

Linezolid is a type of oxazolidinone antibiotic that disrupts protein synthesis by attaching to the 50S ribosomal subunit, thereby hindering the initiation complex for protein formation. Resistance to linezolid occurs through mutations that alter this ribosomal subunit. For treating MDR-TB, it is recommended to administer linezolid once daily with the total daily dose reduced by 50% or more (e.g., 10–15 mg/kg/day instead of the typical 30 mg/kg/day used for other infections such as osteoarticular infections or pneumonia). This lower dosage generally improves tolerability and reduces adverse effects such as peripheral neuropathy, cytopenias, lactic acidosis, and optic neuropathy. Children usually experience fewer side effects than adults, though peripheral neuropathy may be challenging to detect in children and could be irreversible. Other significant side effects include diarrhea, headache, nausea, and pancreatitis. If toxicity is a concern, therapeutic drug monitoring is an option if it is available. Adjusting the daily dose to achieve a target trough level of <2 μg/mL has been shown to mitigate side effects.[6] In certain clinical situations such as in patients with HIV or malnutrition, coadministration of pyridoxine with linezolid might be considered. While some reports suggest that pyridoxine can help reverse cytopenias, there is no current WHO guideline recommending its routine coadministration in pediatric TB cases.

DEVELOPING A TREATMENT PLAN FOR PEDIATRICS WITH DRUG-RESISTANT TUBERCULOSIS

When developing a treatment regimen for pediatric MDR-TB, it is crucial to be familiar with the latest drugs available and to consult resources such as WHO guidelines, the Sentinel Project on Pediatric Drug-Resistant Tuberculosis, and the Curry International Tuberculosis Center. These resources assist clinicians in optimizing treatment regimens, including deciding on the combination of drugs and the duration of treatment.

Recently, significant advancement has been made with short, all-oral regimens that include BPaL or BPaLM. The WHO currently approves these regimens for children aged 14 years or older. Key studies supporting these regimens include the TB-PRACTECAL, Nix-TB, and ZeNix trials, which included some adolescent participants. In particular, the TB-PRACTECAL study employed an innovative design for patients with rifampin-resistant TB.[7] The Nix-TB trial reported a 90% favorable outcome rate in adults (the youngest participant being 17 years old) treated with BPaL, though side effects such as peripheral neuropathy and myelosuppression were noted, primarily due to linezolid at a 1,200 mg daily dose. The subsequent ZeNix trial found that reducing the linezolid dose to 600 mg daily maintained high efficacy with lower toxicity and side effects. There is currently no formal guidance for using BPaL/M in children under 14, but preteens or early teens with adult-like body weight might be considered for this regimen, especially if it is the safest or most effective option available. However, for younger children, especially without understanding the correct dosing for pretomanid, BPaL should not be used until more conclusive data is available. That being said, preliminary PK and safety studies may eventually support the use of these shorter, all-oral regimens in younger children, potentially without waiting for full clinical trial outcomes.

According to the 2022 WHO guidelines,[1] MDR-TB treatment in children unsuitable for a short BPaL or BPaLM regimen involves two primary approaches. The preferred method is a standardized, all-oral 9-month regimen. This involves 6 months of bedaquiline combined with a fluoroquinolone, ethambutol, high-dose isoniazid, pyrazinamide, clofazimine, and either ethionamide or linezolid for the first 2 months. For the remaining 5 months, the regimen includes a fluoroquinolone, clofazimine, ethambutol, and pyrazinamide. Clinical evidence from South Africa supports this approach, indicating bedaquiline-based regimens are safer and more effective than injectable ones. If the preferred regimen is not suitable, a longer, individualized treatment plan is recommended. This involves choosing drugs based on susceptibility from three groups: Group A (including bedaquiline, levofloxacin/moxifloxacin, and linezolid), Group B (clofazimine and cycloserine/terizidone), and Group C (ethambutol, delamanid, pyrazinamide, imipenem-cilastatin, amikacin/streptomycin, ethionamide/prothionamide, and p-aminosalicylic acid). Ideally, treatment begins with drugs from Group A, adding from Group B if necessary, and then Group C. A minimum of four effective drugs should be used, extending treatment over 18–24 months, with the possibility of shortening for less severe cases.

The Sentinel Project on Pediatric Drug-Resistant TB recommends a similar approach in drug selection but emphasizes using at least four drugs, or five for severe cases, and favors delamanid from Group C. Treatment duration for nonsevere cases can be as short as 6 months.

Pediatric TB formulations can be sourced through Stop TB's Global Drug Facility (GDF) for over 100 countries. However, obtaining these medications is more restrictive in some high-income countries due to stringent regulatory requirements. For instance, in the US, delamanid is available only through compassionate use programs, and clofazimine is classified as an orphan drug, available for children only under a single-patient emergency investigational new drug application through the FDA.

CONCLUSION

Despite advancements in the global fight against MDR-TB in children, numerous challenges still remain. Research involving pediatric patients continues to lag significantly behind studies focused on adults. A prime example is pretomanid: although it has received US FDA approval for adult use and has shown efficacy in short, all-oral treatment regimens in multiple trials and investigations into appropriate dosing and safety for children are only now starting. While new diagnostic tools and treatments are becoming available, their accessibility varies greatly depending on region and population vulnerability. Moreover, the quest for an effective TB vaccine that could make a major dent in the global disease burden remains unfulfilled. This chapter aims to equip clinicians with the latest actionable insights for better management of children suspected or confirmed to have MDR-TB.

REFERENCES

1. WHO. (2022). Global Tuberculosis Report 2022. [online] Available from https://www.who.int/teams/global-tuberculosis-programme/tb-reports/global-tuberculosis-report-2022 [Last accessed September, 2024].
2. Koirala S, Shah NP, Pyakurel P, Khanal M, Rajbhandari SK, Pun T, et al. High success and low recurrence with shorter treatment regimen for multidrug-resistant TB in Nepal. Public health action 2021;11(Suppl 1):38-45.
3. Garcia-Prats AJ, Frias M, van der Laan L, De Leon A, Gler MT, Schaaf HS, et al. Delamanid Added to an Optimized Background Regimen in Children with Multidrug-Resistant Tuberculosis: Results of a Phase I/II Clinical Trial. Antimicrob Agents Chemother. 2022;66(5):e0214421.
4. Boekelheide K, Olugbosi M, Nedelman J, Everitt D, Smith E, Betteridge M, et al. Male reproductive hormones in patients treated with pretomanid. Int J Tuberc Lung Dis. 2022;26(6):558-65.
5. World Health Organization. (2019). WHO consolidated guidelines on drug-resistant tuberculosis treatment. [online] Available from https://iris.who.int/bitstream/handle/10665/311389/9789241550529-eng.pdf [Last accessed September, 2024].
6. Song T, Lee M, Jeon HS, Park Y, Dodd LE, Dartois V, et al. Linezolid Trough Concentrations Correlate with Mitochondrial Toxicity-Related Adverse Events in the Treatment of Chronic Extensively Drug-Resistant Tuberculosis. EBioMedicine. 2015;2(11):1627-33.
7. Nyang'wa BT, Berry C, Kazounis E, Motta I, Parpieva N, Tigay Z, et al; TB-PRACTECAL Study Collaborators. A 24-Week, All-Oral Regimen for Rifampin-Resistant Tuberculosis. N Engl J Med. 2022;387(25):2331-43.

Section 3: Clinical

CHAPTER 14

Closing the Gap between Evidence and Implementation in Multidrug-resistant Tuberculosis Management

Kaushal Kumar Dwivedi, Kamal Chopra

Abstract

Multidrug-resistant tuberculosis (MDR-TB) is a critical global health issue that hampers TB control efforts. The gap between evidence and its practical application undermines treatment effectiveness, strains healthcare systems, and impacts patient outcomes. Despite advances in research and evidence-based practices, implementing these findings remains challenging. There is a need to bridge gaps through healthcare system strengthening, better diagnostic access, and patient-centered care. Addressing these issues requires sustained investment, policy advocacy, and collaboration among various stakeholders to enhance infrastructure, resource access, and adherence to evidence-based practices.

Keywords: MDR-TB, evidence-based practices, diagnostic and treatment access, patient-centered care, healthcare system strengthening

INTRODUCTION

Multidrug-resistant tuberculosis (MDR-TB) represents a dreaded global health challenge, with its perseverance posing significant barrier to TB control efforts worldwide. The discrepancy between evidence and its practical application in MDR-TB management constitutes a significant challenge, influencing treatment efficacy, imposing strain on healthcare systems, and impacting health outcomes for affected individuals. In spite of notable advancements in research and evidence-based practices, translating these findings into effective and widespread treatment remains an intricate and multifaceted challenge. So, it is imperative to explore these gaps and propose strategies to bridge them, drawing on the latest research and case studies.

THE BURDEN OF MULTIDRUG-RESISTANT TUBERCULOSIS

Globally, MDR-TB is a major public health concern. According to the World Health Organization (WHO), there were an estimated 410,000 new cases of MDR-TB in 2022, with over 160,000 deaths attributed to this condition.[1] The burden of MDR-TB is unevenly distributed, with high incidence rates reported in countries with weak healthcare systems and high rates of TB transmission.

EVIDENCE-BASED PRACTICES IN MULTIDRUG-RESISTANT TUBERCULOSIS MANAGEMENT

Diagnostic Advances

Accurate diagnosis and timely management are key parts of the management of MDR-TB. Technologies such as rapid molecular assays, such as GeneXpert, and rapid culture techniques like mycobacteria growth indicator tube (MGIT) have changed diagnosis for TB. GeneXpert provides results within 2 hours and detecting rifampicin resistance, a surrogate marker for MDR-TB.[2] Despite these advances, the roll-out of diagnostic tools remains very heterogeneous. The latest global TB report outlined that in 2022 rapid tests accounted for only 47% (3.5 million) of the 7.5 million new cases, of TB diagnosis.[1] Challenges such as high costs, limited availability in resource-poor areas, and insufficient training hinder widespread use of these rapid tests. Addressing these issues requires substantial investments in healthcare infrastructure and training to ensure broader access to these advanced diagnostic tools.

Treatment Regimens

In contrast to drug-sensitive TB, MDR-TB is more complicated to treat, often with 18–24 months of second-line drugs. Newer regimens have opened the way for shorter, more effective treatment pathways; among these are the BPaL regimen, consisting of bedaquiline, pretomanid, and linezolid.[3] However, due to high-drug costs and other obstructions, this progress has not been implemented very fast; most countries stay locked into ancient regimens, still dogged by bureaucracy and price.

Drug Availability and Accessibility

Ensuring the availability and accessibility of second-line drugs is a crucial aspect of managing MDR-TB. The patterns of drug resistance and the availability of effective medications can differ greatly across different geographical regions. The prequalification program of WHO, the Global Fund, and Stop TB Partnership are currently leading activities that involve increased access to quality-assured drugs.[4] However, barriers remain including procurement problems, drug stock-outs, and high costs. Generic versions of the essential MDR-TB medicines, including bedaquiline, are at an affordable cost and just as good as the original brands. Promoting the use of generics drugs and strengthening of supply chain management become very critical in translating evidence to practice.

Infrastructure and Human Resources

Effective MDR-TB management requires strong healthcare infrastructure and skilled personnel. Many low- and middle-income countries struggle with TB and MDR-TB due to inadequate facilities, a shortage of trained workers, and poor infection control measures. Strengthening healthcare systems involves investing in both physical infrastructure and human resources, including specialized training for healthcare workers. Intersectoral collaboration between levels of government, NGOs, and international agencies is essential to overcome these challenges and enhance MDR-TB management.

Patient-centered Care

The MDR-TB treatment is lengthy and challenging; therefore, a patient-centered strategy is necessary to improve adherence and success. The adherence is often impaired by the high cost and side effects of the second-line drugs.[5] In this regard, financial and psychosocial support, patient education, and directly observed therapy are very important. Community-based support and integration of MDR-TB services into primary healthcare improve accessibility and reduce pressure on specialized facilities.

National Guidelines and Policy Implementation

National TB programs are crucial in translating the global recommendations into local implementation; yet, the revision of guidelines by new evidence can be delayed by administrative red tape, a lack of funding, and limited political commitment.[6] Advocacy has had a significant role in effecting policy change. Stakeholder engagement and intersectoral collaboration between national governments and international organizations are paramount for adopting new practices and guidelines.

Funding and Resource Allocation

Adequate funding is essential for effective MDR-TB management, covering infrastructure, laboratory capacity, and healthcare worker training. Financial constraints can restrict access to diagnostics, drugs, and treatment. Although initiatives such as the Global Fund and Gavi have made huge contributions to filling these gaps,[4] sustained funding is crucial for maintaining and expanding MDR-TB programs.

Strategies for Bridging the Gap

Bridging the gap between evidence and implementation in MDR-TB management involves several key approaches such as healthcare system strengthening, access to diagnostics and treatments, patient support programs, policy advocacy and reform, stakeholder collaboration, monitoring and evaluation, etc. If these and some other approaches could be harmoniously integrated, MDR-TB management is significantly more evidence-based and effective. Brief overviews of such approaches are mentioned in the **Table 1**.

TABLE 1: Comprehensive approaches to bridge the gap between evidence and implementation in the multidrug-resistant tuberculosis (MDR-TB) management.

Approaches	Steps to achieve
Enhancing the capability of **health systems**	• *Infrastructure*: Developing/upgrading infrastructures for advanced and rapid diagnostics. Establishing specialized MDR-TB treatments facility within healthcare setup so as to provide comprehensive care • *Human resource development*: Providing training programs for healthcare professionals on the newer evidence-based guidelines related to diagnosis/ treatment along and provision for continuous education and refreshers training courses for latest developments and practices
Turning evidence into effective policy and practice	• *Development of guidelines*: Latest evidence-based guidelines which should be practical and applicable be developed • *Policy advocacy*: Various stakeholders such as policymakers, organizations, or advocacy groups be brought together for making of evidence based guidelines/ policies. Sufficient resources in terms of funding, etc., should also be provided for the implementation of drug resistant TB management program
Improving implementation strategies	• *Pilot initiatives*: New strategies or interventions should be done in the selected areas before scaling up. Stringent monitoring and evaluation systems should be used to assess the effectiveness of pilot study. Findings should be used based on local needs and challenges • *Incorporation into existing systems*: MDR-TB management should be integrated with broader health services such as HIV care to ensure comprehensive patient management. Coordination between different levels of the health systems from national/state to local should be ensured for the consistent implementation of MDR-TB guidelines

Continued

Continued

Approaches	Steps to achieve
Enhancing data systems and utilization of evidence	• *Healthcare information systems*: Comprehensive health information systems should be established to gather data on MDR-TB incidence, treatment outcomes, and drug resistance patterns. This data can then be used for decision-making, tracking progress, and pinpointing areas needing improvement • *Advancement through research and innovation*: Operational research should be conducted on the implementation of MDR-TB interventions so as to identify barriers (if any) and using findings to optimize strategies and practices. MDR-TB care can also be improved by investing in research for new diagnostic tools, treatment, and management strategy
Boosting patient and community involvement	• *Patient education*: Patients should be informed through campaigns about MDR-TB, treatment, and importance of treatment adherence. They should also be counseled with respect to treatment, side effects, and role of laboratory tests in treatment monitoring and drug adherence • *Community involvement*: Community health workers should be employed to reach underserved populations, offering education, and support for MDR-TB treatment management. Additionally, local leaders and organizations must be engaged in TB control efforts to boost the uptake of MDR-TB services
Overcoming to challenges implementation	• *Resource limitations*: Obtain funding and resources to support MDR-TB management programs, including drug procurement, training, and infrastructure development • *Healthcare system barriers*: Systemic challenges such as shortages of healthcare personnel, inadequate infrastructure, stockouts, and limited diagnostic capacity should be addressed through targeted interventions and strategic investments
Advancing equity and access	• *Reasonable access*: Ensure MDR-TB services are accessible in all regions, including remote and underserved areas. Overcome financial barriers by offering subsidized or free treatment for individuals who cannot afford it • *Combating stigma*: Launch campaigns to reduce the stigma associated with MDR-TB and encourage timely diagnosis and treatment. Create a supportive environment for patients by providing access to social and psychological support

CONCLUSION

Closing the gap between evidence and implementation in MDR-TB management is complex and ongoing. It requires addressing diagnostics, treatment, healthcare infrastructure, and policy issues. While advancements in research and technology offer promising solutions, barriers to implementation persist. Strengthening healthcare systems, promoting evidence-based practices, and enhancing patient support are crucial. Addressing these challenges demands concerted efforts from governments, international organizations, healthcare providers, and patients. Investing in infrastructure, improving access to diagnostics and treatments, and advocating for policy changes can help bridge the gap and advance the fight against MDR-TB.

REFERENCES

1. World Health Organization. (2023). Global TB report 2023. [online] Available from https://www.who.int/teams/global-tuberculosis-programme/tb-reports/global-tuberculosis-report-2023 [Last accessed September, 2024].
2. Boehme CC, Nabeta P, Hillemann D, Nicol MP, Shenai S, Krapp F, et al. Rapid molecular detection of tuberculosis and rifampin resistance. N Engl J Med. 2010;363(11):1005-15.
3. World Health Organization. (2022). WHO consolidated guidelines on tuberculosis: Module 4: Treatment—drug-resistant tuberculosis treatment, 2022 update. [online] Available from https://www.who.int/publications/i/item/9789240063129 [Last accessed September, 2024].
4. Global Fund. (2021). Global Fund to Fight AIDS, Tuberculosis and Malaria. Annual Report. [online] Available from https://www.theglobalfund.org/en/results/ [Last accessed September, 2024].
5. Vishwakarma D, Gaidhane A, Sweta Sahu S, Rathod AS. Multidrug Resistance Tuberculosis (MDR-TB) Challenges in India: A Review. Cureus. 2023;15(12):e50222.
6. Zumla A, George A, Sharma V, Herbert RH, Oxley A, Oliver M; Baroness Masham of Ilton. The WHO 2014 Global tuberculosis report—further to go. Lancet Glob Health. 2015;3(1):E10-2.

CHAPTER

15

Significance of Inappropriate or Interrupted Treatment in Tuberculosis

Arun Sampath

Abstract

Tuberculosis (TB) is the second leading killer infectious disease in the world and the incidence is alarmingly rising by 3.9% per year from 2020. About 4% develop multidrug resistance TB, wherein the treatment success is about 50–60%. TB has its own unique issues with indolent chronicity, social stigma, need for multiple drugs for longer duration, and intolerant drug side effects which lead to treatment noncompliance. The observed prevalence of treatment interruption varied between <5 and >60% across different studies. Patients are 1.58 times likely to interrupt their treatment in early intensive phase than in the continuation phase. Treatment interruption can lead to treatment failure, drug resistance, and persistence of infection transmission. Directly observed therapy (DOT) is an important way to improve treatment adherence and it has been shown more beneficial when combined with other measures such as patients'/staff education and motivation, psychological support, medication monitoring, and nutritional incentives. Newer digital technologies such as video-observed therapy (VOT), electronic DOT, 99-DOTS strategy, m-health, and short message reminders show promising results. Though the patient's irrational behavior is the reason for poor treatment compliance, the responsibility of ensuring each patient to complete anti-TB treatment should be borne by appropriate healthcare system.

Keywords: Treatment interruption, tuberculosis, directly observed therapy

INTRODUCTION

Despite the fact that effective therapeutic drugs are available for drug susceptible tuberculosis (TB) for more than six decades, we are yet to conquer this dreadful disease. TB is the second leading killer infectious disease in the world and a major cause of deaths related to drug resistance (DR). According to World Health Organization (WHO) estimate in 2022, there were 10.6 million new TB cases with 1.30 million deaths and an alarming rise in TB incidence rate per year by 3.9% between 2020 and 2022 reversing the decline of 2% per year for most of the past two decades.[1] Eight countries (India, Indonesia, China, the Philippines, Pakistan, Bangladesh, Nigeria, and the Democratic Republic of the Congo) account for more than two-thirds of the global total TB cases. About 4% of the cases develop multidrug resistance TB (MDR-TB), wherein the treatment efficacy is still around 50–60%. The persistent high prevalence of this disease could be attributed mostly to irrational patient behavior and improper healthcare system.

WHY DO TB PATIENTS INTERRUPT TREATMENT?

It is inherent human behavior to be nonadherent to medicines especially when given for longer duration. Almost half of patients with chronic illness such as diabetes, hypertension, hyperlipidemia, asthma, and coronary artery disease either skip or stop medicines. No matter whatever be the illness, if a patient feels better with medications, they decide to skip/stop taking prolonged medicines without realizing the ill effects of treatment interruption.

With the rifampicin-based treatment regimen, the efficacy is almost 98% for drug susceptible TB and can render the patient less communicable as early as 2 weeks of treatment. Theoretically such effective treatment should reduce overall TB case burden in the community, but to the contrary the prevalence of TB is still high in endemic countries. TB has its own unique issues with indolent chronicity, social stigma, need for multiple drugs for longer duration, and intolerant drug side effects which lead to treatment noncompliance. The treatment interruption has been observed not only with ambulatory patients but also by sick/hospitalized patients who also skip or throw the medicines. Even prolonged illness, disease severity, functional impairment does not influence the treatment adherence.

There is still no clarity regarding exact duration to define treatment interruption and research studies on treatment interruption in TB used the duration range from 1 day to 2 months. As per WHO, the outcome "lost to follow-up" defines a patient whose treatment was not started or those interrupting treatment for at least 2 consecutive months. This can lead to "huge time gap" between actual interruption and reporting the outcome and hence Indian NTEP (National TB Elimination Program) guideline defines interruption of >1 month as default/lost to follow-up. Due to the disparity in defining "treatment interruption," the observed prevalence across various studies ranged from >5% to almost >60%. In a systematic review[2] of 50 studies in Asian countries, the pooled prevalence of treatment interruption was 17% with higher prevalence of early interruption up to 28%.

There could be different ways of treatment interruption. Patient can either stop all the drugs for a day or skip some drugs in a day; can take lesser number of FDC (fixed-dose combination) drugs per day (hence achieve lower therapeutic concentration for all drug formulations); either take drugs intermittently or stop entirely for few days to months; either interrupt in the early intensive phase or in continuation phase of antituberculosis treatment (ATT).

How much treatment interruption is significant enough to affect the overall outcome is not well defined until date. However, with the possibility of higher bacillary load just prior to treatment, the early interruption during intensive treatment phase will have more impact on treatment outcome and warrants treatment to be restarted if the interruption is >2 weeks. Also, the treatment interruption in early phase can lead to treatment failure, DR, and persistent transmission of infection. TB patients were 1.58 times likely to quit in intensive phase than in continuation phase.[3] As compared to patients who stop the treatment altogether, those who take treatment either intermittently or taking lower dosage (as in FDC, who take lesser number of tablets per day) pose higher risk for poor treatment outcome and development of DR. The irony is that the nonadherent patient requires prolonged treatment and this itself can amplify the noncompliance again. The poorly compliant patient has prolonged ill-health and persistent disease which also affects his family and community by means of continuous infection transmission.

Patient's age, ethnic/social group, socioeconomic status, marital status, and particular religious belief were not observed to consistently influence the treatment compliance. Similarly, studies were controversial in respect to gender, education status, and residing

BOX 1 Common reasons for treatment interruption in tuberculosis.

- Poor patient's knowledge/orientation about TB treatment
- Lower TB symptoms score/feels better with treatment
- Drug side effects; pill burden
- Internalized stigma (shame/blame)
- Feels "always watched/supervised"
- Work/job hindrance
- Migrant population
- Long distance to travel to healthcare
- Social stigma (fear of discrimination from society)
- Unfriendly health service provider/poor staff motivation
- Nonavailability of drugs

area (rural/urban) to predict default. However, current smoker, alcohol/substance abuse, human immunodeficiency virus (HIV) coinfection, migrant, and retreatment case can predict high risk for poor treatment outcome and lost to follow-up. Certain reasons for treatment interruption are given in **Box 1**.

HOW DOES DRUG RESISTANCE DEVELOP WITH TREATMENT INTERRUPTION?

Drug resistance in TB is most often a man-made error, due to improper treatment regimen, inadequate treatment duration, nonadherence, and poor programmatic management. TB bacilli develop resistance due to chromosomal mutations as an effect to counteract the stress due to host defense milieu, reactive oxygen species (ROS) and or due to the inappropriate treatment (drug selection pressure). These mutations are caused mostly by single nucleotide polymorphisms (SNPs), followed by insertions and deletions (INDELs).[4] In general, any microorganism has a survival instinct to tolerate/adapt and resist from the antibiotics by the development of *DR* genes in the presence of drug selection pressure or via horizontal transfer of genes from other microorganism. The TB bacilli lack horizontal gene transfer and hence the DR-TB bacilli need to acquire mutations in their core/promoter genes. Though spontaneous mutations are relatively rare events, the possibility of such mutants to the two most important TB drugs do develop in a proportion of ~1 in 10^6 for isoniazid (INH) and ~1 in 10^8 for rifampicin. Such mutant colonies tend to be higher in areas of higher bacillary load (such as pulmonary cavities which has ~10^8 bacilli). Earlier studies had shown that combination of drugs could reduce the chances of DR [e.g., with INH and rifampin (RIF) combination, spontaneous doubly resistant bacilli expected in ~1 in 10^{14} are extremely unlikely] and in vitro studies had shown that higher the therapeutic serum drug concentration, lesser the resistant bacilli even in a bacillary population of 10^8. Hence, with the presence of either single drug or subtherapeutic drug concentration, the selection pressure for mutation can lead to proliferation of resistant colonies and amplification of DR. Due to the patient's treatment interruption behavior, the chances of developing acquired DR are thus significantly enhanced. This stresses the importance of "appropriate number of drugs" at "appropriate dosage" for "appropriate duration" in any TB treatment regimen. In a retrospective analysis[5] between 1996 and 2009, Liu CH et al. observed that the DR was more in retreatment cases, and poor treatment outcome was observed more among migrant patients (who tend to interrupt often) and in those who took lesser number of active drugs.

Epigenetics denote chemical modifications in DNA without altering its nucleotide sequence and such modifications affect chromatin superstructure, DNA-histone interactions, and either up or down regulate gene expression. DNA methylation, acetylation, and phosphorylation are the key types of epigenetics by *Mycobacterium tuberculosis* (MTB). Epigenetic processes help MTB to survive in myriad host environment; evade immune system; enhance its virulence and/or emergence of DR. Inappropriate or interrupted treatment can lead to drug selection pressure that may increase the possibility of TB bacilli developing such epigenetic mechanisms.

WAYS TO IMPROVE TREATMENT ADHERENCE

Since TB is highly prevalent in individuals with low-economic status or in low-income countries, the main hindrance could be treatment cost. However, despite free-TB medicines by most of the nationalized program supported by WHO, the treatment adherence was still poor. A landmark Madras study in 1960s showed that long-course treatment (1 year) at home settings (but with intermittent direct supervision of patients by a healthcare provider) was as effective as sanatorium (hospital)-based treatment. This study also observed that the sanatorium patients, despite receiving better healthcare facilities, good environment, and nutrition still skipped their medications. Dr Karel Styblo of the International Union Against Tuberculosis and Lung Disease (IUATLD) in mid 1970s, pioneered the idea of using the basic healthcare unit at district level for integrating the TB control with the existing general health services. He was instrumental in developing DOTS (directly observed treatment-short course) strategy in Tanzania national TB control program and emphasized simplifying the TB program to focus on core aspects of treatment adherence.

In 1993, WHO adopted directly observed therapy (DOT) and by definition DOT means all the dose has been supervised. DOT as compared with SAT (self-administered treatment) had improved treatment adherence, higher 2-month sputum conversion and slightly lower rates of acquired DR. Systematic reviews did not show consistent benefit with DOT as compared to SAT.[6] However, subgroup analysis showed DOT was particularly beneficial for patients with TB-HIV coinfection and those with risks for nonadherence. Randomized controlled trials (RCTs)/observational studies showed that DOT in conjunction with other measures to improve treatment adherence (patient/staff education about disease, material and psychological support to patient, and use of medication monitor) was superior to DOT alone. Though DOT provider can be either a healthcare worker or local community-based lay provider or a close family member/relative, evidences favor nonfamily DOT provider. The preferred DOT facility should be either community or home-based location as compared to healthcare DOT facility so as to be more convenient to patient. Even with DOT, patient still feels that he is always being watched and hence can avoid taking complete treatment. Treatment interruption is a human behavior and hence simple education of patient is not enough. The DOT provider should be socially acceptable by the patient and also should provide psychological support. He/she should be compassionate, communicate in patient's language, bridge intellectual/cultural barriers, and motivate constantly to change the patient's belief/attitudes toward the disease and treatment.

DIGITAL HEALTH TECHNOLOGY IN IMPROVING TREATMENT ADHERENCE

With the Covid-19 pandemic, there was a great realization about the benefits of digital communication methods. Video-observed therapy (VOT) through smart phone apps is being found to be effective. Digital health technology [SMS text reminders, electronic directly observed therapy (e-DOT), medication event reminder monitor (MERM), and mHealth (mobile health)] can be effectively utilized to significantly improve disease management.[7] Digital adherence technology (smart pill box) is another way of monitoring the patients' adherence. Though these digital technologies are promising, they still require a proper internet connectivity and smart phones and hence are not widely available in low-income countries. NTEP has already implemented certain initiatives in India such as nutrition incentives (Nikshay Poshan Yojana), 99DOTS strategy (IT-enabled "pill-in-hand" adherence monitoring system) to enhance treatment compliance. With the rapid evolution of artificial intelligence (AI), deep learning in AI can guide the next level of integrated monitoring of medication adherence in near future.[8]

CONCLUSION

Since the reasons for treatment default in TB are not only patient related, but the responsibility should be borne by healthcare to ensure all the patients to complete their treatment. The overall treatment success can be improved by a standardized national guideline (based on their local efficacy data and social structure); appropriate healthcare service; decentralization of treatment from healthcare facilities to community/home based with utmost preference to patients' convenience; preference to FDC drugs; ensuring adequate delivery of standard drugs and ensuring supervision of the entire treatment for each patient by DOT. The end TB strategy by WHO aims to end the TB epidemic by 2030 by setting targets of 80% reduction in TB incidence and a 90% reduction in TB deaths. In order to achieve these goals, all the partners including patient, family, community worker, healthcare provider, and nationalized program should take due responsibilities and work together for a better humanity.

REFERENCES

1. WHO. (2023). Global Tuberculosis report 2023. [online] Available from www.who.int/teams-global-tuberculossi-programme/tb-reports [Last accessed September, 2024].
2. Oh AL, Makmor-Bakry M, Islahudin F, Wong IC. Prevalence and predictive factors of tuberculosis treatment interruption in the Asia region: a systematic review and meta-analysis. BMJ Glob Health. 2023;8:e010592.
3. Kimani E, Muhula S, Kiptai T, Orwa J, Odero T, Gachuno O. Factors influencing TB treatment interruption and treatment outcomes among patients in Kiambu county, 2016-2019. PLoS ONE. 2021;1(4):e0248820.
4. Dookie N, Rambaran S, Padayatchi N, Mahomed S, Naidoo K. Evolution of drug resistance in *Mycobacterium tuberculosis*: a review on the molecular determinants of resistance and implications for personalized care. J Antimicrob Chemother. 2018;73(5):1138-51.
5. Liu CH, Li L, Chen Z, Wang Q, Hu YL, Zhu B, et al. Characteristics and treatment outcomes of patients with MDR and XDR tuberculosis in a TB referral hospital in Beijing: a 13-year experience. PLoS ONE. 2011;6(4):e19399.
6. World Health Organization. (2017). Guidelines for treatment of drug susceptible tuberculosis and patient care, 2017 update. [online] Available from www.who.int/publications/i/item/9789241550000 [Last accessed September, 2024].
7. Lee S, Rajaguru V, Baek JS, Shin J, Park Y. Digital Health Interventions to enhance tuberculosis treatment adherence: Scoping review. JMIR Mhealth Uhealth. 2023;11:e49741.
8. Sekandi JN, Shi W, Zhu R, Kaggwa P, Mwebze E, Li S. Application of Artificial Intelligence to the monitoring adherence for tuberculosis treatment in Africa. Algorithm development and validation. JMIR AI. 2023;2(1):e40167.

CHAPTER

16

Nonadherence to Medication Regimens: Impact on Drug Resistance

Shanker Matta, Sanjay Rajpal, Kamal Chopra, VK Arora

Abstract

The chapter highlights importance of adherence and its linkage with drug resistance. Nonadherence and drug resistance are also linked with factors such as educational status, poverty, smoking, and alcohol. The chapter also highlights the problem of multidrug resistance (MDR) in India and the urgent efforts such as expansion of rapid molecular tests and development of new shorter regimens needed to curb tuberculosis (TB) problem.

Keywords: Nonadherence, drug resistance, noncompliance

INTRODUCTION

Adherence means when a patient's behavior corresponds with the medication and drug dose. Nonadherence of medication is prevalent in all countries and involves high costs especially in chronic conditions requiring long-term therapies. A study from Nigeria has reported 30% nonadherence to tuberculosis (TB) medication.[1] Adherence is important for achieving outcomes but is often low. As per data, nonadherence among TB patients may lead to multidrug-resistant (MDR)/extended drug-resistant (XDR) TB.[2]

For MDR patients and other chronic conditions, adherence to medication is the most important step. A similar term "noncompliance" is also used for patients not following medical advice. Though there is a direct link between noncompliance and treatment failure, but noncompliance has also been linked with factors such as increased death rates, increased medical costs, and increase in number of hospital visits along with poverty and malnutrition. Taking into account all the factors, noncompliance of medication may further lead to drug resistance.[3-6] There are patient-related factors and therapy-related factors associated with noncompliance. Patient-related factors may be education levels of the individual, smoking, tobacco consumption, alcohol intake, etc. Factors related to therapy may be type and route of medication, treatment duration, side effects of medicines, and taste of medication.

- Epidemiologist
- Director
- Former Director
- Chairman, TB Association of India Red Cross road, New Delhi

Contributory factors such as accessibility, travel time for treatment access, and lack of support may also result in noncompliance.

FACTORS ASSOCIATED WITH NONADHERENCE

A study reported nonadherence of 23.7% among patients' contacts on TB preventive therapy (TPT). Another study[7] reported nonadherence rate of 27.2%.[1] People with drug-resistant (DR) TB face significant economic and social costs and only one out of three have access to quality care. A study quoted that most frequently mentioned reason for nonadherence was feeling better or cured.[1,8] Another study from India quoted that smokers were at 2.4 times higher risk of not adhering to treatment when compared with nonsmokers. The study also associated low education level with nonadherence to TB treatment. Another study concluded that first-time TB treatment seekers, who opted for private clinics for treatment were at 2.24 times higher risk of nonadherence when compared with first-time treatment seekers at public Health facility.[7]

DRUG RESISTANCE

As per World Health Organization (WHO)[9,10] globally, the estimated proportion of new TB cases with MDR/rifampicin-resistant (RR)-TB was 3.6% in 2021 and India had 26% of global case load of MDR cases. As per available data, case load for MDR/RR-TB cases with pre-XDR was 20%. With availability of new molecular tests, countries have started with surveillance systems based on routine drug susceptibility testing (DST) of *Mycobacterium tuberculosis* (MTB) isolates for rifampicin, and for at least 80% of patients with bacteriologically confirmed pulmonary TB. 151 countries have continuous surveillance systems and 31 rely on epidemiological surveys of bacterial isolates.

COVID-19 experience has shown the hesitancy to accept vaccination in the general population. This suggests that patients' decisions are driven by emotions, leading to nonadherence.[11] Research is ongoing with availability of new innovation such as smart inhalers, electronic pill dispensers with varied effectiveness. Health system innovations which improve adherence could benefit various stakeholders in the long run. Nonadherence remains a complex challenge. Moreover efforts to reduce costs along with out of pocket expenditure is obstructed by the emergence of DR-TB cases as a result of mutations of the MTB strain. Social innovations, research and development of affordable test for TB infection and disease, and development of shorter and effective TB regimens for TB/DR-TB management along with a shift in strategies to address issues such as poverty and malnutrition are some of the areas which can impact medication adherence and better patient outcomes. The global tide of noncommunicable chronic conditions and aging of societies urges us to take this problem seriously.[1]

CONCLUSION

Development of shorter regimens to reduce TB resistance is a high priority area that can eliminate all populations of *Mycobacterium*, while also limiting bacterial metabolic processes that drive drug tolerance, mutagenesis, and the ultimate emergence of resistance. Known interventions such as contact tracing, post-treatment follow-up along with active mapping of contacts and TPT prophylaxis are essential to curb spread of DR strains.[11] All interventions when adopted will lead to improved adherence and better management and control of MDR-TB.

REFERENCES

1. Iweama CN, Agbaje OS, Umoke PCI, Igbokwe CC, Ozoemena EL, Omaka-Amari NL, et al. Nonadherence to tuberculosis treatment and associated factors among patients using directly observed treatment short-course in north-west Nigeria: A cross-sectional study. SAGE Open Med. 2021;9:2050312121989497.
2. Jain A, Dixit P. Multidrug resistant to extensively drug resistant tuberculosis: What is next? J Biosci. 2008;33:605-16.
3. Anley DT, Akalu TY, Dessie AM, Anteneh RM, Zemene MA, Bayih WA, et al. Prognostication of treatment non-compliance among patients with multidrug-resistant tuberculosis in the course of their follow-up: A logistic regression-based machine learning algorithm. Front Digit Health. 2023;5:1165222.
4. Jin J, Sklar GE, Min Sen Oh V, Chuen Li S. Factors affecting therapeutic compliance: a review from the patient's perspective. Ther Clin Risk Manag. 2008;4(1):269-86.
5. O'Boyle SJ, Power JJ, Ibrahim MY, Watson JP. Factors affecting patient compliance with anti-tuberculosis chemotherapy using the directly observed treatment, short-course strategy (DOTS). Int J Tuberc Lung Dis. 2002;6(4):307-12.
6. Ogundele OA, Moodley D, Pillay AW, Seebregts CJ. An ontology for factors affecting tuberculosis treatment adherence behavior in sub- Saharan Africa. Patient Prefer Adherence. 2016;10:669-81.
7. Lolong DB, Aryastami NK, Kusrini I, Tobing KL, Tarigan I, Isfandari S, et al. Nonadherence to anti-tuberculosis treatment, reasons and associated factors among pulmonary tuberculosis patients in the communities in Indonesia. PLoS One. 2023;18(8):e0287628.
8. Bagchi S, Ambe G, Sathiakumar N. Determinants of poor adherence to anti-tuberculosis treatment in mumbai, India. Int J Prev Med. 2010;1(4):223-32.
9. WHO. (2022). Drug-resistant TB. [online] Available from https://www.who.int/teams/global-tuberculosis-programme/tb-reports/global-tuberculosis-report-2022/tb-disease-burden/2-3-drug-resistant-tb [Last accessed September, 2024].
10. WHO. (2021). Guidance for the surveillance of drug resistance in tuberculosis: Sixth edition. [online] Available from https://www.who.int/publications/i/item/9789240018020 [Last accessed September, 2024].
11. Liebenberg D, Gordhan BG, Kana BD. Drug resistant tuberculosis: Implications for transmission, diagnosis, and disease management. Front Cell Infect Microbiol. 2022;12:943545.

CHAPTER 17

Strategies to Prevent Mortality and Severe Illness in Multidrug-resistant Tuberculosis

PS Sarma, D Bhima Sankar, T Pratyusha

Abstract

Multidrug-resistant tuberculosis (MDR-TB), though preventable and curable, presents significant challenges due to limited treatment options, complexity, and high costs. Mortality rates can exceed 20–30% in some settings. In India, these rates are particularly concerning, underscoring the urgent need for improved healthcare infrastructure, research, and treatment innovations to enhance outcomes for drug-resistant TB patients.

Active interventions aiming for elimination of TB are the only way forward to curtail this menace.

Keywords: Limited treatment options, research innovation, equitable healthcare, tailored treatment

INTRODUCTION

Despite being a preventable and curable disease, dealing with multidrug-resistant tuberculosis (MDR-TB) is challenging due to limited treatment options, increased complexity, duration, and cost of the treatment compared to drug-susceptible TB. Mortality rates can range widely depending on the specific context. Still, in some settings, mortality rates for MDR-TB[1] have been reported to be as high as 20–30% or even higher in certain subpopulations.

Though efforts are being made to improve the situation, the mortality rate in India remains a significant concern, highlighting the need for continued investment in healthcare infrastructure, research, and treatment innovations to reduce mortality and improve outcomes for patients with drug-resistant TB.

This discussion will explore current strategies and interventions aimed at improving outcomes for individuals with MDR-TB.

VARIOUS CONCERNS TO ADDRESS

- *Delay in diagnosis and treatment initiation*: The disease is often diagnosed late and this allows it to progress unchecked, leading to more severe forms of TB that are harder to treat effectively.
- *Limited treatment options*: Treatment for MDR-TB requires longer durations with second-line drugs that can be more toxic, less effective, and more expensive. Limited access to these drugs can compromise treatment outcomes.

- *Drug toxicity and side effects*: Second-line TB drugs used in MDR-TB treatment can cause significant side effects, such as hepatotoxicity, nephrotoxicity, and psychiatric disorders. Severe side effects may necessitate discontinuation of treatment or adjustment of drug regimens, impacting treatment efficacy.
- *Coinfections and comorbidities*: MDR-TB patients may also suffer from other infections or medical conditions that complicate treatment and contribute to poor outcomes.
- *Treatment nonadherence*: Adherence to lengthy and complex treatment regimens is crucial for successful outcomes. Poor adherence occurs due to various factors such as drug toxicity, socioeconomic challenges, and lack of patient education which lead to treatment failure and disease progression.
- *Disease complications*: MDR-TB can lead to severe complications such as pulmonary hemorrhage, respiratory failure, and disseminated TB, which can be life-threatening if not managed promptly and effectively.
- *Healthcare access and quality*: Disparities in access to healthcare services, including diagnostics, treatment facilities, and supportive care, can affect treatment outcomes.

CURRENT STRATEGIES UNDER NATIONAL TUBERCULOSIS ELIMINATION PROGRAM/PROGRAMMATIC MANAGEMENT OF DRUG-RESISTANT TUBERCULOSIS

In India, under national TB elimination program (NTEP), timely detection is done through rapid diagnostic tests like cartridge-based nucleic acid amplification test (CBNAAT). A pre-evaluation is done before initiation of the regimen as per programmatic management of drug resistant tuberculosis (PMDT) guidelines and identifies the chronic disease. Appropriate second-line drugs for MDR-TB treatment based on LPA and liquid culture patterns are provided under NTEP as per PMDT guidelines and are tailored to ensure that the prescribed drugs are effective. Regular periodic monitoring supports patient adherence to the full course of treatment with directly observed treatment short course (DOTS) under NTEP. Financial assistance is provided through the Nikshay Poshan Yojana (NPS), which is a direct benefit transfer scheme that offers support every month to notified TB patients for nutritional support during the treatment period.[2]

FUTURE DIRECTIONS

Moving forward with Canadian Consortium method of FAST (Fast diagnosis, Active case finding, Safe separation and infection control, Tailored therapy with rapid drug susceptibility testing) aiming for zero deaths, zero transmission, and zero suffering.

Case Finding

Active case finding improves the case detection and tracing close contacts helps in curbing further spread and treating at the earliest.

Monitoring

Close monitoring of active cases for treatment adherence, drug toxicities, and therapeutic drug monitoring (TDM) promotes better treatment outcomes.

Research Innovation

Tuberculosis resist is a global consortium working on whole-genome sequencing (WGS) for better understanding of TB genioplasty and resistance pattern which helps in newer drug and vaccine development.[3]

Fostering international partnerships and collaborations for research in newer drugs to decrease treatment duration, alternate drugs for drug toxicity, newer vaccines, and laboratory techniques for early identification.

Integrated Care for Comorbidities/Coinfections

Newer integrated approaches and special focus on comorbid conditions such as human immunodeficiency virus (HIV), diabetes, and other immunocompromised states are to be designed.

Societal Impact

As TB is a disease of poverty, ameliorating poverty and improving socioeconomic factors such as overcrowding, ventilation, and health seeking behavior will have impact on outcomes.

Empowering and educating the communities against the TB stigma.

High-level Political Commitment

Strong political commitment and involvement of policy makers, industrialists, and governmental organizations are needed.

International and interstate collaboration and cooperation at individual level are needed.

Accessible and Equitable Healthcare to all

Access to high-quality healthcare services, including diagnostics, treatment facilities, and supportive care, yields positive treatment outcomes.

- Holistic approach targeting the treatment of TB disease rather than TB resistance is the need of the hour.
- Strategies aiming toward optimistic approach rather than minimalistic approach need to be designed to envision a world free of TB.

CONCLUSION

Multidrug-resistant tuberculosis is a severe health problem because of its complicated treatment, high costs, and late diagnosis. Despite efforts under the NTEP, high mortality rates persist, particularly in resource-limited places. Achieving zero deaths requires improved healthcare, research and innovation, and global collaboration. Strong political commitment and fair access to high-quality healthcare are essential for eliminating MDR-TB and establishing a TB-free society.

REFERENCES

1. WHO. (2023). WHO Global Tuberculosis Report. [online] Available from https://www.who.int/publications/i/item/9789240083851 [Last accessed September, 2024].
2. WHO consolidated guidelines on tuberculosis. Module 4: treatment - drug-resistant tuberculosis treatment, 2022 update.
3. Forum on Drug Discovery, Development, and Translation; Board on Health Sciences Policy; Institute of Medicine. The Global Crisis of Drug-resistant Tuberculosis and Leadership of China and the BRICS: Challenges and Opportunities: Summary of a Joint Workshop by the Institute of Medicine and the Institute of Microbiology, Chinese Academy of Sciences. Washington (DC): National Academies Press (US); 2014.

CHAPTER

18

Therapeutic Drugs Monitoring in Multidrug-resistant Treatment

Judo J Vachaparambil

Abstract

Therapeutic drug monitoring (TDM) is a clinical technique which measures the drug concentrations from the patient to have better therapy and to avoid treatment failure by increasing the therapeutic drug concentration while minimizing the drug toxicity. It typically includes drug concentration measurements in serum specimens collected between 2 and 6 hours following dosage of the drug or drugs in concern. TDM is most commonly used serum or plasma to assess drug concentration in order to individualize drug therapy and maximize the time drugs stay within therapeutic range. The dried blood spot analysis (DBSA) method which collects a drop of blood from a finger prick on a card that can be shipped by mail at room temperature has made sample collection easier. While techniques such as high-performance liquid chromatography (HPLC) with triple quadrupole mass spectrometry (LC-MS/MS) are desirable for measuring concentrations, HPLC with dual wavelength ultraviolet detection is an affordable alternative for most tuberculosis (TB) drugs. In the case of coinfection of TB and human immunodeficiency virus (HIV), early use of TDM in the course of treatment is recommended.

Keywords: TDM, MDR-TB, LC-MS/MS, HPLC

INTRODUCTION

Multidrug-resistant tuberculosis (MDR-TB) is due to MTB with resistance to at least isoniazid and rifampin, two potent TB drugs. With the advent of new regimens such as bedaquiline, pretomanid and linezolid (BPaL) and BPaL and moxifloxacin (BPaLM), therapeutic drug monitoring (TDM) is an important tool that can be used to minimize interpatient variability to TB drug exposure, maximizing the benefit of the drug to a patient and reducing the risk of treatment failure and relapse.[1-3] It also reduces the danger of developing drug-resistant mutants. Those adjustments following TDM will decrease the time to sputum sterilization and the period where patients are infectious to others.

THERAPEUTIC DRUG MONITORING OVERVIEW

Therapeutic drug monitoring is one tool that may individualize TB pharmacotherapy. It typically includes drug concentration measurements in serum specimens collected between 2 and 6 hours following dosage of the drug or drugs in concern.[1,4] TDM most commonly used serum or plasma to assess drug concentration in order to individualize drug therapy and maximize the time drugs stay within therapeutic range.[1] The dried blood spot analysis (DBSA) method which collects a drop of blood from a finger prick on a card that can be shipped by mail at room temperature has made sample collection easier.[1,2] The ranges are derived from population-based averages where the majority of patient would be expected to respond to drug therapy with minimal to acceptable side effects. Inter patient variability can occur due to pharmacokinetic (PK) differences including bioavailability, body size and composition, distribution through fluid compartments, gastrointestinal absorption, binding to inactive sites, and also on drug metabolization and excretion. Performing TDM requires an understanding of the PK/pharmacodynamics (PD) target that will be optimized. There are three main antimicrobial PK/PD targets.[1,2]

1. The peak drug concentration relative minimum inhibitory concentration (C_{max}/MIC)
2. The percentage of time within a dosing interval that concentrations exceed MIC (%T > MIC)
3. The area under the concentration time curve of MIC ($AUG_{0\ to\ t}$/MIC)

For most TB drug, AUC/MIC ratio been predicted as the index for efficacy. Some exceptions include C_{max}/MIC as the primary efficacy target for aminoglycosides and %T > MIC for carbapenems and cycloserine. PK parameters of drugs used for MDR-TB is summarized in **Table 1**.[2]

THERAPEUTIC DRUG MONITORING INDICATIONS

In general, the indications for TDM is mainly for compliance monitoring, individualizing therapy, avoidance of drug concentration-related toxicities, avoidance of under dozing, and managing drug interactions. Preforming TDM in all MDR-TB patients looks reasonable, but as the resources are limited priority should be given to patients at risk of treatment failure from drug underexposure or patient at risk for drug toxicities.[1,2,5]

The at risk patients include *human immunodeficiency virus* (HIV) patients, type 2 diabetic, gastrointestinal complications, renal and hepatic impairment, and those who are severely ill. Patients with comorbidities such as diabetes and HIV are at risk for malabsorption from the gastrointestinal tract, increasing the risk of treatment failure. Those patients showing adverse effects and slow response to drug treatment are excellent candidates for TDM.[2]

Renal Dysfunction

Those patients with comprised renal function are at risk of drug accumulation and overexposure, leading to adverse effects. Special considerations should be given to MDR-TB therapies with renal clearance including aminoglycosides, carbapenems, cycloserine, ethambutol, and levofloxacin. Patients on hemodialysis, drawing pre- and postdialysis samples can be used to assess the impact of dialysis on drug concentrations.[2]

Hepatic Dysfunction

Hepatic function and its impact on drug clearance cannot be estimated based on tests such as aspartate transaminase, alanine aminotransferase, alkaline phosphatase, or bilirubin, unlike renal function's relationship with serum creatinine. Liver test abnormalities have occurred in up to 30% of patients treated with multiple drug regimens. The MDR-TB drug undergoing hepatic metabolism (may contribute to hepatotoxicity) includes bedaquiline, pyrazinamide, pretomanid, and moxifloxacin. Therefore, liver test should be measured throughout therapy and TDM is recommended.[2]

TABLE 1: Pharmacokinetic parameters of drugs used for MDR-TB.

Drug	Typical adult dose	Average C_{max} and C_{min} (mg/L)	T_{max} (h)	Recommended sampling strategy
Bedaquiline	400 mg daily or 200 mg TIW	C_{max}: • Week 2: 2.8–3.3 • Week 8: 1.7 • Week 24: 1.3 C_{min}: • Week 2 (24 hours): 0.73–0.96 • Week 8 (48 hours): 0.62 • Week 24 (48 hours): 0.36	4–6	Trough, 2 and 5–6 hours
Carbapenems	Varies, ~1,000 mg every 6–8 hours	C_{max}: 30–70	End of infusion	1 hour postinfusion and trough
Clofazimine	100 mg	C_{max}: 0.5–2.0	2–7	2 and 6 hours
Cycloserine	250–750 mg daily, can be divided into two doses	C_{max}: 20–35	2	2–3 and 6–7 hours
Ethambutol	15–25 mg/kg daily 50 mg/kg BIW	C_{max}: 2–6 C_{max}: 4–12	2–3	2–3 and 6–7 hours
Levofloxacin	750–1,000 mg	C_{max}: 8–12	1–2	2 and 6 hours
Linezolid	600 mg	C_{max}: 12–26 C_{min}: • BID: 3–9 • Once daily: <2	2	Trough, 2 and 5–6 hours
Moxifloxacin	400 mg	C_{max}: 3–5	1–2	2 and 6 hours
Pretomanid	200 mg	C_{max}: 2.3–4.3 C_{min}: 1.0–2.4	5	Trough, 2 and 5–6 hours
Pyrazinamide	25 mg/kg daily 50 mg/kg BIW	C_{max}: 20–60* C_{max}: 60–80	2	2 and 6 hours
Amikacin	15 mg/kg daily 25 mg/kg BIW	C_{max}: 35–45 C_{max}: 65–80	0.5–1.5 (IM) or end of infusion (IV)	2 and 6 hours
Streptomycin	15 mg/kg daily	C_{max}: 35–45	0.5–1.5 (IM) or end of infusion (IV)	2 and 6 hours

*Evidence suggests better outcomes when C_{max} values exceed 35 mg/L.

(BID: twice daily; BIW: twice weekly; C_{max}: peak serum drug concentration; C_{min}: minimum serum drug concentration during dosing interval; IM: intramuscular; IV: intravenous; T_{max}: time to C_{max}; TIW: three times weekly)

Source: Adapted from Maranchick NF, Peloquin CA, et al. Role of therapeutic drug monitoring in the treatment of multi-drug resistant tuberculosis. J Clin Tuberc Other Mycobact Dis. 2024;36:100444.

Diabetes Mellitus

High-fasting plasma glucose is a risk factor for drug-resistant TB. Patients with diabetes mellitus (DM) are more likely to be slow responders and have subtherapeutic drug concentrations. In addition to weakening the immune response against TB, DM impacts with PKs of anti-TB drugs, particularly drug absorption phase. Delayed absorption or malabsorption in diabetic patients can be due to polypharmacy interactions or gastropathy. So the second postdose sample (6 hours sample) can rule out whether a diabetic patient is experiencing malabsorption or delayed absorption. It is important to do TDM in diabetic patients as neuropathy and renal damage from diabetics itself can present similarly to the side effects of anti-TB drugs.[2]

Human Immunodeficiency Virus

The coinfection of HIV with TB has a synergistic effect to each other, with both pathogens hastening the deterioration of the immune system. MDR-TB patients coinfected with HIV (especially with low CD4 count) are at high risk for subtherapeutic drug exposures which can be due to gastrointestinal disease, drug interactions, diarrhea, etc. TDM is mandatory to avoid therapy failure and resistance in both diseases.[2]

THERAPEUTIC DRUG MONITORING PROCEDURE

The TDM is primarily performed using blood samples such as serum, plasma, or dried blood spots. Alternative samples such as oral fluid/salvia, urine, or hair have been studied as less invasive ways of measuring drug concentrations. More invasive sample types such as cerebrospinal fluid (CSF) are collected to have a better understanding of drug concentrations at difficult to penetrate sites.[1-3]

The clinician may consider collecting samples once the drug is at steady state or after approximately 5 half-lives. If the patient is critically ill or has a severe infection, sample can be ordered soon. In practice, for nonrifamycin drugs with relatively short half-lives such as pyrazinamide, ethambutol, or fluoroquinolones, TDM can be drawn within days after initiation. Drug with longer half-lives such as bedaquiline or clofazimine can take weeks to achieve steady state concentrations.[2]

Drug concentrations can be quantified with techniques such as high-performance liquid chromatography (HPLC) with triple quadrupole mass spectrometry (LC-MS/MS). LC-MS/MS methods have high specificity for the analyte as well as high sensitivity, enabling quantification of very low drug concentrations, even with low sample volume. In addition, LC/MS/MS has a favorable turnaround time and multiple drugs run on the same assay. More affordable options such as HPLC with dual wavelength ultraviolet detection can be an alternative for most TB drugs less sensitive than (LC-MS/MS).[2,3]

CONCLUSION

The TDM is a very important tool in the management of MDR-TB. It is used to minimize interpatient variability to TB drug exposure, maximizing the benefit of the drug to a patient, reducing the risk of treatment failure. Most TB drugs show concentration dependent killing, meaning that low concentrations are associated with minimal killing. While techniques such as HPLC with LC-MS/MS are desirable for measuring concentrations, HPLC with dual wavelength ultraviolet detection is an affordable alternative for most TB drugs. In the case of coinfection of TB and HIV early use of TDM in the course of treatment is recommended.

REFERENCES

1. WHO. (2023). WHO Global Tuberculosis Report 2023 [online] Available from https://www.who.int/teams/global-tuberculosis-programme/tb-reports/global-tuberculosis-report-2023#:~:text=The%20WHO%20Global%20Tuberculosis%20Report,TB%20commitments%2C%20strategies%20and%20targets [Last accessed September, 2024].
2. MaranchickNF, Peloquin CA. Role of therapeutic drug monitoring in the treatment of multi-drug resistant tuberculosis. J Clin Tuberc Other Mycobact Dis. 2024;36:100444.
3. WHO consolidated guidelines on tuberculosis: Module 4: treatment - drug-resistant tuberculosis treatment, 2022 update. Geneva: World Health Organization; 2022.
4. Anderson G, Vinnard C. Diagnostic Accuracy of Therapeutic Drug Monitoring during Tuberculosis Treatment. J Clin Pharmacol. 2022;62(10):1206-14.
5. Saluzzo F, Maria CD. Mind the gap. Rolling out new drug resistant tuberculosis regimens with limited diagnostic tools. J Clin Tubercul Other Mycobacterial Dis. 2023;32:100350.

Section 4: Treatment

CHAPTER

19

Phytochemicals to Combat Multidrug-resistant Tuberculosis

Rashmi Saxena Pal, MVNL Chaitanya

Abstract

Urgent investigation of other treatment approaches is required in light of the growing danger of *Mycobacterium tuberculosis (M. tb)* strains that are resistant to existing drugs. Potentially useful in the fight against drug-resistant tuberculosis (TB), traditional medicinal herbs are a treasure trove of bioactive phytochemicals. To combat drug-resistant tuberculosis, this study takes a close look at the molecular processes that make some phytochemicals found in traditional medicinal plants effective. By combining findings from different studies, we look at how phytochemicals interact with different molecular targets in *M. tb*. These targets include enzymes involved in cell wall biosynthesis (like mycolic acid synthesis), efflux pumps (like Rv1258c), and regulatory proteins linked to drug resistance (like WhiB7). In particular, we shed light on well-known phytochemicals like berberine, curcumin, and resveratrol, derived from plants like *Berberis* species, and explain how they work, as well as any synergistic effects they may have with traditional anti-TB medications. In addition, we explore phytochemicals' immunomodulatory characteristics, highlighting their capacity to boost host immunological responses against tuberculosis infection. We also go over some new ways of looking at the potential interactions between phytochemicals and *M. tb* targets, including molecular docking and network pharmacology. In order to improve their effectiveness and clinical translation, we also tackle problems with phytochemical bioavailability, pharmacokinetics, and formulation methods. This study offers a thorough framework for using phytochemicals from traditional medicinal plants as adjunctive or alternative therapy against drug-resistant tuberculosis by combining existing information and highlighting knowledge gaps.

Keywords: *Mycobacterium tuberculosis, Berberine*, curcumin, resveratrol, phytochemicals

INTRODUCTION

Tuberculosis (TB) continues to be one of the most lethal contagious diseases worldwide, and the rise of multidrug-resistant (MDR) strains poses a substantial risk to global well-being. Researchers are looking to nature's pharmacy for answers when traditional medicines become useless against these tough bacteria. A potential weapon against MDR-TB is phytochemicals, bioactive molecules taken from plants. Examining their several modes of action and the difficulties in fully exploiting their potential, this chapter investigates the possibilities of phytochemicals in the fight against this aggressive disease.[1]

UNDERSTANDING MULTIDRUG-RESISTANT TUBERCULOSIS

The most effective first-line anti-TB medications, isoniazid and rifampicin, are not effective against *Mycobacterium tuberculosis (M. tb)* strains that are resistant to several treatments. Around 500,000 new instances of TB that was resistant to rifampicin were reported in 2020, with 78% of those cases being multidrug-resistant (MDR). Factors like insufficient treatment regimens, low patient adherence, and the bacterium's incredible resistance-building capabilities have contributed to this concerning trend.

Compared to drug-susceptible TB, MDR-TB poses substantial therapeutic hurdles, necessitating lengthier, costlier, and frequently more toxic medication regimens. When compared to drug-susceptible TB, the success rates for MDR-TB treatment are substantially lower, hovering at 57% globally. This discrepancy highlights the critical requirement for novel, efficient, and tolerably safe treatment choices.

This discrepancy highlights the critical requirement for novel, efficient, and tolerably safe treatment choices. Treatment of MDR-TB is challenging for a number of reasons, including the bacteria's complex cell wall structure, its capacity to remain dormant for long periods of time, and its ability to hijack host immune responses. There has been a surge in interest in exploring alternate treatments, such as chemicals produced from plants with anti-mycobacterial characteristics, due to these considerations and the restricted pipeline of novel antibiotics.[2]

BIOACTIVE PLANT SUBSTANCES: A NATURAL WEAPON

Traditional medicine has made use of phytochemicals, which are non-nutritive plant substances, for countless generations. Plants create these bioactive chemicals to ward off diseases, herbivores, and other environmental threats. From alkaloids and flavonoids to terpenoids and phenolics, the diversity of phytochemicals is immense.

Phytochemicals have gained significant scientific attention in recent years due to their potential therapeutic uses in various diseases, particularly infectious diseases such as TB. The attractiveness of phytochemicals in addressing MDR-TB stems from their wide range of structural diversity, which results in a multitude of different modes of action. The presence of several strains of *(M. tb)* may aid in overcoming the resistance mechanisms that have been established by the bacteria against traditional antibiotics.

Furthermore, some phytochemicals demonstrate immunomodulatory characteristics, which could be especially advantageous in the treatment of TB, considering the crucial role of the host immunological response in managing the illness. The possibility of synergistic interactions between various phytochemicals or between phytochemicals and current antibiotics presents promising opportunities for combining therapy against MDR-TB.[3]

Table 1 details the molecular mechanisms by which several phytochemicals combat MDR-TB, as well as the plants from which they are derived.

TABLE 1: Key phytochemicals with potential anti-MDR-TB activity.

Phytochemical	Biological source	Molecular mechanism
Curcumin	*Curcuma longa*	• By interfering with the integrity of cell membranes, curcumin inhibits the growth of bacteria • Reduces expression of genes that are involved in the production of mycolic acid • Alters the host immune response in a way that makes macrophages more active

Continued

Continued

Phytochemical	Biological source	Molecular mechanism
Berberine	*Berberis vulgaris, Hydrastis canadensis, Mahonia aquifolium*	• Inhibits protein biosynthesis in bacteria • Damages bacterial cell wall and membrane
Resveratrol	*Vitis vinifera, Reynoutria japonica*	• Eliminates NAD+ from bacteria DNA ligase that is reliant, modulates the host immunological response, which in turn reduces inflammation • Decreases the intracellular growth of *Mycobacterium tuberculosis*
Quercetin	*Allium cepa, Malus domestica, Capparis spinosa*	Synergizes with other phytochemicals, inhibits bacterial DNA gyrase, and increases the efficacy of anti-TB medications
Epigallocatechin gallate (EGCG)	*Camellia sinensis*	Enhances host immunological response against tuberculosis; inhibits fatty acid synthase in *Mycobacterium tuberculosis*; disrupts bacterial cell wall integrity
Piperine	*Piper nigrum, Piper longum*	• Modulates the host immunological response • Inhibits efflux pumps in multidrug-resistant tuberculosis strains • Improves the bioavailability of additional anti-TB medications
Allicin	*Allium sativum*	Inhibits bacterial cysteine proteases and disrupts bacterial cell membrane
Plumbagin	*Plumbago zeylanica, Drosera binata*	• Modulates the host immunological response • Inhibits efflux pumps in multidrug-resistant tuberculosis strains • Improves the bioavailability of additional anti-TB medications
Thymoquinone	*Nigella sativa*	When combined with isoniazid, it has a multiplicative impact on bacteria and blocks their NDH-2 enzyme
Ursolic acid	*Ocimum sanctum, Rosmarinus officinalis*	• Eliminates the ability of bacteria to produce biofilms • Modulates the host immunological response
Eucalyptol	*Eucalyptus globulus, Rosmarinus officinalis*	Has anti-inflammatory effects, increases ethambutol's efficacy, and breaks the cell membranes of bacteria
Shikonin	*Lithospermum erythrorhizon*	Potent inhibition of *Mycobacterium* Mt-PTPa

(MDR-TB: multidrug-resistant tuberculosis)

Table 1 presented above in this chapter provides a comprehensive overview of key phytochemicals that have shown promise in combating MDR-TB. These compounds, derived from a wide variety of plant species, represent nature's diverse arsenal against this persistent pathogen. From common culinary herbs like turmeric and garlic to lesser-known medicinal plants like purple gromwell, the sources of these bioactive compounds span the globe. Researchers have investigated several phytochemicals derived from various plants in an effort to combat MDR-TB. A wide variety of bioactive chemicals with anti-mycobacterial activity are available in these natural substances.

ANTITUBERCULAR MECHANISM

Phytochemicals work against MDR-TB because they have different ways of working than traditional antibiotics. The development of resistance mechanisms by *(M. tb)* can be overcome with the use of this diversity.[4] Here are some ways the main modalities of action are classified.

Many phytochemicals, including curcumin, berberine, and eucalyptol, disrupt the bacterial cell wall or membrane. They boost the effectiveness of other antimicrobials and hinder bacterial development by interfering with these crucial structures.

Essential Enzyme Inhibition

Resveratrol and plumbagin are compounds that disrupt important biological processes by inhibiting essential bacterial enzymes. One example is plumbagin, which targets the NDH-2 enzyme, and resveratrol, which inhibits NAD+-dependent DNA ligase. Mycolic acid is an essential component of mycobacterial cell walls, and certain phytochemicals, such as curcumin, can modulate bacterial gene expression by downregulating genes involved in this process.

Supplementation of Standard Antibiotics

A number of phytochemicals have synergistic benefits when used in conjunction with standard anti-TB medications. Thymoquinone increases the efficacy of streptomycin and rifampicin, for instance, whereas piperine increases the bioavailability of other drugs.

Immunomodulation

Numerous phytochemicals influence the immunological response of the host in addition to their direct antibacterial actions. The host's capacity to manage the infection may be improved by compounds such as curcumin and resveratrol, which increase macrophage activity while decreasing inflammation.

Antioxidant

The production of bacterial biofilms is essential in the development of medication resistance and chronic infections; ursolic acid and thymoquinone both possess anti-biofilm activities. Inflammatory responses to infections can damage host cells, but compounds with antioxidant characteristics, such as gallic acid and ellagic acid, can prevent this damage.[5]

CHALLENGES AND FUTURE DIRECTIONS

While phytochemicals offer promising avenues for MDR-TB treatment, several challenges must be addressed, including poor bioavailability and stability of some compounds, the need for standardization of plant extracts, potential drug interactions, and the lack of comprehensive clinical trials. Future research should focus on elucidating precise molecular mechanisms, developing semisynthetic derivatives with improved pharmacokinetic properties, investigating optimal phytochemical-antibiotic combinations, exploring preventive applications, and conducting large-scale clinical trials.

Additionally, the potential for *(M. tb)* to develop resistance to phytochemicals, although less likely due to their multiple mechanisms of action, should be monitored. Overcoming these hurdles will be crucial in translating the promising laboratory findings into clinical applications, potentially leading to shorter treatment durations, reduced side effects, and improved outcomes for MDR-TB patients. The integration of traditional medicinal knowledge with modern scientific approaches in phytochemical research exemplifies a holistic strategy in drug discovery, offering hope not only in the battle against MDR-TB but also in addressing the broader challenge of antimicrobial resistance.

CONCLUSION

The global health epidemic of MDR-TB requires new treatments. One intriguing, treatment for this resilient sickness is phytochemicals, which have numerous action pathways and may supplement traditional antibiotics. MDR-TB's natural enemies go beyond chemicals. Although translating these encouraging discoveries into clinical practice will be difficult, phytochemical research may generate new MDR-TB treatments. When we learn more about phytochemicals and solve their development issues, they could revolutionize TB treatment.

By combining conventional medical understanding with cutting-edge phytochemical research methods, drug creation can be more complete. This method gives MDR-TB fighters hope, but it also emphasizes the need to protect biodiversity and traditional knowledge while searching for new treatments. As TB research advances, phytochemicals may become more important in the global pandemic fight. They may also treat other drug-resistant illnesses besides MDR-TB.

REFERENCES

1. Schito M, Migliori GB, Fletcher HA, McNerney R, Centis R, D'Ambrosio L, et al. Perspectives on Advances in Tuberculosis Diagnostics, Drugs, and Vaccines. Clin Infect Dis. 2015;61(Suppl 3):S102-18.
2. Antoun F, Véziris N. Managing multidrug-resistant tuberculosis. Revue Des Maladies Respiratoires. 2011;28(8), 956-7.
3. Fatima S, Kumari A, Dwivedi VP. Advances in adjunct therapy against tuberculosis: Deciphering the emerging role of phytochemicals. Med Comm. 2021;2(4):494.
4. Sakallioglu IT, Barletta RG, Dussault PH, Powers R. Deciphering the mechanism of action of antitubercular compounds with metabolomics. Comput Struct Biotechnol J. 2021;19:4284-99.
5. Soh AZ, Chee CBE, Wang YT, Yuan JM, Koh WP. Dietary Intake of Antioxidant Vitamins and Carotenoids and Risk of Developing Active Tuberculosis in a Prospective Population-Based Cohort Study. Am J Epidemiol. 2017;186(4):491.

CHAPTER

20

Revolutionizing Drug-resistant Tuberculosis Care: The Global BPaL Implementation Experience

Sandeep Juneja, Aastha Gupta, Maria Diachenko, Sunil Khaparde

Abstract

The advent of the BPaL (bedaquiline, pretomanid, and linezolid) regimen marks a transformative shift in the treatment of drug-resistant tuberculosis (DR-TB), treatment for which has so far been characterized by ineffective, lengthy, and costly regimens. Prior to BPaL, DR-TB treatments were arduous, spanning 18–24 months with low success rates and high costs. Since 2019, BPaL has emerged as a simpler, more effective, shorter regimen, that is significantly cheaper. This new regimen is now endorsed by the World Health Organization (WHO) as the new standard care for most forms of DR-TB. The rollout of BPaL has been notable for its rapid global adoption, with more 85,000 treatments procured by more than 85 countries within 1½ years of WHO's endorsement. Key factors in this swift implementation include strategic early engagement with high-burden countries, generation of robust field evidence through initiatives like LIFT-TB, effective pricing strategies, and the establishment of supportive platforms like the PeerLINC Knowledge Hub for sharing of information and best practices among countries. The BPaL experience also highlights effectiveness of collaborations, offering a hopeful precedent for addressing other global health challenges.

Keywords: Drug-resistant TB, BPaL, BPaLM, access, global implementation, evidence generation, adoption, implementation

INTRODUCTION

Tuberculosis (TB) continues to be one of the world's deadliest infectious diseases, with an estimated 10 million cases annually. While drug-susceptible TB (DS-TB) accounts for most cases and can be treated effectively with a well-established regimen, most drug-resistant forms of TB (DR-TB) have traditionally been very challenging to treat effectively, easily, and affordably. However, the recent introduction of new regimens like BPaL (bedaquiline, pretomanid, and linezolid) offers new hope by changing the landscape of DR-TB treatment for the better.

BACKGROUND

For the last half century, the treatment landscape for DR-TB was bleak and advances in new drugs were scant. As recently as 10 years ago physicians had to cobble together treatments from decades old antibiotics, most of which were highly toxic and with passage of time, a high degree of resistance to them had become prevalent. People treated with such regimens struggled with brutal adverse effects, crippling expenses, long duration, and still low success rates.

For instance, the treatment duration for some of the most resistant forms of TB such as XDR TB (extensively drug-resistant) or pre-XDR-TB could last 18–24 months, with full treatment cost ranging up to US $15,000 (₹12.5 Lakhs) with average efficacy as low as 43% globally (36% in India) in 2018. The situation was not much better for multidrug-resistant TB (MDR-TB) at that time, with global average success rate of 58% (49% in India).[1] So, someone treated for MDR-TB had slightly <50% chance of successful therapy after 18–24 months.

That changed in 2019, when a new regimen called BPaL was approved for use in pre XDR-TB. BPaL comprised three relatively new drugs: pretomanid—first approved in 2019, linezolid—first recommended by the World Health Organization (WHO) for use in TB in 2016, and bedaquiline—first approved in 2012. BPaL offered a shorter, 6-month duration treatment at a much lower cost and higher efficacy (~90%).[2,3] In 2022, WHO endorsed the regimen as the first-line standard of care for almost all of DR-TB, including MDR-TB, to be used programmatically and globally, also recommending use of moxifloxacin (M) with BPaL (or, BPaLM regimen) if there was no resistance to fluoroquinolones.[4]

As pretomanid was developed by a nonprofit research organization—TB Alliance—its price was at a historical low for a new drug, allowing BPaL to be highly cost saving and cost-effective from the beginning with medicines cost at approximately US $1,000 per treatment for pre-XDR-TB. Following WHO guidelines of 2022 which expanded use of BPaL to almost all DR-TB, cost economies and negotiations with manufacturer lowered the price of pretomanid. That, with reduction in cost of other drugs, reduced price of BPaL to below US $500—the long-demanded ceiling by the TB community.

TREATING DRUG-RESISTANT TUBERCULOSIS WITH BPAL/BPALM

Unlike older treatments, BPaL and BPaLM regimens provide a more effective, shorter, and less burdensome user experience. This is particularly relevant for India, which faces a high burden of DR-TB. By offering a shorter duration, lower pill burden, more effective, and more affordable treatment option, BPaL significantly improves treatment outcomes and reduces the financial burden on healthcare systems and people.

ENSURING BPAL/BPALM REACH ALL IN NEED

The successful implementation of BPaL and BPaLM globally required strategic planning and proactive and early measures. To date, the global roll out of BPaL/BPaLM has been the most robust and rapid in modern TB treatment history, with >85,000 treatments procured by over 85 countries in the 1½ years since the WHO guidelines update of December 2022. Although additional work is still needed to further expand access—including in India—the developer, TB Alliance has undertaken several key initiatives to achieve access globally:

- *Early country engagement and market studies*: During clinical trials, TB Alliance engaged with several high-burden countries to understand need-gaps and prerequisites to implement a new treatment. Systematic feasibility and value proposition studies for BPaL were conducted in multiple countries. These helped to understand the treatment environments in which the regimen could potentially be used and ensure the regimen's attributes and rollout were aligned with the priorities of stakeholders including WHO, and country stakeholders such as National TB Programs (NTPs), policy makers, clinicians, nurses, laboratory experts, and community members.

- *Generation of field evidence*: Consistent with WHO guidelines and to encourage adoption, TB Alliance conceptualized and secured funding for projects like the LIFT-TB (www.lifttb.org), enabling operational research (OR) on BPaL in seven countries. LIFT-TB ORs generated early real-world experience and evidence, confirming clinical trial outcomes. Interim data from LIFT-TB shows 93.6% success rate and lost to follow-up rate of about 1.8%. Further, most adverse events for BPaL observed in OR were related to linezolid, whose use in TB and side effects are well known. The LIFT-TB experience helped countries understand how to transition from complex regimens to simpler, shorter BPaL/BPaLM treatments, facilitating early and widespread adoption. Currently, all seven LIFT-TB countries use BPaL/BPaLM programmatically. This experience also aided other countries, like Pakistan, in rapidly piloting, adopting, and scaling up the regimens.
- *Capacity building and knowledge sharing*: To make the experience of LIFT-TB and other early adopter countries available to others, TB Alliance launched a peer-to-peer learning platform called PeerLINC Knowledge Hub in March 2024 in collaboration with the Tropical Disease Foundation and the Department of Health Philippines (https://www.peerlinc.org/). PeerLINC provides technical assistance, capacity building, and training to countries on clinical, laboratory, programmatic use, and community engagement aspects of DR-TB care. Such knowledge transfer avoids reinventing the wheel when implementing new treatments in "new" countries, speeding the process. In the first 4 months since inception, four countries—Peru, Rwanda, Democratic Republic of Congo, and Nigeria—have obtained technical assistance from PeerLINC, and several others are in the pipeline. PeerLINC provides its services free of charge to countries or specific states within countries wanting to implement BPaL/BPaLM. TB Alliance intends to expand the services of PeerLINC to other TB treatments as well, once they are recommended by WHO.
- *Commercialization and pricing*: During development of BPaL, TB Alliance executed a strategy to ensure worldwide accessibility and affordability of the drug for people who need it. A key element of this approach was licensing five high-quality, low-cost manufacturers to produce pretomanid, the new drug in BPaL/BPaLM. The first manufacturer is producing pretomanid in India for global supply. Four other companies, including two based in India, will soon start supplying pretomanid. This strategy will ensure competition and supply security. The maximum price of pretomanid at launch in 2019 was $364 per course in 150 developing countries, about 60% below the lowest launch price of bedaquiline for similar countries and similarly, 79% less than price of delamanid. This made pretomanid the most affordable new DR-TB drug at launch, though the drug was then meant only for use in a small number of people—those affected by pre-XDR-TB, and hence had virtually no economies of scale. However, with expansion of guidelines to almost all DR-TB, the price was further reduced by 34% to $240 per course in 2022 through negotiations with the manufacturer and a volume guarantee agreement, which has enabled the BPaL/BPaLM regimens to be priced at around $400, well under the long-standing price target of $500 of the TB community.[5] Price improvements have served as a catalyst for the rapid global adoption of BPaL. A recent study suggests that implementing BPaL could save up to $740 million per year.[6] A model for calculating cost savings and cost-effectiveness, SLASH-TB, recently published estimated savings for four countries due to BPaL/M, ranging from 23 to 51%, with 11–19% lives saved.[7]
- *Stakeholder support*: Recognizing the importance of BPaL/BPaLM in saving lives and ending TB, the global TB community has rallied to support implementation of the regimens. On World TB Day in March 2023, WHO's Global TB Program noted that

the BPaL/BPaLM regimen represents a "historic change" in the management of drug-resistant TB and issued a call to action urging NTPs, healthcare providers, and partners to accelerate the transition to these regimens. WHO has also launched a platform called "BPaLM Accelerator" which facilitates a monthly dialogue among countries and stakeholders on speeding up access to BPaL/BPaLM.

Two advocacy initiatives, 1/4/6×24 campaign (146x24) and the Fast Track the Cure initiative (FTTC) were also established by stakeholders in TB. 1/4/6×24, launched by Treatment Action Group and others urges countries to implement the shortest available regimens for TB including BPaL/BPaLM, by the end of 2024. FTTC, supported by TB Alliance and the Stop TB Partnership, has a growing list of 30 endorsing partners and community implementing partners who advocate for rapid access to BPaL/BPaLM and capacitate communities to support NTPs toward the same.

- *Current status of implementation of BPaL/BPaLM*: Many among top 20 high DR-TB burden countries were early adopters of BPaL notably South Africa, Ukraine, Indonesia, Philippines, Vietnam, Nigeria, Myanmar, and Uzbekistan. These, as also many other top 20 countries who have caught up rapidly such as Pakistan, Peru, and Democratic Republic of Congo, are rolling out BPaL/BPaLM nationwide. At the time of writing, over 85 countries had procured >85,000 course of pretomanid in the 1½ years since WHO's recommendation for establishing the regimens as the new standard of care for DR-TB, marking the fastest uptake of any new treatment in TB. Consequently, countries that are currently not implementing BPaL/BPaLM are exceptions.

STATUS IN INDIA

Among all high-burden countries, India has perhaps the most to gain from BPaL/BPaLM having about a third of all people globally currently treated for DR-TB. In 2021–2022, a local study, called the mBPaL trial, was conducted by ICMR's National Institute of Research in Tuberculosis with the NTEP to evaluate the effectiveness and safety of varying doses of linezolid in the BPaL regimen. Interim results were presented at the Union conference in 2023 and showed 95% culture conversion by the end of 26 weeks.[8] India was the second country after USA to approve pretomanid in July 2020. India has recently announced that the country is getting ready to roll out the regimen.

CHALLENGES, LESSONS LEARNED, AND CONCLUSION

Despite rapid adoption of BPaL/BPaLM by most high DR-TB burden countries, implementation of the regimen has not been without challenges. Key obstacles included shortage of technical assistance providers, limited financing for implementation particularly in early years following regulatory approval, slow issuance of local guidelines and variable national regulatory requirements, often necessitating additional local data. However, leadership of NTPs in early adopter countries helped overcome many such these barriers. The BPaL/BPaLM experience has also demonstrated that while WHO endorsement is critical for policy change in most countries, active involvement of the developer (TB Alliance in this case) is crucial: by proactively engaging countries, sharing knowledge, generating field evidence, and demonstrating the value proposition early on, often at risk, and ensuring knowledge sharing between countries, the developer can play a key role in global access. This approach facilitates coordination, rapid and open exchange of best practices among countries and stakeholders. While some high DR-TB burden countries have yet to implement these regimens, the overwhelming global acceptance and available evidence offer a strong impetus. With continued collaboration and knowledge sharing, BPaL/BPaLM can become universally accessible, ensuring more effective and manageable TB treatment for all in need.

REFERENCES

1. World Health Organization. Global tuberculosis report 2023. Geneva: World Health Organization; 2023.
2. Conradie F, Diacon AH, Ngubane N, Howell P, Everitt D, Crook AM, et al. Treatment of highly drug-resistant pulmonary tuberculosis. N Engl J Med. 2020;382(10):893-902.
3. Conradie F, Bagdasaryan TR, Borisov S, Howell P, Mikiashvili L, Ngubane N, et al. Bedaquiline–pretomanid–linezolid regimens for drug-resistant tuberculosis. N Engl J Med. 2022;387(9):810-23.
4. World Health Organization. WHO consolidated guidelines on tuberculosis. Module 4: treatment - drug-resistant tuberculosis treatment, 2022 update. Geneva: World Health Organization; 2022.
5. MedAccess Viatris, Alliance TB. (2022). Price reduction paves the way for expanded access to highly effective multidrug-resistant tuberculosis treatment. [online] Available from https://medaccess.org/news/price-reduction-paves-the-way-for-expanded-access-to-highly-effective-multidrug-resistant-tuberculosis-treatment/ [Last accessed September, 2024]
6. Gupta A, Juneja S, Sahu S, Yassin M, Brigden G, Wandwalo E, et al. Lifesaving, cost-saving: Innovative simplified regimens for drug-resistant tuberculosis. PLOS Glob Public Health. 2022;2(11):e0001287.
7. Auer C, Gupta A, Malbacius C, Ghafoor A, Kock Y, Medvedieva O, et al. 2024. Savings from the introduction of BPaL and BPaLM regimens at the country level. IJTLD Open. 2024;1(7):314-9.
8. Padmapriyadarsini C, Devaleenal B, Ponnuraja C, Ramraj B, Singla R, Parmar M, et al. Randomised trial to evaluate the effectiveness and safety of varying doses of linezolid with bedaquiline and pretomanid in adults with pre-XDR or treatment intolerant/non-responsive multidrug-resistant pulmonary tuberculosis: study protocol. BMJ Open. 2022;12(8):e058606.

CHAPTER

21

Poor Drug Quality: Impact on Drug Resistance

Chandragiri Pranay Sai, Tejas Menon Suri

Abstract

Multidrug-resistant tuberculosis (MDR-TB) is an important cause of adverse outcomes in patients with tuberculosis. While poor drug quality could be a significant contributor to multidrug resistance in the context of tuberculosis, it is often neglected. Poor quality may be either due to substandard medicine or counterfeit medicine. The prevalence of poor-quality antitubercular medication may range between 10 and 15% and is likely to be a common occurrence, particularly in low- and middle-income countries. In this chapter, we explore the mechanisms by which poor-quality medication leads to decreased treatment success and the emergence of drug resistance. We also discuss the methods for quality assessment of drugs. Finally, we suggest some remedial measures that can be implemented, including patient education, clinician vigilance, and regulatory measures to mitigate the problem of poor-quality antitubercular drugs.

Keywords: Tuberculosis, drug resistance, poor-quality drugs, antitubercular drugs, substandard medicines

INTRODUCTION

Tuberculosis (TB) has been a significant public health problem with a total incidence rate of 199 per one lakh population. Multidrug-resistant (MDR)-TB has an incidence rate of 8 per one lakh population in India, according to the World Health Organization (WHO) Global Tuberculosis Report 2023. In India, nearly 80% of TB patients are diagnosed and initiated on treatment from the private sector, and almost 50% of patients continue to take their treatment there. Poor patient adherence to the long duration of treatment, side effects, drug–drug interactions, lack of awareness of dangers of monotherapy, poor prescribing practices, treatment interruptions, inappropriate drugs, dosing, and duration impact patient quality of life, leading to treatment failure and the emergence of drug resistance and increased morbidity and mortality.[1] While the focus remains on the aforementioned causes regarding treatment failure and the emergence of drug resistance, a factor of uncertain importance is the quality of antitubercular medicine that the patients take.[1] According to a global survey conducted by the WHO, 1 in 10 medicines in low- and middle-income countries (LMICs) is of poor quality.[2] Out of 7,682 anti-tubercular drug samples collected from 22 countries, 1,170 (15.2%) failed at least one quality test.[1] In this chapter, we will analyze the impact of poor-quality antitubercular medication on patient management and its role in the emergence of drug resistance.

POOR-QUALITY MEDICATION

Poor-quality medicine includes substandard and falsified medicinal products (WHO definitions).

- Substandard medicines are authorized medical products that fail to meet either quality standards or specifications.
- Falsified medical products (counterfeit) deliberately or fraudulently misrepresent the original drugs' identity, composition, or source.

Often, the differentiation between these two entities is not possible without referring to the packaging or regulatory status of the sampled medication.[1]

In India, as per the Drug and Cosmetic (D and C) Act, 1940, under Sections 17, 17A, 17B and its 2008 amendment of the D and C Act, the Indian drug regulatory authority, i.e., the Central Drugs Standard Control Organization (CDSCO), has classified poor-quality drugs into categories A, B, and C:[3]

- *Category A*: Spurious and adulterated drug products that conceal the real identity of the product or formulation and are similar to some well-known brands (may or may not contain active ingredients).
- *Category B*: Grossly substandard drugs in which the product fails the disintegration or dissolution test and where active ingredient assay gets below 70% and 5% of the permitted limit for thermolabile and thermostable products, respectively, for tablets or capsules.
- *Category C*: Products with minor defects like emulsion cracking, change in color, a slight variation in net content, sedimentation in a clear liquid preparation, failing of weight variation test, spot or discoloration on the product, uneven coating, presence of foreign matter, and labeling errors.

The majority of quality issues with anti-TB medicines were due to inadequate content of the active pharmaceutical ingredient (API). A further problem has been identified with poor bioavailability of anti-TB drugs, primarily rifampicin, both in monocomponent products and fixed-dose combinations (FDCs).[1]

MECHANISM OF DRUG RESISTANCE

Poor-quality antitubercular medicines contribute to prolonged infection duration and antimicrobial resistance.[2] Mutant TB bacilli emerge as they replicate inside the host as a part of natural evolution. Still, their concentration remains low because they must compete with the wild variants to survive. High concentrations of the API during the early stages of infection will kill susceptible microbes and may kill partially resistant mutants. However, poor-quality medicines containing subtherapeutic concentrations of the anti-infective substance may not be adequate to achieve this, and thus mutant microorganisms will overproliferate while "wild type" ones will perish.[2] While falsified medication allows a false sense of security to the patient, it contributes indirectly to the development of drug resistance through increasing infective periods, i.e., the more the number of replication cycles, the more the chance of mutants. Genetic mutations of genes encoding synthesis of mycobacterial enzymes (KatG and InhA), RNA polymerase (rpoB), and type 2 topoisomerase (DNA gyrase) confer resistance to isoniazid (H), rifampicin (R), and fluoroquinolones, respectively. Additionally, the production of efflux pumps to pump out the penetrated drug also remains a cause of resistance to fluoroquinolones.[2]

ASSESSING THE QUALITY OF MEDICINES

Quality assessment of a drug includes testing for the identity and appearance and assays for the content of the active ingredient, dissolution, uniformity of mass, pH value, sterility, and the presence of bacterial endotoxins.[4] The most common methods used for determining API are high-performance liquid chromatography (HPLC), either alone or coupled with UV-spectrophotometry, differential scanning calorimetry (DSC), Fourier-transform infrared spectroscopy (FTIR), and liquid chromatography coupled with mass spectrometry (LC-MS).[1] The limits for the content of the active ingredient(s) applied to the individual products were 90.0–110.0% according to the specifications in the pharmacopeia monographs.[4] Appearance includes physical signs of instability like container, cracks, chipping in the tablet surfaces or coating, swelling, mottling, discoloration, fusion between tablets, appearance of crystals on the container walls, injection, solutions for infusion, and reconstituted solutions should be clear and free from visible particulate matter. The storage conditions of the drugs, especially the temperature, affect their activity, and inappropriate storing temperatures can lead to treatment failures. In general, capsules and tablets are stored at 15–24°C, powders for solution for injection at 5–24°C, solutions for infusion at 18–19°C, and solutions for injection at 4–7°C.[4] Bioavailability is often considered a surrogate of the quality of the medicine. Usually, the bioavailability is measured through its concentration time profiles in plasma or urinary excretion data.[1] Apart from the studies mentioned above, assessing the medicine's accelerated stability is crucial, i.e., its stability under stress conditions like temperature and humidity simulating a patient's home environment. These assays are called accelerated stability assays and are an integral part of quality assessment.[1]

INDIAN SCENARIO

India is the largest manufacturer of generic drugs, and poor quality remains a significant concern as it affects both domestic and global markets. India is one of the largest manufacturers of antitubercular medicines. While most are consumed domestically, a small proportion is exported internationally. In a survey conducted by WHO in the newly independent states of the former Soviet Union, out of 33 manufacturers supplying antitubercular medicines, 10 manufacturers were from India.[4] The European Commission and US Pharmacopeia blame that the majority of the poor-quality medicines in global markets originate in India and China; on the other hand, India extensively interacts with other LMICs, like African countries, in providing quality medicine at an affordable price. As per Indian government official statements and data, substandard medicine in India was 10.6% in 1995–1996 and 5.75% in 2008–2009.[3] India has worked significantly to reduce this number, showing it is more concerned with public health and safety. The CDSCO strives to eradicate this issue by increasing its workforce and strengthening the government establishments dedicated to providing various services, from quality control measures to providing immediate legal aid and punishment to offenders. The CDSCO publishes a monthly list of drugs, medical devices, and cosmetics that are evaluated and declared as not of standard quality, spurious, adulterated, or misbranded.[3] No large-scale studies show the exact prevalence of poor-quality antitubercular medicines. We could find only one pilot study reporting the extent of substandard and counterfeit drugs available in the market in two major cities (Delhi and Chennai). About 12% of the isoniazid samples and 9% of the rifampicin samples failed the quality tests.[5] We could not find any data regarding the prevalence of substandard quality among other first- or second-line antitubercular drugs in India.

REMEDIAL MEASURES FOR THE PROBLEM

The solution to this problem must be dealt with at the level of patient, clinician, and regulatory bodies. Patient education is most important; they should be educated regarding

India's national program to deal with both drug-sensitive and drug-resistant TB, along with the provision of both medical and financial aid to them as needed. Lack of finances should not be a reason for the patient to resort to an unreliable source of medicine. Patients should be educated regarding proper storage conditions to safeguard the functionality of the medicine. As clinicians, we must ensure that the patient takes the prescribed drugs. A visual inspection of the medicine blister can give us an idea regarding the appearance and sterile packing conditions. Inspection for color changes, manufacturers' labels, and uniformity of shape and size can help identify counterfeit medications. This measure will only take a few extra minutes during a clinical visit and can impact patient care and help build an excellent patient–clinician relationship. Reporting your findings of a suspected substandard or counterfeited medicine to the health authorities, if encountered, will aid the regulatory bodies to act accordingly. A "Whistle Blower" scheme has been initiated to encourage attentive public participation in exploring the detection of spurious drug products. Under this scheme, informers are suitably rewarded if accurate information on the movement of spurious drug products is provided to the regulatory authorities.[3] Mandatory drug serialization combined with authentication has a good potential to bridge the gap in fake medicines detection standards.[2] The application of new technologies to track and trace the manufactured medication and user perception of authentic medicine by means of verification via a scratch-off serial number has been an effective method.[2] The WHO stresses strict legislation and stringent laws ensuring punishments for offenders. The Indian government, through its Drugs and Cosmetics Act, has made provisions that make certain offenses nonbailable to prevent illegal practices. If adulterated or spurious drugs cause death, punishment ranges from a minimum of 10 years and up to life imprisonment with a penalty of not less than 1 million Indian Rupees (INR) or three times the value of the drugs confiscated, whichever is more.[3]

CONCLUSION

Poor-quality medication is a major problem with little awareness among patients or clinicians. Among antitubercular medications, the prevalence of substandard quality has been most widely studied for isoniazid and rifampicin. Substandard medication adversely impacts treatment outcomes and increases the morbidity and mortality of TB. It also contributes to the development of antimicrobial resistance. Surveillance of the quality of TB medicines needs to be an integral part of treatment programs. Research on the quality of other first-line and second-line antitubercular drugs and its impact on the development of drug resistance is urgently required.

REFERENCES

1. Tabernero P, Newton PN. Estimating the prevalence of poor-quality anti-TB medicines: a neglected risk for global TB control and resistance. BMJ Glob Health. 2023;8(7):e012039.
2. Akpobolokemi T, Martinez-Nunez RT, Raimi-Abraham BT. Tackling the global impact of substandard and falsified and unregistered/unlicensed anti-tuberculosis medicines. J Med Access. 2022;6:23992026211070406.
3. Khan AN, Khar RK. Current Scenario of Spurious and Substandard Medicines in India: A Systematic Review. Indian J Pharm Sci. 2015;77(1):2-7.
4. World Health Organization. (2012). Survey of the quality of anti-tuberculosis medicines circulating in selected newly independent states of the former Soviet Union [Internet]. [online] Available from https://www.who.int/news/item/04-02-2012-survey-of-the-quality-of-anti-tuberculosis-medicines-circulating-in-selected-newly-independent-states-of-the-former-soviet-union [Last accessed September, 2024]
5. Bate R, Tren R, Mooney L, Hess K, Mitra B, Debroy B, et al. Pilot Study of Essential Drug Quality in Two Major Cities in India. PLoS One. 2009;4(6):e6003.

CHAPTER

22

Surgical Modalities in Multidrug-resistant/Extensively Drug-resistant Tuberculosis

Pallavi Purwar

Abstract

There is increasing incidence and prevalence of drug-resistant tuberculosis. Newer drugs and guideline-based regimens have improved the treatment success rate that is 50–75% with best medical therapy. Surgical interventions in select patients have the potential to improve the cure rates and possibly prevent sequelae in this difficult to treat subset of patients. Surgery as an adjunct to medical therapy has been associated with high treatment success, trend toward better outcomes, and lesser morbidity. Further with advancements in technology and protocols, surgical interventions are associated with minimal morbidity and must be considered early in the course of the disease.

Keywords: Lobectomy, surgery, MDR-TB, VATS lobectomy

INTRODUCTION

The reported global number of estimated cases of tuberculosis (TB) was 10.6 million people (95% UI: 9.9–11.4 million) in 2022, people newly diagnosed with TB 7.5 million and India accounts for 28% of the global burden. The proportion who had multidrug-resistant TB (MDR-TB)/rifampicin-resistant TB (RR-TB) was 3.3% (95% UI: 2.6–4.0%) in newly detected TB and 17% (95% UI: 11–23%) patients previously treated. For MDR-/XDR (multidrug-resistant-/extensively drug-resistant)-TB, the treatment success rate with the best medical therapy is 50–75%. Adjunctive surgery has the potential to improve outcomes based on emerging evidence and advances in thoracic surgery.[1]

TUBERCULOSIS AND THORACIC SURGEONS: HISTORICAL PERSPECTIVE

The development of thoracic surgery dates to the era of the Ancient Greeks when Hippocrates described the first procedure for the chest for a patient of tubercular empyema. Subsequently collapse therapy, iatrogenic pneumothorax, plombage procedures, phrenic nerve crushing, cavernostomy, thoracoplasty, thoracostoma, and lung resections were all developed in the late 19th to 20th centuries for patients of TB. The first minimally invasive procedure of the chest was also developed by Jacobeus for a TB patient. Soon with the advent of effective antitubercular therapy, the role of surgery in TB diminished drastically. However, with advancements in technology, thoracic surgery continued to develop in the lung cancer patients. Currently, we are in a unique position to offer the advantages of the safe lung resections with minimal morbidity and mortality using minimally invasive techniques to tackle the patients with MDR/XDR TB wherein the outcomes are 75% success rates for a benign pathology.[2,3]

RATIONALE, INDICATIONS, AND CONTRAINDICATIONS FOR SURGERY FOR MULTIDRUG-RESISTANT/EXTENSIVELY DRUG-RESISTANT TUBERCULOSIS

Patients with pulmonary TB generally have disease confined to the upper lobes generally with necrotic, nonviable lung portions harboring up to 10^7–10^{12} bacilli. Further with persistent nonviability, there is cavity formation, and these cavities are not just sites for no drug penetration but also sites for drug resistance development or progression. Removal of this focus of infection teaming with bacteria can improve the response to medical therapy. Further, the immune response to the residual infection also improves after removal of the major focus of disease in a segment/lobe of the lung.[4]

Selection criteria for lung resection were established by Isseman et al. in 1990[2-4] and included:

1. Drug resistance so extensive that there is a high probability of failure or relapse.
2. Disease sufficiently localized that most of the disease can be resected with the expectation of adequate cardiopulmonary capacity post-surgery.
3. Sufficient drug activity to diminish the mycobacterial burden enough to facilitate probable healing of the bronchial stump.

The indications for adjuvant surgery in MDR-/XDR-TB are evolving and the major indications currently are the following:[2-6]

1. *Refractory to medical therapy*: Failure to achieve culture conversion at 3–4 months
2. *High risk of relapse*: Resistance to all known drugs; previous nonadherence to therapy (missed doses > 20%); high bacillary load; cavitary forms of disease; intolerance to antitubercular therapy
3. Localized disease
4. *Life-threatening complications*: Massive hemoptysis/recurrent significant hemoptysis
5. Unilateral empyema

Fitness criteria for patients to tolerate the procedure have been extrapolated from data for studies based on surgery for cancer and the rough guidelines constitute the following:

1. Vital capacity of <50%, forced expiratory volume in 1 second (FEV1) <800–2,000 mL
2. Cardiac insufficiency diagnosed by a cardiologist as exclusion criteria
3. Predicted postoperative FEV1/carbon monoxide lung diffusion capacity (DLCO) > 30%
4. Adequate nutritional status and ECOG status 0/1

Contraindications to offer the surgery are the following for TB, MDR-/XDR-TB as well as sequelae of TB are similar and the basic tenet to avoid morbidity and mortality of these complex thoracic procedures. The following are:

1. Bilateral extensive disease
2. Military TB
3. Disseminated TB
4. Active bronchial TB

While these are criteria, indications and contraindications are evolving, this complex disease must be evaluated in multidisciplinary team (MDT) of thoracic surgeons, TB physicians, as well as anesthesiologist.

SURGICAL PROCEDURES FOR MULTIDRUG-RESISTANT/ EXTENSIVELY DRUG-RESISTANT TUBERCULOSIS

The preferred procedures for localized disease are lobectomy (removal of a lobe), segmental lung resection (anatomical segmentectomy/nonanatomical wedge resection), cavernostomy with thoracoplasty, and decortication for empyema. In exceptional cases for life-threatening hemoptysis, pneumonectomy and thoracostoma for recalcitrant bronchopleural fistula are recommended.

The unique features for technical challenges in MDR surgery include dense adhesions **(Fig. 1)** that may be addressed by extrapleural dissection. Further, there is intense desmoplasia and the lymph nodes of TB are especially sticky **(Fig. 2)**, and the dissection of these nodes is likely to lead to intraoperative complications especially during hilar dissection. Another significant technical challenge is the nonpliability of the remanent

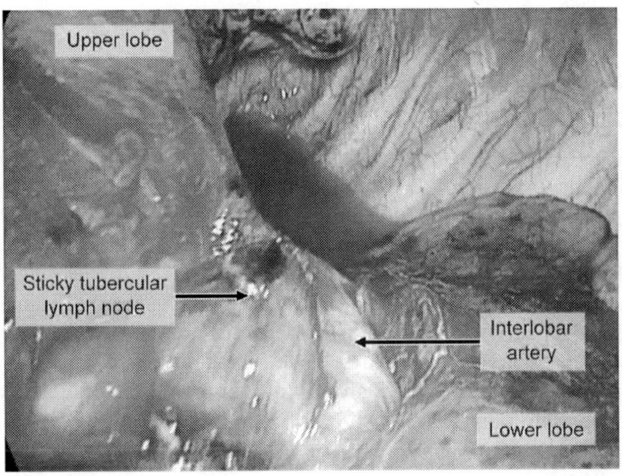

FIG. 1: Adherent sticky lymph node on the interlobar artery ***(For color version, see Plate 1)***.

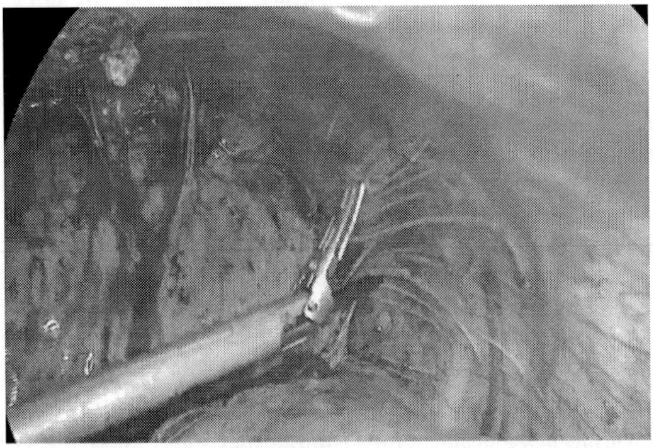

FIG. 2: Adhesions in tuberculosis surgery ***(For color version, see Plate 1)***.

lung tissue which increases the possibility of space problems and must be dealt with expertise during surgery with options such as pleural tenting, muscle flap, thoracoplasty, and temporary nerve paralysis.

Minimally Invasive Thoracic Surgery

The approach to surgery has also revolutionized in the 21st century with most centers offering minimally invasive surgery that include both video-assisted thoracic surgery (VATS) and robot-assisted thoracic surgery (RATS). While decortication is universally performed by VATS currently, most centers are offering other procedures as well with better precision and reduced postoperative morbidity and mortality. This has improved both the patient acceptability of the procedure and less exposure to the surgical team of these resistant bacteria. As per latest published data, nearly 50% of lobectomy for MDR-/XDR-TB are currently completed by the minimally invasive approaches. VATS/RATS reduces pain and complication rates and better preserves postoperative respiratory function, immune function, quality of life, and shoulder mobility and should be considered in all patients at centers of excellence.[2-4]

Outcomes of Surgery for Multidrug-resistant/Extensively Drug-resistant Tuberculosis

While medical therapy is the established modality for MDR-/XDR-TB, the outcomes are much worse than drug-sensitive TB. It has been proposed that adjunctive surgery improves outcomes in both case series and reports, but there are no randomized trials that compare surgery with medical therapy versus medical therapy alone. In 18 case series, 964 patients with drug-resistant pulmonary TB had surgical resection. Postoperative culture conversion was noted in 47–100% from positive to negative. Perioperative morbidity rates were 0–39% (median 23%) and mortality rates were (0–5%) regardless of the surgical approach.[2,3]

There have been several reports of achieving bacteriological cure or improvement in MDR-TB patients. The factors predictive of poor outcome in patients that underwent surgical resection were poor lung function, primary resistance, resistance to ofloxacin, preoperative hemoptysis, low body mass index, and cavitary lesions not amenable to complete resection.[4]

The effect of surgery on outcome of treatment for MDR/XDR TB was assessed in a meta-analysis by Harris et al.[7] The total pooled subjects were 9,513 and the proportion of patients that underwent surgery was 5.5–13.4%. In the surgery group, the WHO-defined successful outcome of cured/treatment completion was 81.9% (371/453) versus 59.7% (1,197/2,006) in the medical treatment group. The odds ratio summary comparing surgery versus nonsurgery was 2.62 (95% CI 1.94–3.54). Similar results were reported by review done by Marrone et al. (OR 2.24; 95% CI 1.68–2.97) and Falzon et al. (OR 1.5; 95% CI 0.9–2.6).[7]

The above evidence is based on the studies done on patients without the newer drugs like bedaquiline and delamanid. In a study published by Borisov et al., the authors studied the impact of surgery in patients that underwent bedaquiline-based therapy. The combination of surgery and bedaquiline was responsible for a 40% additional bacteriological conversion (at the end of treatment >90% of the cases were bacteriologically negative). These results are consistent with the outcomes published by Calligara et al. They had reported a lower odds of treatment failure when bedaquiline-based regimen was used in postoperative period OR 0.06 (0.00–0.48).[8]

Timing of Surgery

Currently, there is no clear consensus on the timing for surgery for MDR-/XDR-TB. Ideally, surgery should be performed at culture conversion to minimize the risk of postsurgical complications as it allows time for nutritional supplementation and control of coexisting medical conditions. However, most patients, especially those of XDR-TB are unlikely to achieve culture conversion. In such cases, delay in surgery and continuation of the ineffective chemotherapy may lead to progression of disease and, therefore, promote the development of drug resistance. It may also make certain patients who are initially amenable unfit to tolerate the procedure. Hence, the timing of adjuvant surgery is best decided by a MDT keeping the likelihood of potential culture conversion based on the resistance profile of the TB isolate. In general, a minimum of 3–6 months of preoperative chemotherapy is preferable when feasible. Patients with massive hemoptysis are offered emergency surgery with poorer outcomes and this should be considered in the decision-making process.[2-8]

Early Recovery after Surgery in Tuberculosis Surgery

Standardized early recovery after surgery (ERAS) protocols have been shown to reduce cost, complications, and length of stay, without sacrificing quality of care. This is particularly true after thoracotomy, though the impact may not be as great after VATS. The basic key guidelines for ERAS[9] in thoracic surgery are as follows:

1. Perioperative venous thromboembolism prophylaxis
2. Routine intravenous antibiotics administered within 60 minutes of, but prior to, the skin incision
3. Prevention of intraoperative hypothermia
4. Lung-protective strategies during one-lung ventilation
5. Combination of regional and general anesthesia
6. Nonpharmacological approach to decrease postoperative nausea and vomiting
7. Restrictive or liberal fluid regimens avoided in favor of euvolemia
8. If a thoracotomy is required, a muscle-sparing technique should be performed.
9. *Minimally invasive surgery*: VATS approach is recommended.

CONCLUSION

Surgical resection has both historical precedence and can be a key element in the management of MDR-/XDR-TB until more research and better drugs improve cure rates. Adjunctive surgery is safe and effective means of achieving culture conversion in selected patients with localized disease. There are several reports of improved outcomes with lobar and sublobar resections for patients with MDR-/XDR-TB with both the older and newer regimens and surgery should be considered until the discovery of more effective medical therapy. The quality of data is not based on randomized studies, but it can be considered early during treatment especially at centers of excellence. Further studies are needed to further define and optimize the role of surgical resection in treatment of drug-resistant TB and a consensus document of practices in our country can generate a guideline document for the same as we have a large global burden of TB.

REFERENCES

1. World Health Organization. Global tuberculosis report 2023. Geneva: World Health Organization; 2023.
2. Sihoe ADL. Role of Surgery in the Diagnosis and Management of Tuberculosis. Microbiol Spectr. 2017;5(2):159-86.
3. Calligaro GL, Moodley L, Symons G, Dheda K. The medical and surgical treatment of drug-resistant tuberculosis. J Thorac Dis. 2014;6(3):186-95.
4. Kempker RR, Vashakidze S, Solomonia N, Dzidzikashvili N, Blumberg HM. Surgical treatment of drug-resistant tuberculosis. Lancet Infect Dis. 2012;12(2):157-66.

5. World Health Organization. The role of surgery in the treatment of pulmonary TB and multidrug- and extensively drug-resistant TB. Copenhagen: WHO Regional Office for Europe; 2014.
6. Nahid P, Mase SR, Migliori GB, Sotgiu G, Bothamley GH, Brozek JL, et al. Treatment of drug-resistant tuberculosis. An official ATS/CDC/ERS/IDSA clinical practice guideline. Am J Respir Crit Care Med. 2019;200(10):e93-e142.
7. Harris RC, Khan MS, Martin LJ, Allen V, Moore DA, Fielding K, et al. The effect of surgery on the outcome of treatment for multidrug-resistant tuberculosis: a systematic review and meta-analysis. BMC Infect Dis. 2016;16:262.
8. Calligaro GL, Singh N, Pennel TC, Steyn R, Brink A, Esmail A, et al. Outcomes of patients undergoing lung resection for drug-resistant TB and the prognostic significance of pre-operative positron emission tomography/computed tomography (PET/CT) in predicting treatment failure." EClinicalMedicine. 2022;55:101728.
9. Medbery RL, Fernandez FG, Khullar OV. ERAS and patient reported outcomes in thoracic surgery: a review of current data. J Thorac Dis. 2019;11(Suppl 7):S976-86.

CHAPTER

23

Recent Advances in Management of Drug-resistant Tuberculosis

MM Puri, Prabhpreet Sethi, Ajantha Panneerselvam, Lokender Kumar

Abstract

Drug-resistant tuberculosis (DR-TB) remains a significant global health challenge, characterized by its complex treatment regimens and high mortality rates. However, recent years have witnessed substantial progress in the development of novel diagnostic and therapeutic strategies. Advancements in diagnostic techniques have enabled earlier detection and more accurate identification of drug resistance patterns. New drugs, such as bedaquiline (Bdq), delamanid (Dlm) and pretomanid (PA) have been introduced for management of drug-resistant tuberculosis in particular. In this chapter rapid diagnostic tests and treatment regimens that have emerged to treat drug-resistant tuberculosis are discussed. A short note on the key advancements in TB preventive treatment among contacts exposed to multidrug- or rifampicin-resistant tuberculosis is also included.

Keywords: BPaL, BPaLM DR-TB, MDR-TB, RR-TB, XDR-TB, CBNAAT, LPA, Truenat

INTRODUCTION

Drug resistance threatens global efforts to curb an otherwise curable disease. The blueprint for the resistance to anti-tuberculosis (TB) drugs was laid out in the clinical literature with the development of streptomycin, the first effective drug for the treatment of TB in 1943 by Selman Waksman. In 1948, the British Medical Research Council (BMRC)[1] conducted the world's first published large-scale modern randomized, controlled, clinical drug trial with streptomycin. Although a significant number of patients were successfully treated, a substantial proportion experienced recurrence; mycobacterial isolates cultured from these patients exhibited resistance to streptomycin. In the same year, thiacetazone and para-amino salicylic acid (PAS) were introduced to the market. When either of these agents was administered in conjunction with streptomycin, cure rates increased and acquired antibiotic resistance decreased. In 1951, isoniazid (INH) underwent clinical trials and demonstrated a significant improvement in clinical outcomes, leading to its prompt introduction for wider use. Isoniazid was subsequently followed by the development of pyrazinamide (1952), cycloserine (1954), ethionamide (1956), rifampicin (1965), and ethambutol (1961). The introduction of each new drug resulted in the selection of mutations conferring resistance to it. Observations of rapid development of isoniazid resistance among patients receiving monotherapy and the suppression of resistance when isoniazid was administered in combination with streptomycin or para-amino salicylic acid led to the establishment of the principle to utilize multidrug treatment regimens for TB management. Rifampicin revolutionized the treatment of TB and short-course chemotherapy was born with the backbone of isoniazid and rifampicin given for 6–9 months. Ultimately empirical regimen with four-drugs (2HRZE/4HR) for patients with newly diagnosed TB was recommended by BMRC. World Health Organization (WHO) promoted the directly observed therapy, short-course strategy (DOTS) which was an important development in global TB policy. With implementation of the DOTS approach, many lives were saved and many new cases averted. Despite the implementation of a powerful disease-control strategy, *Mycobacterium tuberculosis* remained resilient, with resistant strains continuing to emerge and spread. This was due to the ineffectiveness of empirical treatment using first-line anti-TB drugs for patients infected with resistant strains. The HIV epidemic further exacerbated TB outbreaks. In the late 1980s and early 1990s, the United States witnessed outbreaks of multidrug-resistant tuberculosis (MDR-TB), with genetic analysis revealing that airborne transmission of undetected and untreated strains played a significant role.[1] To address drug-resistant TB, New York City employed a strategy that included diagnosis through mycobacterial culture and rapid drug-susceptibility testing, provision of second-line anti-TB medications, proper infection control measures, and directly observed medication administration. This approach differed from the DOTS strategy introduced by WHO in 1994–1995, which relied solely on smear microscopy for diagnosis—despite its lack of sensitivity and inability to detect drug resistance—and empirically used only first-line anti-TB agents for treatment.[1] In DOTS strategy, prevention was promoted as the main tool for combating drug-resistant TB until 2006 when the guidelines for the programmatic management of drug-resistant TB were provided to integrate the management of MDR-TB into comprehensive national TB control plans. These guidelines were subsequently updated in 2008 and 2011. In December 2010, WHO first recommended the use of the Xpert MTB/RIF assay to improve case-detection and to detect cases earlier, including cases of smear negative disease and to enhance the capacity to diagnose MDR-TB. Simultaneously the landscape of TB drug development evolved and considering the global MDR-TB crisis and the limited therapeutic options available for this life-threatening MDR-TB, WHO provided Interim policy guidance for newer drugs bedaquiline (Bdq) and delamanid (Dlm) in 2013 and 2014, respectively. In 2022, WHO Consolidated Guidelines on Tuberculosis includes two new recommendations—one for the use of a 6-month bedaquiline, pretomanid, linezolid, and moxifloxacin (BPaLM) regimen, in patients with MDR-/rifampicin-resistant TB (RR-TB) and those with additional resistance to fluoroquinolones (pre-XDR-TB) and another for a 9-month all oral regimen in patients with MDR/RR-TB and in whom resistance to fluoroquinolones has been excluded. In this article, we will discuss the definitions, diagnosis, newer drugs, and regimens for treatment of drug-resistant TB.

DEFINITIONS[2]

- *Mono-resistant TB (MR-TB)*: A TB patient, whose biological specimen is resistant to one first-line anti-TB drug only.
- *Poly-drug-resistant TB (PDR-TB)*: A TB patient, whose biological specimen is resistant to more than one first-line anti-TB drug, other than both H and R.
- *MDR/RR-TB*: Refers to either MDR-TB or RR-TB.
- *Rifampicin-resistant TB (RR-TB)*: TB disease caused by a strain of *M. tuberculosis* complex that is resistant to rifampicin. These strains may be susceptible or resistant to isoniazid [i.e., multidrug-resistant TB (MDR-TB)], or resistant to other first-line or second-line TB medicines.

- *Multidrug-resistant TB*: TB disease caused by a strain of *M. tuberculosis* complex that is resistant to rifampicin and isoniazid.
- *Rifampicin-susceptible, isoniazid-resistant TB (Hr-TB)*: TB disease caused by a strain of *M. tuberculosis* complex that is resistant to isoniazid but susceptible to rifampicin. Also called H-mono resistant or INH-resistant TB (Hr-TB), i.e., a TB patient, whose biological specimen shows resistance to isoniazid and susceptibility to rifampicin.
- *Pre-extensively drug-resistant TB (pre-XDR-TB)*: TB disease caused by a strain of *M. tuberculosis* complex that is resistant to rifampicin (and may also be resistant to isoniazid), and that is also resistant to at least one fluoroquinolone (either levofloxacin or moxifloxacin).
- *Extensively drug-resistant TB (XDR-TB)*: TB disease caused by a strain of *M. tuberculosis* complex that is resistant to rifampicin (and may also be resistant to isoniazid), and that is also resistant to at least one fluoroquinolone (levofloxacin or moxifloxacin) and to at least one other "Group A" drug (Bdq or linezolid).

DIAGNOSIS OF DRUG-RESISTANT TUBERCULOSIS[3]

Initial Diagnostic Tests for Diagnosis of Tuberculosis and Detection of Drug Resistance

The Xpert MTB/RIF assay marked a crucial advancement in enhancing TB diagnosis and identifying rifampicin resistance worldwide. Nevertheless, the sensitivity of Xpert MTB/RIF is less than optimal, especially for patients with smear-negative and HIV-associated TB. To address these shortcomings, the Xpert MTB/RIF Ultra, henceforth referred to as Xpert Ultra, was created as a more advanced version. This new assay operates on the same GeneXpert® platform as its predecessor, the Xpert MTB/RIF.

Xpert MTB/RIF test is recommended for:

- *Pulmonary TB*: Xpert MTB/RIF *should be used* as an initial diagnostic test for TB and rifampicin-resistance detection in patients with signs and symptoms of pulmonary TB:
    - In adults, rather than smear microscopy/culture and phenotypic DST, Xpert MTB/RIF test is performed on sputum.
    - In children, sputum collection is difficult and hence Xpert MTB/RIF can be performed on sputum, gastric aspirate, nasopharyngeal aspirate, and stool.
- *TB meningitis*: Any patient (adult or children) presenting with clinical signs and symptoms of TB meningitis. Adults and children with signs and symptoms of TB meningitis, Xpert MTB/RIF *should be performed* in cerebrospinal fluid (CSF) as an initial diagnostic test, rather than smear microscopy/culture.
- *Extrapulmonary TB*: Xpert MTB/RIF *may be used* as an initial diagnostic test for TB with signs and symptoms of extrapulmonary TB *in the adults and children* rather than smear microscopy/culture in following situations:
    - Lymph node aspirate
    - Lymph node biopsy
    - Pleural fluid
    - Peritoneal fluid
    - Pericardial fluid
    - Synovial fluid
    - Urine specimens

(Conditional recommendation, moderate certainty of evidence for test accuracy for pleural fluid; low certainty for lymph node aspirate, peritoneal fluid, synovial fluid, urine; very low certainty for pericardial fluid, lymph nodes biopsy)

- *Extrapulmonary TB*: Xpert MTB/RIF *should be used for rifampicin-resistance detection* in adults and children with signs and symptoms of extrapulmonary TB.

- *Disseminated TB*: In HIV-positive adults and children with signs and symptoms of disseminated TB, *Xpert MTB/RIF may be used* in blood, as an initial diagnostic test for disseminated TB.

Xpert Ultra Test

Endorsed by WHO in 2011 and recommended for use where available as a replacement for Xpert in all settings. The Xpert Ultra test was designed to enhance the sensitivity of the Xpert MTB/RIF platform. It uses the same analyzer as the Xpert test but incorporates a new specimen cartridge and updated software. Overall, Xpert Ultra shows improved sensitivity compared to Xpert, particularly in detecting *M. tuberculosis* in smear-negative culture-positive specimens, pediatric samples, extrapulmonary specimens (especially CSF), and samples from HIV-positive individuals.

Xpert Ultra test is recommended for:

- *Pulmonary TB*: For adults showing signs and symptoms of pulmonary TB who either have no history of TB within the past 5 years or have a past history of TB treatment that ended >5 years ago, the Xpert Ultra test should be used as the first diagnostic tool for TB and for detecting rifampicin resistance in sputum. This approach is preferred over smear microscopy, culture, and phenotypic drug susceptibility testing (DST).
- *Pulmonary TB*: For adults with signs and symptoms of pulmonary TB who have a history of TB treatment completed within the past 5 years, the Xpert Ultra test can be utilized as an initial diagnostic tool for TB and for detecting rifampicin resistance in sputum. This is an alternative to using smear microscopy, culture, and phenotypic DST.
- *Pulmonary TB*: For children showing signs and symptoms of pulmonary TB, the Xpert Ultra test should be used as the primary diagnostic tool for TB and for identifying rifampicin resistance in sputum or nasopharyngeal aspirate. This is preferred over smear microscopy, culture, and phenotypic DST.
- *TB meningitis*: *In adults and children with signs and symptoms of TB meningitis, Xpert Ultra should be* used in CSF as an initial diagnostic test for TB meningitis.
- *Extrapulmonary TB (lymph node TB)*: *In adults and children with signs and symptoms of lymph node TB, Xpert Ultra may* be used in lymph node aspirate and lymph node biopsy as the initial diagnostic test.

Repeat testing in adults and children with signs and symptoms of pulmonary TB. Recommendations on Xpert MTB/RIF and Xpert Ultra:[3]

- *In adults* with signs and symptoms of *pulmonary TB* who have an *Xpert Ultra trace positive result on the initial test, repeated testing with Xpert Ultra may not be used.*
- In children with signs and symptoms of pulmonary TB in settings with *pretest probability below 5%* and an *Xpert MTB/RIF negative result on the initial test, repeated testing* with Xpert MTB/RIF in sputum, gastric fluid, nasopharyngeal aspirate or stool specimens *may not be used.*
- In children with signs and symptoms of pulmonary TB in settings with *pretest probability 5% or more and an Xpert MTB/RIF negative result on the initial test, repeated testing* with Xpert MTB/RIF (for total of two tests) in sputum, gastric fluid, nasopharyngeal aspirate, and stool specimens *may be used.*
- In children with signs and symptoms of pulmonary TB in settings with *pretest probability below 5% and an Xpert Ultra negative result on the initial test,* repeated testing with Xpert Ultra in sputum or nasopharyngeal aspirate specimens may not be used.
- In children with signs and symptoms of pulmonary TB in settings with *pretest probability 5% or more and an Xpert Ultra negative result on the first initial test, repeated one Xpert Ultra test* (for a total of two tests) in sputum and nasopharyngeal aspirate specimens *may be used.*

Xpert MTB/RIF and Xpert Ultra as initial tests for pulmonary TB in adults in the general population either with signs and symptoms of TB or chest radiograph with lung abnormalities or both:[3]

- In adults in the general population who had either signs or symptoms of TB or chest radiograph with lung abnormalities or both, the *Xpert MTB/RIF or Xpert Ultra may replace culture as the initial test for pulmonary TB.*
- In adults in the general population who had either a positive TB symptom screen or chest radiograph with lung abnormalities or both, *one Xpert Ultra test may be used rather than two Xpert Ultra tests as the initial test for pulmonary TB.*

Truenat MTB, MTB Plus and MTB-RIF Dx assays:[3] Molbio Diagnostics, Goa, India developed new molecular assays—the Truenat MTB, MTB Plus, and MTB-RIF Dx assays, hereafter referred to as *Truenat.*

Truenat tests are utilized at the same health system level as Xpert MTB/RIF. Truenat MTB and MTB Plus are used as initial diagnostic tests for TB, while MTB-RIF Dx is employed as a follow-up test to detect rifampicin resistance in individuals with positive results from the initial Truenat tests.

- For diagnosing pulmonary TB in adults with symptoms, Truenat MTB has a low certainty of evidence for sensitivity but a high certainty for specificity when compared to the microbiological reference standard (MRS).
- For diagnosing pulmonary TB in adults with symptoms, Truenat MTB Plus also has low certainty of evidence for sensitivity and high certainty for specificity compared to the MRS.
- For detecting rifampicin resistance in adults with pulmonary TB symptoms, Truenat MTB-RIF Dx shows serious concerns about indirectness regarding specificity. This is due to the low number of rifampicin-resistant cases and the fact that most cases were reported from India and Peru.

Recommendations for using Truenat MTB, MTB Plus, and Truenat MTB-RIF Dx in adults and children with pulmonary TB symptoms:

- For adults and children exhibiting signs and symptoms of pulmonary TB, Truenat MTB or MTB Plus can be used as the initial diagnostic test for TB instead of smear microscopy or culture.
- For adults and children with signs and symptoms of pulmonary TB who have a positive result on Truenat MTB or MTB Plus, Truenat MTB-RIF Dx can be used as the initial test to detect rifampicin resistance, replacing culture and phenotypic DST.

The Truenat MTB and MTB Plus tests, along with the rifampicin-resistance detection reflex assay, utilize real-time micropolymerase chain reaction (PCR) to detect *M. tuberculosis* and rifampicin resistance from DNA extracted from a patient's sputum sample. These assays are conducted using automated, battery-operated devices that handle the extraction, amplification, and confirmation of specific genomic DNA regions, enabling quick TB diagnosis with minimal user intervention. Designed for use in peripheral laboratories with basic infrastructure, these tests can be easily performed by technicians with minimal training, providing results in under an hour. Additionally, these devices allow for PCR testing to be initiated directly at the field level. If the Truenat MTB test yields a positive result, the extracted DNA can then be used with the MTB-RIF Dx assay to identify specific mutations associated with rifampicin resistance.

Loop-mediated isothermal amplification (TB-LAMP):[3] This technology relies on DNA amplification at a constant temperature, unlike PCR, which needs a thermocycler. The detection of the amplified product is performed visually using an ultraviolet (UV) lamp directly in the reaction tubes. It requires only basic equipment, making it feasible for implementation at the lowest levels of the laboratory network. However, the current technology does not support the detection of mutations in resistance-associated genes. For antigen detection, the lateral flow assay (LF-LAM) is used. Although the current urinary LAM assay has less than optimal sensitivity and specificity, making it unsuitable as a universal diagnostic tool for TB, it shows improved sensitivity for diagnosing TB in individuals coinfected with HIV compared to traditional methods.

Follow-on Diagnostic Tests for Detection of Additional Drug Resistance after Tuberculosis Confirmation[3]

First-line Line Probe Assays

In 2008, the WHO approved the use of commercial line probe assays (LPAs) for detecting *Mycobacterium tuberculosis* complex (MTBC) and assessing resistance to rifampicin and isoniazid. This approval covered both direct testing of sputum smear-positive specimens and indirect testing of cultured MTBC isolates. Two commercially available LPAs that supported this endorsement were the INNO-LiPA Rif.TB assay (by Innogenetics, Ghent, Belgium) and the GenoType® MTBDRplus (version 1), referred to as Hain version 1. Both tests demonstrated excellent accuracy in detecting rifampicin resistance, although their sensitivity for isoniazid resistance was lower, despite high specificity. WHO's recommendations for using LPAs were initially confined to culture isolates or smear-positive sputum specimens.

Since then, newer versions of LPA technology have been developed, including Hain GenoType MTBDRplus version 2 (Hain version 2), and other manufacturers have introduced their own products. By 2015, FIND showed that the three commercially available LPAs were equivalent in detecting TB and resistance to rifampicin and isoniazid.

World Health Organization recommendation: For persons with a sputum smear-positive specimen or a cultured isolate of MTBC, commercial molecular LPAs may be used as the initial test instead of phenotypic culture-based DST to detect resistance to rifampicin and isoniazid (conditional recommendation, moderate certainty in the evidence for the test's accuracy).

Remarks:

- These guidelines pertain to the use of LPAs for testing both sputum smear-positive specimens (direct testing) and cultured MTBC isolates (indirect testing) from pulmonary and extrapulmonary sites.
- Line probe assays are not recommended for direct testing of sputum smear-negative specimens.
- These guidelines focus on detecting MTBC and diagnosing MDR-TB, but they recognize that the accuracy in detecting rifampicin and isoniazid resistance varies, which can affect the overall accuracy of MDR-TB diagnosis.
- These recommendations do not replace the need for traditional culture-based DST, which remains essential for identifying resistance to other anti-TB drugs and for monitoring the development of additional drug resistance.

Second-line Line Probe Assays

Second-line line probe assays (SL-LPAs) offer significant advantages for rapid diagnosis and detection of drug resistance in TB. The MTBDRsl (version 1.0) was the first commercial SL-LPA designed to identify resistance to second-line TB drugs. In 2015, Hain Lifescience, Nehren, Germany, released version 2.0 of the MTBDRsl assay, which not only detects the mutations associated with resistance to fluoroquinolones and second-line injectable drugs (SLIDs) identified by version 1.0 but also additional mutations. After diagnosing MDR or rifampicin-resistant (RR) TB, an SL-LPA can be employed to identify further resistance to second-line drugs (SLDs). The MTBDRsl assay includes probes for detecting mutations in genes related to resistance, such as gyrA and rrs in version 1.0, and adds gyrB and the eis promoter in version 2.0.

World Health Organization recommendation:

- For patients with confirmed MDR/RR-TB, SL-LPA may be used as the initial test, instead of phenotypic culture-based DST, to detect *resistance to fluoroquinolones*.
- For patients with confirmed MDR/RR-TB, SL-LPA may be used as the initial test, instead of phenotypic culture-based DST, to detect *resistance to the SLIDs*.

Remarks:

- These recommendations apply to the use of SL-LPA for testing sputum specimens (direct testing) and cultured isolates of *M. tuberculosis* (indirect testing) from both pulmonary and extrapulmonary sites. Direct testing on sputum specimens allows the earlier initiation of appropriate treatment.
- These recommendations apply to the direct testing of sputum specimens from MDR-/RR-TB, irrespective of the smear status, while acknowledging that the indeterminate rate is higher when testing smear-negative sputum specimens than with smear-positive sputum specimens.
- These recommendations do not eliminate the need for conventional phenotypic DST capacity, which will be necessary to confirm resistance to other drugs and to monitor the emergence of additional drug resistance.
- Conventional phenotypic DST can still be used in the evaluation of patients with negative SL-LPA results, particularly in populations with a high pretest probability for resistance to fluoroquinolones or SLID (or both).
- These recommendations apply to the use of SL-LPA in children with confirmed MDR-/RR-TB, based on the generalization of data from adults.
- Resistance-conferring mutations detected by SL-LPA are highly correlated with phenotypic resistance to ofloxacin and levofloxacin.
- Resistance-conferring mutations detected by SL-LPA are highly correlated with phenotypic resistance to SLID.
- Given the high specificity for detecting resistance to fluoroquinolones and SLID, the positive results of SL-LPA could be used to guide the implementation of appropriate infection control precautions.

Low Complexity Automated Nucleic Acid Amplification Tests for the Detection of Resistance to Isoniazid and Second-line Anti-TB Agents

Xpert® MTB/XDR (Cepheid).

Moderate Complexity Automated Nucleic Acid Amplification Tests for Detection of TB and Resistance to Rifampicin and Isoniazid

Abbott RealTime® MTB and Abbott RealTime MTB RIF/INH (Abbott) BD MAX™ MDR-TB (Becton Dickinson) cobas® MTB and cobas MTB-RIF/INH (Roche) FluoroType® MT. The tests belonging to this class are faster and less complex to perform than phenotypic culture-based DST and line probe assays (LPA). They have the advantage of being largely automated following the sample preparation step. Moderate complexity automated nucleic acid amplification tests (NAATs) may be used as an initial test for detection of TB and resistance to rifampicin and isoniazid simultaneously. They offer the potential for the rapid provision of accurate results and for testing efficiency where high volumes of tests are required daily. Hence, these technologies are suited to areas with a high population density and rapid sample referral systems. GenoType® MTBDRplus v1 and v2; GenoType MTBDRsl (Hain Lifescience/Bruker), Genoscholar™ NTM + MDRTB II; Genoscholar PZA-TB II (Nipro).

Although these new technologies are excellent at detecting resistance to selected drugs, conventional culture-based phenotypic DST remains important to determine resistance to other anti-TB agents, particularly the new and repurposed medicines such as Bdq and linezolid. Regulatory approval from national regulatory authorities or other relevant bodies is required before implementation of new diagnostic tests.

Targeted Next-generation Sequencing[3]

Next-generation sequencing (NGS) technologies: NGS technologies offer the ability to detect resistance to a broader range of drugs by amplifying selected genes and using NGS to identify specific mutations associated with resistance. This approach may provide greater accuracy compared to existing WHO-recommended diagnostic tests. Additionally, targeted NGS can identify resistance to new and repurposed drugs not covered by current molecular assays, offering the potential for comprehensive resistance detection aligned with modern treatment regimens. However, these tests require regulatory approval from national authorities before they can be implemented.

World Health Organization recommendations:

- For individuals with bacteriologically confirmed pulmonary TB, targeted next-generation sequencing (NGS) can be used on respiratory samples to diagnose resistance to rifampicin, isoniazid, fluoroquinolones, pyrazinamide, and ethambutol, instead of relying on culture-based phenotypic DST. This recommendation is conditional with moderate certainty of evidence for isoniazid and pyrazinamide, and low certainty for rifampicin, fluoroquinolones, and ethambutol.
    - *Remarks*: Priority should be given to individuals at higher risk of resistance to first-line treatments, such as those who remain smear or culture positive after 2 or more months of treatment, have previously received TB treatment, are in contact with someone known to have drug-resistant TB, or live in areas with high rates of resistance. The conditional nature of this recommendation reflects limited data on health benefits, variable diagnostic accuracy, and the newness of the technology, which results in limited information on costs, cost-effectiveness, and implementation feasibility.
- For individuals with bacteriologically confirmed rifampicin-resistant pulmonary TB, targeted NGS technologies can be used on respiratory samples to diagnose resistance to isoniazid, fluoroquinolones, Bdq, linezolid, clofazimine, pyrazinamide, ethambutol, amikacin, and streptomycin, instead of culture-based phenotypic DST. This recommendation is conditional with high certainty of evidence for isoniazid, fluoroquinolones, and pyrazinamide; moderate for ethambutol; low for Bdq, linezolid, clofazimine, and streptomycin; and very low for amikacin.
    - *Remarks*: Priority should be given to those at higher risk of resistance to SLDs, including individuals who continue to test positive after 2 months or more of treatment, have a history of TB treatment, are in contact with someone with known drug resistance, or have pre-XDR-TB with fluoroquinolone resistance. The recommendation remains conditional due to suboptimal drug accuracy and limited evidence on costs, cost-effectiveness, and feasibility. The following products meet class-based performance criteria:
        - *Deeplex® Myc-TB (Genoscreen, France)*: Covers rifampicin, isoniazid, pyrazinamide, ethambutol, fluoroquinolones, Bdq, linezolid, clofazimine, amikacin, and streptomycin
        - *AmPORE-TB® (Oxford Nanopore Diagnostics, United Kingdom)*: Covers rifampicin, isoniazid, fluoroquinolones, linezolid, amikacin, and streptomycin
        - *TBseq® (Hangzhou ShengTing Medical Technology Co., China)*: Covers ethambutol

For drugs not yet covered by available products, further product development and evidence review are necessary before clinical use.

Drug-resistant TB case finding under NTEP (National Tuberculosis Elimination Programme): The vision of NTEP is to provide early diagnosis to all persons with any form of DR-TB through universal access to DST. Rapid identification of DR-TB is achieved by using a combination of NAAT (CBNAAT/Truenat), first- and second-line LPA and liquid C&DST for specific drugs, using a step-wise approach elaborated in integrated DR-TB diagnostic algorithm.

NEWER DRUGS TO TREAT DRUG-RESISTANT TUBERCULOSIS

Development of new drugs to treat drug-resistant TB is most important in the fight against TB. Prior to 2010, no new class of drug was introduced to treat TB for over 40 years. Although rifapentine was introduced, it was rarely used and is not effective for multidrug-resistant TB. In the past decade, however, three new drugs (Bdq, Dlm, and pretomanid) have been introduced to combat multidrug-resistant and extensive drug-resistant TB.

Bedaquiline

Bedaquiline is an oral diarylquinoline drug with bactericidal activity approved by the US Food and Drug Administration (FDA) in 2012 for treatment of MDR-TB. It is an important option for the treatment of drug-resistant pulmonary TB. Bdq specifically targets mycobacterial adenosine triphosphate (ATP) synthase, an enzyme essential for the supply of energy to *M. tuberculosis*. It has strong bactericidal and sterilizing activities against *M. tuberculosis*. Bdq has significant benefits in improving the time to culture conversion in MDR-TB patients and is now well incorporated within NTEP as a part of standard longer oral MDR-/XDR-TB regimen for eligible patients. This drug can cause QT prolongation, leading to cardiac arrhythmia and/or death. However, in larger clinical studies, Bdq appeared to be safer than in the initial trials. Patients on Bdq should be monitored for symptoms of cardiac toxicity and by electrocardiogram (ECG). Discontinuation of Bdq is warranted in the setting of clinically significant ventricular arrhythmia or QTc F > 500 ms. Serum potassium, calcium, and magnesium should be obtained at baseline and monitored until fully corrected. Bdq is a cytochrome P450 substrate; therefore, coadministration with strong CYP3A4 inducers (such as rifampin, rifapentine, and rifabutin) or inhibitors should be avoided whenever possible. WHO 2020 guidelines concluded no major safety concerns for Bdq (>6 months' duration), the use of Bdq with Dlm, or Bdq use during pregnancy. It is important to take drug-drug interactions into account when administering TB and HIV medications in combination, including the documented interactions between Bdq and efavirenz. The drug has a high volume of distribution, with extensive tissue distribution, highly bound to plasma proteins and is hepatically metabolized. It has an extended half-life, which means that it is still present in the plasma up to 5.5 months post stopping the drug. *To minimize the likelihood of Bdq resistance, it is recommended to discontinue the drug prior to other active drugs; at least three other agents should be included for the remainder of treatment.* Cross-resistance between Bdq and clofazimine has been observed via mutation in the *Rv0678* regulatory gene, resulting in upregulation of an efflux pump.

Delamanid

Delamanid was first approved by the European Medicines Agency (EMA) in November 2014. It is an oral drug first in the class of nitro-dihydro-imidazooxazole class approved for the treatment of MDR-TB. It is bactericidal drug with 36 hours of half-life and acts with two different mechanisms of action. It blocks the synthesis of mycolic acids (i.e., stopping the bacteria from creating building blocks important for their cell walls) as well as poison the bacilli with nitric oxide, which the drugs release when metabolized. In a clinical study involving patients with pulmonary MDR-TB or extensively drug-resistant TB, treatment of Dlm in combination with WHO-recommended optimized background treatment regimen was associated with improved treatment outcomes and reduced mortality rate. It is used in the treatment of MDR- and extensively drug-resistant TB in a combination regimen. WHO advised to only add Dlm to a longer MDR-TB regimen when it cannot be composed according to WHO recommendations. When an effective and well-tolerated longer MDR-TB regimen can be otherwise composed, the addition of Dlm may not be warranted. Use of Dlm in the shorter MDR-TB regimen under programmatic conditions is not recommended by WHO given the lack of data. Spontaneous resistance to Dlm was observed during treatment, where mutation in one of the *5 F420 coenzymes* responsible for bioactivation of Dlm contributes to this effect. Its oral bioavailability in humans is enhanced when administered with a standard meal, by about 2.7-fold compared to fasting conditions because it exhibits poor water solubility. It is a substrate of CYP3A4; therefore, caution should be exercised in patients receiving CYP3A4 inducers (such as rifampin) and inhibitors (such as ritonavir). It can cause QT prolongation, leading to cardiac arrhythmia and/or death; caution is warranted when administering Dlm with other agents that may cause QT prolongation. The WHO 2020 guidelines concluded no major safety concerns for use of Bdq with Dlm.

Pretomanid

Pretomanid (PA) previously known as PA-824 was developed by TB Alliance and approved in 2019 by the US Food and Drug Administration (FDA). It is a new antimycobacterial oral drug derived from nitroimidazole with both solid bactericidal and bacteriostatic effect, and with an excellent effectiveness and tolerability profile. Currently, it is in the spotlight for its use in BPaLM and bedaquiline, pretomanid, and linezolid (BPaL) regimens to treat patients at least 14 years old with pulmonary RR, MDR, or pre-XDR-TB.

Efavirenz significantly reduces the exposure levels of PA, so an alternative antiretroviral agent should be considered if PA is included in the BPaLM/BPaL regimen. The recommended antiretroviral therapy (ART) regimens to use alongside BPaLM/BPaL are those based on dolutegravir combined with two nucleoside reverse transcriptase inhibitors. The safety of PA during pregnancy and breastfeeding is not well established due to unknown effects on fetal development. Therefore, breastfeeding is not advised for women taking PA. The available data on the central nervous system (CNS) penetration are limited.

NEWER TREATMENT REGIMEN

Six-month Bedaquiline, Pretomanid, Linezolid, and Moxifloxacin Regimen[2]

Bedaquiline, Pretomanid, and Linezolid Regimen

- The BPaL regimen was first investigated as part of the Nix-TB study. The study was conducted in South Africa from 2015 to 2017, and investigated the safety, efficacy, tolerability, and pharmacokinetic properties of a 26-week treatment regimen with BPaL to treat MDR-/RR-TB and MDR-/RR-TB that was resistant to any fluoroquinolone and any second-line injectable drugs, or MDR-TB patients intolerant or nonresponsive to the previous MDR-TB treatment.
- In 2019, WHO convened a Guideline Development Group (GDG) that recommended the use of the BPaL regimen under operational research for the treatment of MDR-TB patients with fluoroquinolone resistance and <2-week exposure to Bdq and linezolid.

- World Health Organization recommends that this regimen should be the initial choice for all eligible patients diagnosed with MDR-/RR-TB. The recommendation in the updated 2022 WHO guidelines states: WHO suggests the use of a 6-month treatment regimen composed of Bdq, PA, linezolid (600 mg), and moxifloxacin (BPaLM) rather than the 9-month or longer (18-month) regimens in MDR-/RR-TB patients. The recommended dose of linezolid is 600 mg once daily, both for the BPaLM and the BPaL regimen.
- *Drug susceptibility testing for fluoroquinolones is strongly encouraged in people with MDR-/RR-TB, and although it should not delay initiation of the BPaLM, results of the test should guide the decision on whether moxifloxacin can be retained or should be dropped from the regimen*—in cases of documented resistance to fluoroquinolones, BPaL without moxifloxacin would be initiated or continued. *In cases of possible fluoroquinolone resistance* (e.g., a history of >4 weeks of fluoroquinolone use or close contact with a person infected with a fluoroquinolone-resistant strain), it is best to initiate a BPaLM regimen until DST for fluoroquinolones is available, to decide whether moxifloxacin should be continued. If the result of fluoroquinolone DST is never determined or not done, the BPaLM regimen should be used throughout. This is often done even if fluoroquinolone resistance is suspected, because the toxicity of adding moxifloxacin is low and some patients with past use of a fluoroquinolone or contact cases may still be infected with susceptible strains. If resistance is highly likely (i.e., a treatment with a fluoroquinolone failed or the patient is a close contact of a fluoroquinolone-resistant case and was unlikely to get TB from another source, or in a setting with a high prevalence of fluoroquinolone resistance and in the absence of DST), it is reasonable to omit the moxifloxacin and use the BPaL.
- Although not readily accessible, if DST is available for Bdq or linezolid, it is highly desirable that this is also carried out at baseline. DST for PA is being developed. Patients with strains resistant to Bdq, PA, or linezolid should commence treatment with a longer, individualized MDR-TB regimen.
- For patients who submit a sputum sample for culture-based second-line DST at the beginning of treatment, results may not be available until after treatment has started. If resistance to any of the regimen component drugs (except moxifloxacin) is discovered after treatment is initiated, the regimen needs to be discontinued.

Two further studies, the ZeNix trials and TB-PRACTECAL, have confirmed the efficacy and safety of BPaL and BPaL-based regimens for a wider group of DR-TB patients.

- *Nix-TB study:*[2]
  - *The Nix-TB* was a single-arm uncontrolled unblinded intervention study, in South Africa, with 108 participants, which investigated the BPaL regimen with high-dose linezolid (1,200 mg daily).
  - *ZeNix study*: The ZeNix study was a partially blinded randomized controlled trial (RCT) of 181 patients, conducted in Georgia, Republic of Moldova, the Russian Federation and South Africa, investigating four different arms of the 26-week BPaL regimen with different doses (1,200 mg or 600 mg) and durations (9 or 26 weeks) of linezolid. Both the Nix-TB and ZeNix trials were conducted by TB Alliance.
- *The TB-PRACTECAL:*[2]
  - This was a phase 2–3, open-label RCT of 419 patients, investigating three different 24-week regimens containing a backbone of BPaL against the locally approved standard of care (SoC) that was based on WHO recommendations at the time of the study. The trial was conducted by Médecins Sans Frontières and the London School of Tropical Medicine and Hygiene, in Belarus, South Africa and Uzbekistan. A total of eight BPaL-based regimens were investigated by these trials:
    - *Nix-TB study*: BPaL for 26 weeks with 1,200 mg of linezolid for the entire duration
    - *ZeNix trial*: BPaL for 26 weeks with 1,200 mg of linezolid for the entire duration

- *ZeNix trial*: BPaL for 26 weeks with 1,200 mg of linezolid for 9 weeks
- *ZeNix trial*: BPaL for 26 weeks with 600 mg of linezolid for the entire duration
- *ZeNix trial*: BPaL for 26 weeks with 600 mg of linezolid for 9 weeks
- *TB-PRACTECAL*: BPaL for 24 weeks with 600 mg linezolid for 16 weeks, followed by 300 mg for 8 weeks
- *TB-PRACTECAL*: BPaL with moxifloxacin (BPaLM) for 24 weeks with 600 mg linezolid for 16 weeks, followed by 300 mg for 8 weeks
- *TB-PRACTECAL*: BPaL with clofazimine (BPaLC) for 24 weeks with 600 mg linezolid for 16 weeks, followed by 300 mg for 8 weeks.

A successful treatment outcome was achieved in >80% of participants, at the end of treatment, for all eight investigational regimens, with 89% treatment success in the BPaLM arm of the TB-PRACTECAL. The treatment success rates were 52% in the SoC regimens in TB-PRACTECAL, 66% in the 2019 South Africa cohort, 69% in the 2017 South Africa cohort, and 75% in the multicountry cohort. Based on programmatic data, 59% treatment success rates are reported globally to WHO for MDR-/RR-TB.

Eligibility:

- People with MDR-/RR-TB or with MDR-/RR-TB and resistance to fluoroquinolones (pre-XDR-TB)
- People with confirmed pulmonary TB and all forms of extrapulmonary TB except for TB involving CNS, osteoarticular and disseminated (miliary) TB
- Adults and adolescents aged 14 years and older
- All people regardless of HIV status
- Patients with <1 month previous exposure to Bdq, linezolid, PA, or Dlm. When exposure is >1 month, these patients may still receive these regimens if resistance to the specific medicines with such exposure has been ruled out.
- All people regardless of HIV status
- No XDR-TB according to the 2021 WHO definitions
- Patient is not pregnant or breastfeeding or if the patient is a premenopausal woman, is willing to use effective contraception. This recommendation does not apply to pregnant and breastfeeding women owing to limited evidence on the safety of PA.

Other considerations when initiating the BPaLM/BPaL regimen include the following:

- Linezolid is associated with anemia and thrombocytopenia, and care should be taken in patients with anemia. Care should also be taken for patients who have a hemoglobin level of <8 g/dL or a platelet count <75,000/mm^3. Consideration of a linezolid-sparing 9-month or longer regimen may be a safe option. Patients with a very low body mass index (BMI) should be monitored. Although the ZeNix-TB trial excluded those with a BMI of <17 kg/m^2, TB-PRACTECAL had no such exclusion criteria and 167 (40%) of those in TB-PRACTECAL had a BMI of <17 kg/m^2. *Low BMI should not be an absolute contraindication in commencing the BPaLM/BPaL regimen, but patients should be monitored closely*. Patients with liver enzymes at levels three times greater than the upper limit of normal were excluded from both the ZeNix and TB-PRACTECAL trials because Bdq and PA are both associated with increases in liver enzymes.
- Linezolid is associated with *peripheral neuropathy*; therefore, those with pre-existing peripheral neuropathy of grade 3–4 should be treated with caution when commencing the BPaLM/BPaL regimen. Alternatively, to decrease the risk of peripheral neuropathy exacerbation, the 9-month regimen with ethionamide (and no linezolid) could be used.
- Patients who are moribund or with advanced disease should have considerations made for symptoms control and palliative care over initiation of treatment. Decisions should be guided by clinical judgement and the patient's preferences. Vigilance or,

preferably, drug substitution should be considered when certain medications are prescribed concurrently with the BPaLM/BPaL regimen, for example:
  - Efavirenz may induce the metabolism of Bdq and alternative antiretroviral therapy regimen for treatment.
  - The safety of PA during pregnancy and breastfeeding is unclear, other treatment options need to be used pregnant and lactating women were excluded from the ZeNix and TB-PRACTECAL trials owing to unknown effects of the new medicine, PA, on fetal development; breastfeeding is not recommended for women taking PA.
  - The available data on the CNS penetration of Bdq or PA are limited.
- The GDG felt that extrapolation to extrapulmonary TB and other forms of TB was warranted except in cases involving severe forms of TB that may require special treatment arrangements and decisions, particularly TB involving the CNS, osteoarticular and disseminated forms of TB. Thus, the recommendation of the BPaLM/BPaL regimen applies to people with pulmonary TB and all forms of extrapulmonary TB except for TB involving the CNS, and osteoarticular and disseminated (miliary) TB.

World Health Organization 9-month All-oral Regimen[2]

World Health Organization suggests the use of the 9-month all-oral regimen rather than longer (18-month) regimens in patients with MDR-/RR-TB and in whom resistance to fluoroquinolones has been excluded *(conditional recommendation, very low certainty of evidence)*.

The 9-month all-oral regimen comprises Bdq (used for 6 months), in combination with levofloxacin/moxifloxacin, ethionamide, ethambutol, isoniazid (high dose), pyrazinamide, and clofazimine (for 4 months, with the possibility of extending to 6 months if the patient remains sputum smear positive at the end of 4 months), followed by treatment with levofloxacin/moxifloxacin, clofazimine, ethambutol, and pyrazinamide (for 5 months). Ethionamide can be replaced by 2 months of linezolid (600 mg daily). Following review of the data presented from the South African NTP, the GDG judged the benefits of the 9-month regimen with linezolid to be small and the undesirable effects to be moderate compared with the 9-month regimen with ethionamide. The certainty of evidence was judged to be very low. Based on this, the GDG judged that the *balance of health effects does not favor either the 9-month regimen with linezolid or the 9-month regimen with ethionamide. Therefore, WHO has updated its conditional recommendation* that, in eligible patients with MDR-/RR-TB, the 9-month all-oral regimen may be used, and that *2 months of linezolid can be used as an alternative to 4 months of ethionamide* within this shorter regimen.

Eligibility: In settings where the 6-month MDR-/RR-TB regimen is not yet available, or implementation of the regimen is not yet feasible, or for patients who are not eligible, selected patients with MDR-/RR-TB may benefit from a 9-month all-oral regimen. Several eligibility criteria must be considered for this regimen, with additional considerations for the use of linezolid instead of ethionamide. The 9-month all-oral regimen (with either ethionamide or linezolid) may be offered to the following patients with MDR-/RR-TB *(where resistance to at least rifampicin has been confirmed and resistance to fluoroquinolones has been ruled out)*:

- Those with no documented resistance or suspected ineffectiveness of Bdq, clofazimine, or ethionamide or linezolid (whichever is considered for inclusion in the regimen)
- Those with no exposure to previous treatment with Bdq, fluoroquinolones, clofazimine, or ethionamide or linezolid (whichever is considered for inclusion in the regimen) for >1 month—when prior drug exposure is >1 month, patients may still receive this regimen if resistance to the specific medicine with such exposure has been ruled out
- Those with no extensive or severe TB disease and no severe extrapulmonary TB

- All people living with or without HIV
- *Women who are pregnant or breastfeeding*: These patients may be considered eligible for the linezolid-containing 9-month regimen, but they should not receive the 9-month regimen containing ethionamide
- Children and adults without bacteriological confirmation of TB or resistance patterns but who require MDR-/RR-TB treatment based on clinical signs and symptoms of TB (including radiological findings) and history of contact with someone with confirmed MDR-/RR-TB: these patients may be eligible for this regimen based on the drug resistance profile of the isolate obtained from the most likely index case.

Linezolid is associated with considerable toxicity, which necessitates close monitoring for signs of bone marrow suppression and neuropathies. Optic neuritis and peripheral neuropathies tend to be reported beyond 2 months of treatment with linezolid, whereas myelosuppression is significantly dose dependent and is more likely to occur during the first 2 months of exposure to the drug. Nevertheless, linezolid is far more effective than ethionamide and helps to maintain a relatively effective regimen, particularly in cases of MDR-/RR-TB where phenotypic DST results are awaited to confirm fluoroquinolone susceptibility. Therefore, the 9-month all-oral regimen containing linezolid (instead of ethionamide) should be offered wherever possible to patients who fulfil the eligibility criteria above, as well as the following:

- Serum hemoglobin above 8 g/dL, neutrophils above 0.75×10^9/L, and platelets above 150×10^9/L at the start of treatment
- No evidence of severe peripheral neuropathy, or any sign or suspicion of optic neuritis, at the start of treatment

The 9-month all-oral regimen with ethionamide instead of linezolid, or a longer regimen without linezolid, may be more appropriate options for patients with very low hemoglobin, neutrophils or platelets, severe peripheral neuropathy, or concerns regarding vision. Mild or moderate peripheral neuropathy (grade 1 or 2) may also be sufficient reason to offer a 9-month regimen that uses ethionamide, based on the patient's preference after discussing the risks and benefits of not including linezolid. However, the ethionamide-containing regimen must be avoided in individuals who are pregnant or breastfeeding. If the 9-month all-oral MDR-/RR-TB regimen (with either linezolid or ethionamide) cannot be used, the patient must be reassessed for their eligibility for another appropriate regimen, either BPaLM/BPaL or a longer MDR-TB regimen.

Drug susceptibility testing:[2] *The 9-month all-oral regimen is not adequate for the treatment of patients with pre-XDR-TB or XDR-TB; it is also not adequate to treat MDR-/RR-TB that has both inhA and katG mutations.* It is recommended that *samples be submitted for susceptibility testing to at least fluoroquinolones before the start of this regimen.* In settings without access to the Xpert MTB-XDR cartridge, a line probe assay (LPA: MTBDRplus) can be used to detect the two most common mutations that confer resistance to isoniazid. These mutations are found in the inhA promoter and katG regions, and they confer resistance to isoniazid at different levels. *Low-level isoniazid resistance is conferred when only inhA mutations are present, and high-level resistance is conferred when mutations in the katG gene are present. Mutations at the inhA promoter region are also associated with resistance to ethionamide and prothionamide.* High doses of isoniazid (15–20 mg/kg) are generally considered to be effective in the presence of low-level isoniazid resistance when used as part of combination therapy, but the efficacy of high doses of isoniazid in the presence of katG mutations remains unclear. Nevertheless, high-dose isoniazid is always included in the 9-month all-oral regimen if either (but not both) of the mutations is present. *The presence of mutations in both regions (i.e., inhA promoter and katG genes) suggests that neither isoniazid at a high dose nor thioamides may be effective and, therefore, the 9-month all-oral regimen is not appropriate in these cases.*

In the absence of information on isoniazid resistance or mutation patterns in the case of an individual patient, knowledge of the prevalence of both mutations among locally circulating RR-TB strains (e.g., from DRS in the relevant epidemiological setting) may also inform decisions as to which treatment regimen would be most appropriate. *DST for pyrazinamide and ethambutol is not carried out routinely in most settings and these results do not affect eligibility for the 9-month all-oral regimen.* There are no rapid methods to detect *M. tuberculosis resistance to clofazimine, linezolid, and Bdq*; however, the critical concentrations for mycobacterial growth indicator tube (MGIT) have been established, enabling NTPs to perform phenotypic DST. *If resistance to these drugs is detected in isolates obtained from patients with MDR-/RR-TB, the 9-month all-oral regimen should not be offered, or the patient must switch to a longer individualized treatment regimen.* In the absence of DST for Bdq, linezolid, and clofazimine, treatment decisions will rely on the likelihood of effectiveness of these medicines, based on an individual patient's clinical history and surveillance data from the country or region. This should be considered a last resort and an interim measure until the capacity for DST for these drugs becomes available.

World Health Organization Longer Regimens[2]

The design of longer regimens (18–20 months) is founded on grouping of medicines recommended for use in longer regimens based on the drug-resistance profile. In ideal conditions, only a small proportion of MDR-/RR-TB patients should opt for longer regimens, because this indication is mainly for those who cannot benefit from either BPaLM/BpaL or the 9-month all-oral regimen. Reasons for not using the shorter regimens may be related to the age of the patients, additional resistance (including fluoroquinolone resistance and other group A medicines; i.e., XDR-TB), intolerance to key medicines used in shorter regimens, severity of disease, pregnancy, certain types of extrapulmonary TB, or other complications needing an individualized approach.

In multidrug- or rifampicin-resistant tuberculosis (MDR-/RR-TB) patients on longer regimens, *all three group A agents and at least one group B agent should be included to ensure that treatment starts with at least four TB agents likely to be effective, and that at least three agents are included for the rest of treatment if Bdq is stopped. If only one or two group A agents are used, both group B agents are to be included. If the regimen cannot be composed with agents from groups A and B alone, group C agents are added to complete it (conditional recommendation, very low certainty of evidence).*

Eligibility: World Health Organization states that a longer treatment regimen should be proposed mainly when the BpaLM/BpaL or 9-month all-oral regimen cannot be used as described above. A longer regimen is expected to be used in the following situations:

- Severe extrapulmonary TB
- Additional resistance to key medicines of the BPaLM/BPaL regimen (except moxifloxacin) or the 9-month all-oral regimen
- Lack of response to shorter treatment regimens (e.g., treatment failure due to no bacteriological conversion, no clinical response, emerging resistance or loss to follow-up)
- Drug intolerance to the component medicines of the BPaLM/BPaL regimen (except moxifloxacin) or 9-month shorter all-oral treatment regimen
- Pregnant and lactating women who could not benefit from the 9-month shorter all-oral regimen owing to certain clinical conditions or children aged below 14 years who could not be treated with BpaLM/BpaL or who, for any reason, cannot opt for a 9-month regimen. There is limited or no evidence of BpaLM/BpaL use in some patient groups; thus, a longer regimen could also be considered as an option for patients with low BMI (<17 kg/m^2), altered hepatic enzymes (three times greater than the upper limit of normal), baseline anemia (hemoglobin <8 g/dL), thrombocytopenia (platelet count $<150{,}000$/mm^3), or pre-existing peripheral neuropathy of grade 3–4.

World Health Organization recommendation for composition and duration of the regimens:

- *Kanamycin and capreomycin* are not to be included in the treatment of MDR-/RR-TB patients on longer regimens *(conditional recommendation, very low certainty of evidence).*
- *Levofloxacin or moxifloxacin* should be included in the treatment of MDR-/RR-TB patients on longer regimens *(strong recommendation, moderate certainty of evidence).*
- *Bedaquiline* should be included in longer MDR-TB regimens for patients aged *18 years or more (strong recommendation, moderate certainty of evidence).*
- *Bedaquiline* may also be included in longer MDR-TB regimens for patients aged *6–17 years (conditional recommendation, very low certainty of evidence).*
- In *children* with MDR-/RR-TB aged below 6 years, an all-oral treatment regimen containing *Bdq may be used (conditional recommendation, very low certainty of evidence).*
- *Linezolid* should be included in the treatment of MDR-/RR-TB patients on longer regimens *(strong recommendation, moderate certainty of evidence).*
- *Clofazimine and cycloserine or terizidone* may be included in the treatment of MDR-/RR-TB patients on longer regimens *(conditional recommendation, very low certainty of evidence).*
- *Ethambutol* may be included in the treatment of MDR-/RR-TB patients on longer regimens *(conditional recommendation, very low certainty of evidence).*
- *Delamanid* may be included in the treatment of MDR-/RR-TB patients aged 3 years or more on longer regimens (conditional recommendation, moderate certainty of evidence). *In children with MDR-/RR-TB aged below 3 years, Dlm may be used as part of longer regimens (conditional recommendation, very low certainty of evidence).*
- *Pyrazinamide* may be included in the treatment of MDR-/RR-TB patients on longer regimens (conditional recommendation, very low certainty of evidence). 3.10 Imipenem–cilastatin or meropenem may be included in the treatment of MDR-/RR-TB patients on longer regimens (conditional recommendation, very low certainty of evidence).
- *Amikacin* may be included in the treatment of MDR-/RR-TB patients aged 18 years or more on longer regimens when susceptibility has been demonstrated and adequate measures to monitor for adverse reactions can be ensured. If amikacin is not available, streptomycin may replace amikacin under the same conditions *(conditional recommendation, very low certainty of evidence).*
- *Ethionamide or prothionamide* may be included in the treatment of MDR-/RR-TB patients on longer regimens only if Bdq, linezolid, clofazimine, or Dlm is not used, or if better options to compose a regimen are not possible (*conditional recommendation against use, very low certainty of evidence).*
- *P-aminosalicylic acid* may be included in the treatment of MDR-/RR-TB patients on longer regimens only if Bdq, linezolid, clofazimine, or Dlm is not used, or if better options to compose a regimen are not possible *(conditional recommendation against use, very low certainty of evidence).*
- *Clavulanic acid* should not be included in the treatment of MDR-/RR-TB patients on longer regimens 10 (*strong recommendation against use, low certainty of evidence*).

World Health Organization Regimen for Rifampicin-susceptible and Isoniazid-resistant Tuberculosis[2]

World Health Organization released its first evidence-based guidance for the treatment of *Hr-TB* using the GRADE approach in 2018. The guidance is based on these two recommendations:

1. In patients with confirmed rifampicin-susceptible, isoniazid-resistant TB, treatment with rifampicin, ethambutol, pyrazinamide, and levofloxacin is recommended for

duration of 6 months *(conditional recommendation, very low certainty in the estimates of effect).*

2. In patients with confirmed rifampicin-susceptible, isoniazid-resistant TB, it is not recommended to add streptomycin or other injectable agents to the treatment regimen *(conditional recommendation, very low certainty in the estimates of effect).*

   The recommendations made were conditional and had very low certainty of evidence.

The basic regimen can be summarized as:

- *Hr-TB regimen: 6 RZE-Lfx*—All medicines in this regimen are to be used daily for 6 months. When fixed-dose combination (FDC) formulations are used, isoniazid is included but it is not obligatory for the regimen. If levofloxacin cannot be used because there is fluoroquinolone resistance or intolerance or other contraindications to the use of fluoroquinolone, then 6(H) RZE may be prescribed daily for 6 months.
- *NTEP newer treatment regimen for DR-TB:*[4] The NTEP provides simplified regimen for various types of DR-TB including *shorter oral bedaquiline-containing MDR-/RR-TB regimen and longer oral MDR-/XDR-TB regimen* based on DST/DRT results with scope in difficult patients to extend Bdq beyond 6 months, combined use of Bdq and Dlm, and Bdq use in pregnancy. As the fully oral regimens get scaled up nationwide, the shorter MDR-TB regimen with injectable SLDs will be phased out.

  Injectable SLDs will be available for use under PMDT to substitute oral SLDs based on DST and ADR. Guidance is also provided for using Bdq for children above 5 years and Dlm for children above 6 years. Use of BPaL regimen consisting of Bdq, PA, and linezolid (Lzd) is ongoing in select group of patients on a research mode.
- *NTEP: Integrated drug-resistant TB algorithm:*[4] Effective management of DR-TB relies on detection of drug resistance followed by appropriate treatment. Genotypic testing is much faster than phenotypic methods. As these are not growth-based tests, timely diagnosis and prompt treatment initiation is possible. These include—NAAT which includes CBNAAT and Truenat. These tests detect R resistance, and line probe assay (LPA) which detects resistance to R, H, FQ, and SLI drugs. *Rapid molecular tests such as NAAT are the preferred method for initial detection of RR. This is followed with LPA for detection of resistance to FQ and SLI drugs.* MGIT system is the preferred method for phenotypic DST. The following drugs are tested by this method:
  - *Group A*: Levofloxacin, moxifloxacin, Bdq, and linezolid
  - *Group B*: Clofazimine
  - *Group C*: Delamanid, pyrazinamide, amikacin, and streptomycin

The first tier of the integrated diagnostic algorithm begins with three groups of patients classified as all presumptive TB or key population, all TB patients and nonresponders to treatment, who are all subjected to NAAT. Upfront NAAT will be offered to all presumptive TB patients in areas that have transitioned from smear microscopy to molecular tests for diagnosis of TB. Key population includes PLHIV, children, EP-TB, smear-negative/NA with CXR suggestive of TB, contacts of DR-TB patients, and other vulnerable groups. While presumptive TB and key population as well as nonresponders to treatment are offered upfront NAAT for TB/RR-TB detection respectively, all TB patients in whom an appropriate specimen can be collected are to be offered NAAT for bacteriological confirmation of TB and RR-TB and further test for FQ.

The subsequent time points when NAAT is offered for determining additional/acquired rifampicin resistance are:

- bacteriologically positive during the course of DS-TB or H mono/poly DR-TB treatment;
- failure to respond to treatment;
- patients who are retrieved after loss to follow-up; and
- any other reason as per treating physician's advice.

The algorithm is designed to segregate patients based on NAAT results as *RR detected or RR not detected* and offer DST-guided treatment. For patients with NAAT result as MTB detected (irrespective of R status), the second specimen will by reflexly be transported in cool chain from the NAAT facility to the C&DST laboratory. In rare circumstances, if the second specimen is used at the NAAT facility itself to repeat the test, a fresh specimen will be collected from the patient and transported in cool chain to the concerned C&DST laboratory. However, this will not always be possible for EP specimens.

When rifampicin resistance is detected, the patient is offered first-line (FL) and second-line (SL) LPA. RR detected in a new case with no risk factors for DR-TB needs to be retested if only *M. tuberculosis* detected was very low as that could be false positive. If there is a *discordance in rifampicin resistance between NAAT and LPA*, a second NAAT is performed at the C&DST laboratory using the decontaminated deposit and microbiologist will provide the final decision. *Direct LPA* can be performed only on smear positive specimen. In instances where the smear is negative, a culture is set up and if the culture is positive, an *indirect LPA* is performed on the isolate. While FL LPA provides information on InhA mutations associated with Eto resistance, SL LPA provides information on resistance to Lfx, Mfx, and Am. LC DST would be set up for Z, Mfx (if resistance detected by LPA), Lzd, Cfz, Bdq, and Dlm. Treatment is initiated based on the results of LPA and if required modified based on the LC DST results which would be available later. If FQ resistance is not detected and H resistance is detected due to mutations either in katG or InhA (but not both), the patient is eligible for shorter oral Bdq-containing MDR-/RR-TB regimen described in detail below. If FQ resistance is detected or H resistance is due to mutations in both katG and InhA, the patient is eligible for longer oral MDR-/XDR-TB regimen, again described in detail below.

When rifampicin resistance is not detected, the patient is offered FL LPA for detecting resistance to H. If there is a discordance in rifampicin resistance between NAAT and LPA, a second NAAT is performed at the C&DST laboratory using the decontaminated deposit and microbiologist will provide the final decision. Direct LPA can be performed only on smear-positive specimen. In instances where the smear is negative, a culture is set up and if the culture is positive, an indirect LPA is performed on the isolate. *If H resistance is not detected, the patient is continued on a DS TB regimen.* If H resistance is detected, the patient is eligible for *H mono-/poly-DR-TB regimen*. SL LPA will be performed for detecting resistance to FQ and LC DST will be performed for Mfx (if resistant by SL LPA), Z, Lzd, and Cfz. Treatment is initiated based on LPA results and modified based on the LC DST results which would be available later.

- *NTEP: Regimen for drug-resistant TB:*[4]

Shorter oral bedaquiline-containing MDR-/RR-TB regimen:

Eligibility criteria: Shorter oral Bdq-containing MDR-/RR-TB regimen is recommended for those MDR-/RR-TB patients in whom resistance to the component drugs has been excluded or those who have not been previously treated for more than 1 month with SLDs used in shorter oral Bdq-containing MDR-/RR-TB regimen and have no other exclusion criteria.

The criteria to include or exclude the patients from offering shorter oral Bdq-containing MDR-/RR-TB regimen are given below.

Inclusion criteria:

- *DST-based inclusion criteria*:
  - Rifampicin resistance detected/inferred
  - MDR-/RR-TB with H resistance detected/inferred based on InhA mutation only or based on KatG mutation only (not both)
  - MDR-/RR-TB with FQ resistance not detected
- *Other inclusion criteria*:
  - Children, aged 5 years to <18 years of age and weighing at least 15 kg, given their special needs, in consultation with the pediatrician

- No history of exposure to previous treatment with second-line medicines in the regimen (Bdq, Lfx, Eto, or Cfz) for >1 month (unless susceptibility to these medicines is confirmed)
- No extensive TB disease
- No severe extrapulmonary TB
- Women who are not pregnant or lactating

Exclusion criteria:

- *DST-based exclusion criteria*:
  - MDR-/RR-TB patients with H resistance detected with both KatG and InhA mutation
  - MDR-/RR-TB patients with FQ resistance detected
- *Other exclusion criteria*:
  - If result for FL-LPA, SL-LPA and DST to Z, BDQ, and Cfz is not available after pretreatment, evaluation is completed and it is a time to initiate the first dose of the regimen, then, exclude those with history of exposure for >1 month to Bdq, Lfx, Eto, or Cfz
  - Intolerance to any drug or risk of toxicity from a drug in shorter oral Bdq-containing MDR-/RR-TB regimen (e.g., drug–drug interactions)
  - Extensive TB disease found in presence of bilateral cavitary disease or extensive parenchymal damage on chest radiography. In children aged under 15 years, presence of cavities or bilateral disease on chest radiography
  - Severe EP-TB disease where there is a presence of miliary TB or TB meningitis or CNS TB. In children aged under 15 years, extrapulmonary forms of disease other than lymphadenopathy (peripheral nodes or isolated mediastinal mass without compression)
  - Pregnant and lactating women
  - Children below 5 years

Regimen and duration: A shorter oral Bdq-containing MDR-/RR-TB regimen of 9–11 months duration is recommended in eligible patients with confirmed MDR-/RR-TB who have not been exposed to treatment with second-line TB medicines used in this regimen for >1 month, and in whom resistance to fluoroquinolones has been excluded.

Composition of shorter oral bedaquiline-containing MDR-/RR-TB regimen:
(4–6) Bdq (6 m), Lfx, Cfz, Z, E, Hh, Eto (5) Lfx, Cfz, Z, E—
The regimen consists of an initial phase of 4 months that may be extended up to 6 months and a continuation phase of 5 months, giving a total duration of 9–11 months. Bdq is used for a duration of 6 months. The composition or the duration of the initial or continuation phase cannot be changed.

Longer oral MDR-/XDR-TB regimen:[4] The grouping of anti-TB drugs for designing longer MDR regimen are shown in **Table 1**.

Eligibility criteria: Longer oral MDR-/XDR-TB regimen is recommended for:
The MDR-/RR-TB patients who are excluded from shorter oral Bdq-containing MDR-/RR-TB regimen including for the XDR-TB patients.

In case of additional resistance or intolerance or nonavailability of any drug in use or emergence of exclusion criteria to shorter oral Bdq-containing MDR-/RR-TB regimen or any longer regimen, the patient would be re-evaluated and initiated on longer oral MDR-/XDR-TB regimen, if additional resistance to any SLDs especially Lfx, Mfx, Bdq, Lzd, Cfz, Dlm, and Z (whenever available). The regimen modification would be done using replacement sequence. The details of replacement sequence are described in NTEP guidelines for programmatic management of drug-resistant TB in India.

TABLE 1: Grouping of anti-TB drugs and steps for designing longer MDR-TB regimen.[2]		
Groups and steps	**Medicine**	**Abbreviation**
Group A: Include all three medicines	Levofloxacin	Lfx
	Moxifloxacin	Mfx
	Bedaquiline	Bdq
	Linezolid	Lzd
Group B: Add one or both medicines	Clofazimine	Cfz
	Cycloserine	Cs
	Terizidone	Trd
Group C: Add to complete the regimen and when medicines from group A and B cannot be used	Ethambutol	E
	Delamanid	Dlm
	Pyrazinamide	Z
	Imipenem–cilastatin	Ipm-Cln
	Meropenem	Mpm
	Amikacin (*Or* Streptomycin)	Am (S)
	Ethionamide	Eto
	Prothionamide	Pto
	p-aminosalicylic acid	PAS

(MDR: multidrug-resistant; TB: tuberculosis)

Duration and composition of longer oral MDR-/XDR-TB regimen:[4]

NTEP longer oral MDR-/XDR-TB regimen:
(18–20) Lfx Bdq (6 month or longer) Lzd, Cfz, Cs

Composition: In MDR-/RR-TB patients on longer oral MDR-/XDR-TB regimen, all three group A agents and at least one group B agent should be included to ensure that treatment starts with at least four TB agents likely to be effective and that at least three agents are included for rest of the treatment if Bdq is stopped. If only one or two group A agents are used, both group B agents are to be included.If the regimen cannot be composed with agents from groups A and B alone, group C agents are added to complete it as recommended by WHO. However, *in India, the experts concurred to start with all 5 drugs of group A and B and continue with 4 drugs in the latter part of the regimen (beyond 6–8 months) if the patient can tolerate the drugs and for operational ease in the field.*

Duration: Longer oral MDR-/XDR-TB regimen is of 18–20 months with no separate IP or CP. Although standardization in the design of longer regimens is possible, in many cases, the modification of the composition and duration of a regimen to make it individualized could enhance regimen effectiveness or safety (or both). *Once a patient is placed on a longer oral MDR-/XDR-TB regimen for at least 4 weeks, normally that patient can no longer be switched to the shorter oral bedaquiline-containing MDR-/RR-TB regimen because this 4-week treatment would represent an exposure to second-line medicines.*

Replacement sequence:[4] The drugs are replaced according to their efficacy, no demonstrable resistance, prior use, side effects profile, and background resistance to the replacement drug in the country.

- At least 4–5 drugs are to be used in the initial 6–8 months. In situations where no replacement of any drug is required in the first 6 or 8 months of treatment in MDR-TB or XDR-TB patients, continue with at least 3 drugs after this depending upon resistance, tolerability, availability, contraindication, etc. of any one of group A or B drugs.
- If resistance detected, then the drugs to be used in the order of Dlm, amikacin, pyrazinamide, ethionamide, PAS, ethambutol, imipenem–cilastatin or meropenem in combination with amoxiclav.
- Dlm and Am may not be introduced after initial 8 months of treatment and during this later phase, the replacement sequence would be Z, Eto, PAS, and E.
- No replacement required if any one drug is dropped in the last 12 months of treatment.

NTEP BPaL/BPaLM regimen: Six-month BPaLM regimen for MDR-TB/RR-TB was approved for use in India under National TB Elimination Program (NTEP) in September 2024. This regimen includes a new anti-TB drug namely PA in combination with Bdq and linezolid (with/without moxifloxacin) for patients who have either no previous exposure to Bdq and linezolid or have been exposed for no more than 2 weeks.

Tuberculosis preventive treatment to contacts MDR-/RR-TB patients:[5]

World Health Organization recommendation:

World Health Organization: TB preventive treatment: In contacts exposed to multidrug- or rifampicin-resistant TB: 6 months of daily levofloxacin should be used as TB preventive treatment.

Target population: People with HIV, household contacts of people with TB despite HIV status, other people at risk (patients who are to be initiated on antitumor necrosis factor treatment, receiving dialysis, preparing for an organ or hematological transplant or who have silicosis).

Testing: Newer TB antigen skin tests (TBSTs) have been developed, using the specific *M. tuberculosis* antigen ESAT-6 and CFP-10: *Cy-Tb* (Serum Institute of India, India), *Diaskintest®* (Generium, Russian Federation), and *C-TST* (formerly known as ESAT6-CFP10 test, Anhui Zhifei Longcom, China). These tests combine the simpler skin-test platform with the specificity of IGRAs. All these TBSTs use intradermal injection of antigen and are read after 48–72 hours as induration in millimeters, using the method suggested by Mantoux.

NTEP: TB preventive treatment:[6]

Treatment regimen:
- In contacts exposed to rifampicin-resistant FQ-sensitive TB: 6 months of levofloxacin
- In contacts exposed to H-resistant rifampicin-sensitive TB: 4 months of rifampicin

CONCLUSION

The advancements in diagnostic and therapeutic strategies represent a substantial step forward in management of drug-resistant tuberculosis. The success of the therapy depends on the adherence to treatment, results of the diagnostic tests along with the previous medications taken by the patient. Challenges remain for equitable access to treatment, particularly in high-burden countries. In addition to the diagnostics and long-duration treatment, side effects exhibited by the drugs contribute to the inefficiency of the treatment. If a patient develops uncontrolled side effects, the drug regimen should be reassessed and potentially discontinued. Usage of bedaquiline and delamanid, requires electrocardiograph monitoring to prevent the development of unwanted side effects in high-risk patients. Development of drug sensitivity test for newer drugs, continued research, investment, and global collaboration are essential to achieve the ultimate goal of eliminating DR-TB as a public health threat.

REFERENCES

1. Keshavjee S, Farmer PE. Tuberculosis, Drug Resistance, and the History of Modern medicine. N Engl J Med. 2012;367(10):931-6.
2. World Health Organization. (2022). WHO operational handbook on tuberculosis. Module 4: treatment – drug-resistant tuberculosis treatment, 2022 update. [online] Available from https://www.who.int/publications/i/item/9789240065116 [Last accessed September, 2024]
3. World Health Organization. WHO consolidated guidelines on tuberculosis: Rapid diagnostics for tuberculosis detection, 3rd edition. Geneva: World Health Organization; 2024.
4. National Tuberculosis Elimination Programme. (2021). Guidelines for programmatic management of drug resistant TB in India, 2021. [online] Available from https://tbcindia.mohfw.gov.in/wp-content/uploads/2023/05/8368587497Guidelines-for-PMDT-in-India-1.pdf [Last accessed September, 2024].
5. World Health Organization. (2024). WHO consolidated guidelines on tuberculosis. Module 1: prevention – tuberculosis preventive treatment, 2nd edition. [online] Available from https://www.who.int/publications/i/item/9789240096196#:~:text=The%20main%20changes%20from%20the,TB%20infection%3B%20withdrawal%20of%20two [Last accessed September, 2024]
6. Ministry of Health and Family Welfare. (2021). Guidelines for Programmatic Management of TB Preventive Treatment in India, 2021. [online] Available from https://cghealth.nic.in/ehealth/2022/Instructions/NTEP_ProgrammeticMgmt_26092022.pdf [Last accessed September, 2024]

CHAPTER

24

Global Drug Pipeline for Tuberculosis Treatment

Salah Foraida, Zaid Tanvir, Eugene Sun

Abstract

The all-oral, 6-month bedaquiline, pretomanid, and linezolid (BPaL)/moxifloxacin (M) regimen represented a novel and tolerable option with significantly shorter duration and 90% treatment success for eligible drug-resistant tuberculosis (DR-TB) patients. To further improve TB treatment, the current pipeline of anti-TB assets being tested globally has candidates in all stages of development and is marked by several organizations and consortia who are working in this field. This unprecedented pipeline of anti-TB candidates may result in more novel, shorter, and possibly universal regimens for all forms of TB regardless of pre-existing resistance. This article reviews the global pipeline compounds being tested to improve treatment of TB, including DR-TB.

Keywords: Tuberculosis, drug-resistant, DR-TB, TB pipeline, anti-TB candidates, pretomanid, delamanid, bedaquiline, linezolid, oxazolidinones, diarylquinolines, Telacebec (Q203), DprE1 inhibitors

INTRODUCTION

Effective treatment of TB, including its drug-resistant (DR)-TB forms, largely relies on the use of a combination of multiple medicines for an adequate duration. For several decades, conventional treatment regimens for DR-TB were lengthy (often exceeding 20 months), hard to comply with, involved multiple drugs including injections, and associated with numerous toxicities and poor outcomes.[1]

In the early 2000s, TB patients who did not achieve cure by the 6-month standard-of-care for DS-TB (isoniazid, rifampicin, pyrazinamide, and ethambutol) were treated by numerous combinations of medicines, including approved, novel, and repurposed drugs. Health professionals used their own expertise and the World Health Organization (WHO) recommendations that were based on limited evidence.

The first shorter course regimen for DR-TB to be identified in an observational study by Van Deun et al. was the 9-month "Bangladesh Regimen".[2] The WHO recommendations were updated in 2016 to reflect this new regimen based on this and other observational studies.[2] That same year, the first randomized clinical trial conducted to evaluate TB regimens treating MDR-TB was initiated: the STREAM trial. The STREAM successfully provided strong evidence that the Bangladesh regimen was noninferior to previous

20-month long regimens that the WHO had recommended (NCT02409290). In the years since STREAM began, more clinical trials have been initiated with the hope of identifying even shorter TB regimens for DR-TB.

The repurposing of linezolid (first oxazolidinone) in DR-TB treatment, along with the conditional approvals of bedaquiline (first diarylquinoline), delamanid and pretomanid (nitromidazoles) by stringent regulatory authorities over the past 15 years have been major steps forward for DR-TB treatment. Results from TB Alliance's Nix-TB and ZeNix trials, along with Médecins Sans Frontières (MSF) TB-PRACTECAL study paved the way for the all-oral, 6-month BPaL/M regimen to be recommended by the WHO as front-line treatment for all eligible DR-TB patients, offering them a novel and tolerable option with significantly shorter duration and ~90% treatment success.

In this article, we will review the pipeline assets being tested globally that may further improve the treatment of TB, including DR-TB.

Oxazolidinones

Oxazolidinones are a class of antibacterial agents that inhibit the growth of *Mycobacterium tuberculosis (M. tuberculosis)* by inhibiting bacterial protein synthesis.

Linezolid, which was the first oxazolidinone licensed for the treatment of complicated skin infections and hospital-acquired pneumonia (at an adult dose of 600 mg given BID for up to 28 days), has been repurposed to treat difficult cases of DR-TB. In the last decade, linezolid became more important in the management of DR-TB. Based on TB Alliance's Nix-TB trial, pretomanid in combination with linezolid and bedaquiline (BPaL) received United States Food and Drug Administration (USFDA) approval in 2019 and European Medicines Agency (EMA) approval in 2020 for the treatment of patients with pulmonary extensive drug resistant (XDR) (pre-2021 WHO definition) or treatment-intolerant or nonresponsive MDR-TB. Subsequently, the BPaL/M regimen was recommended by the WHO for all eligible DR-TB patients in 2022. In addition to being effective, there is also currently minimal preexisting resistance to the oxazolidinones, or cross-resistance with other TB drug classes.

However, prolonged linezolid use in TB treatment is associated with adverse effects, including myelosuppression, peripheral neuropathy, and optic neuritis. These adverse events are thought to be due to inhibition of mitochondrial protein synthesis (MPS). As such, novel oxazolidinones with less MPS inhibition are being evaluated for potentially better tolerability and safety.

- *Sutezolid:* Sutezolid (PNU-100480) is an oxazolidinone initially investigated by Pfizer in two: Phase 1 studies in healthy subjects and a Phase 2a monotherapy early bactericidal activity (EBA) study in patients with TB (license transferred to Sequella Inc. in 2013). The TB alliance also conducted a Phase 1 single-ascending dose (SAD) study in healthy subjects. There are several Phase 2 studies that have completed recruitment or are recruiting. Different doses of sutezolid [0 mg, 600 mg once daily (OD), 1,200 mg OD, 600 mg twice daily (BD), 800 mg BD] were studied in combination with bedaquiline, delamanid, and moxifloxacin in the Phase 2, 12-week, 75-participant PanACEA-sponsored SUDOCU clinical trial (NCT03959566). A 4-month Phase 2c trial of a pan-TB regimen is currently testing two different doses (1,200 mg OD and 1,600 mg OD) of sutezolid with bedaquiline and pretomanid (NCT05686356). 1,200 mg OD is also being investigated in a two-stage Phase 2 trial, the Gates MRI-TBD06-201 trial, with arms evaluating, the combination of bedaquiline, OPC-167832, and sutezolid with either pretomanid or delamanid in drug-sensitive patients (NCT05971602). Further testing is also planned by the National Institutes of Health (NIH)-funded ACTG in the RAD-TB (A5409: RAD-TB) study, a Phase 2 8-week oxazolidinone dose-ranging study in drug-sensitive patients. The study arms include bedaquiline, pretomanid, and an oxazolidinone–linezolid, two doses of TBI-223, or two doses of sutezolid

(NCT06192160). Clinical experience with sutezolid to date suggests a reduced risk of adverse events due to less potent MPS inhibition compared to linezolid.

- *TBI-223:* TBI-223 is a new, orally available oxazolidinone in development by TB alliance. TBI-223 was identified following a medicinal chemistry program seeking to optimize the anti-*M. tuberculosis* activity and safety of oxazolidinones, by reducing inhibition of MPS while maintaining efficacy against *M. tuberculosis*. TBI-223 was selected due to its anti-*M. tuberculosis* MIC, which is similar to linezolid, together with less potent inhibition of MPS, and a greater safety margin with respect to bone marrow suppression in nonclinical species. Of particular note, TBI-223 was tested in an MPS inhibition assay and found to have a half maximal inhibitory concentration (IC-50) of 126 μM (46 μg/mL). This concentration exceeds the expected maximum clinical TBI-223 concentration by fourfold and suggests a low risk of MPS inhibition. TB alliance has evaluated the safety, tolerability, and pharmacokinetic profile in healthy subjects in Phase 1 studies (NCT04865536 and NCT03758612). Further testing of this investigational compound is planned by ACTG in the Phase 2 RAD-TB (A5409: RAD-TB) study, described above with sutezolid (NCT06192160).
- *Tedizolid:* Tedizolid has been approved in the USA for treatment of acute bacterial and skin structure infections since 2014. Tedizolid is another repurposed oxazolidinone being tested in a 7-day Phase 2 EBA study, compared with linezolid and with HRZE (NCT05534750).
- *Delpazolid:* A novel cyclic amidrazone oxazolidinone in development by LegoChem BioSciences Inc. Delpazolid's bactericidal activity was comparable to linezolid.[3,4] Because of its promising toxicity profile, a 16-week, Phase 2b trial using delpazolid at varying doses in combination with bedaquiline, delamanid, and moxifloxacin is ongoing in smear-positive drug-sensitive pulmonary TB subjects with results expected by the end of 2024 (NCT04550832).
- *Contezolid:* Contezolid is a new oxazolidinone specifically designed to reduce the risk of myelosuppression and monoamine oxidase (MAO) inhibition, with in vitro and in vivo activity against *M. tuberculosis* comparable to that of linezolid. Preclinical and clinical safety studies suggest that it may be less toxic than linezolid, making contezolid a potential candidate to replace linezolid in the treatment of DR-TB.[4,5] Contezolid was used in 25 patients with DR-TB in China, who received linezolid-containing regimen first and then switched to contezolid-containing regimens due to the intolerable linezolid-related adverse events. The linezolid-related adverse events resolved or improved in 90% of cases.[4,6]
- *TBD09 (MK7762):* TBD09 is in development by Bill and Melinda Gates Medical Research Institute and Merck. In vitro and in vivo evaluation of MK-7762 has shown that it has potent antibacterial activity against *M. tuberculosis*. A Phase 1, 2-part blinded, placebo-controlled, combined single ascending dose with a food effect cohort and multiple ascending dose trial is ongoing (NCT05824091).

Oxaboroles

Oxaboroles are a newer type of protein synthesis inhibitors. GSK3036656 (ganfeborole) is a first-in-class benzoxaborole inhibiting the *M. tuberculosis* leucyl-tRNA synthetase. Ganfeborole's EBA, safety, and PK were assessed in a 14-day, Phase 2a, single-center, open-label, randomized trial in DS-TB patients (NCT03557281). Further evaluation is currently underway.[7]

Diarylquinolines

Bedaquiline (BDQ), a mycobacterial respiratory chain inhibitor and first-in-class diarylquinoline that inhibits the proton pump of mycobacterial ATP synthase, received initial approval by US-FDA in 2012 and by EMA in 2014. BDQ is currently listed as a group A drug for DR-TB by the WHO. Despite clinical experience having demonstrated that the BDQ is generally well tolerated, there are safety concerns related to QT prolongation requiring ECG monitoring during therapy. BDQ analogs that are in clinical development will hopefully have less cardiodysrhythmic side effects and more efficacy.

- *TBAJ-876:* TBAJ-876 is a diarylquinoline (DARQ) clinical drug candidate being developed by TB alliance for the treatment of tuberculosis. The goal is to develop a safer, more efficacious DARQ than BDQ, as part of novel TB treatment regimens. TBAJ-876 demonstrates a lower risk of corrected QT (QTc) prolongation, and the in vitro minimal inhibitory concentrations (MICs) against *M. tuberculosis* are ~10-fold lower for TBAJ-876 than they are for BDQ, including strains having mutations. When compared to BDQ in mouse models of *M. tuberculosis* infections, TBAJ-876 demonstrates superior efficacy at lower doses and exposures than are required for BDQ. These attributes may allow TBAJ-876 to safely deliver superior efficacy and better safety than BDQ and may shorten the treatment duration both DS-TB and DR-TB. TBAJ-876 has entered a pan-Phase 2 clinical trial (combining components of Phase 2a, 2b, and 2c) which began enrollment in October 2023–NC-009 trial (NCT06058299).[7]
- *TBAJ-587:* Similar to TBAJ-876, TBAJ-587 is another dialkoxypyridine analog of BDQ being developed by TB alliance. It was selected based on improved safety and reduced potential for QT prolongation. Completed Phase 1 trials demonstrated a generally well tolerated safety profile. Further evaluation is being planned to enter Phase 2 trials.[7]
- *Sudapyridine (WX-081):* WX-081 (sudapyridine) is a BDQ derivative being developed in China by Shanghai Jiatan Biotech. It completed evaluation in a multicenter, randomized, parallel, open-label, positive-controlled Phase 2 clinical trial, which aimed to evaluate the EBA, safety, and tolerability of WX-081 in patients with drug-naïve DS-TB and DR-TB (NCT04608955). This drug candidate entered a Phase 3 clinical trial, in 2022, to demonstrate noninferiority to BDQ when added to a background regimen for treatment of DR-TB (NCT05824871).

Telacebec (Q203)

Telacebec (Q203) targets cytochrome bc1 complex and shows potent activity against DR-TB. It is also active against *Mycobacterium ulcerans*, which causes Buruli ulcer, a chronic, necrotizing disease of skin and soft tissue that can lead to permanent deformity and long-term disability. Telacebec is also highly active against *M. leprae,* the causative agent of leprosy. Telacebec was discovered by Qurient and is being developed by TB alliance.

DprE1 Inhibitors

DprE1 is an essential enzyme for the mycobacterial cell wall. Inhibition of DprE1 leads to cell lysis and bacterial death.

- *TBAJ-7371:* TBA-7371 has completed a Phase 2a, dose escalation, trial to evaluate the safety, EBA, and pharmacokinetics, showing the highest activity with 100 mg three times daily dosing (NCT04176250).
- *Quabodepistat (OPC-167832):* A multicenter, Phase 2b/c, open label, dose-finding trial designed to evaluate the safety and efficacy of a 4-month regimen of quabodepistat in combination with delamanid and BDQ in patients with DS-TB in comparison with 6 months standard treatment is in progress. Full results of this Phase 2b/c, randomized trials are expected by the end of 2024 (NCT05221502)
- *BTZ-043:* BTZ-043 belongs to a novel class of nitrobenzothiazinones which inhibit mycobacterial cell wall formation by covalent binding of an essential cysteine in the catalytic pocket of decaprenylphosphoryl-β-d-ribose oxidase (DprE1). Thus, the

compound blocks the formation of decaprenylphosphoryl-β-d-arabinose, a precursor for the synthesis of arabinans. BTZ-043 showed good safety and strong bactericidal activity in a combined Phase 1b/2a study in patients with pulmonary TB.[8]

- *Macozinone (PBTZ-169):* PBTZ-169 covalently inhibits DprE1. PBTZ-169 is a derivative optimized by medicinal chemistry from the lead BTZ-043. PBTZ-169 has several advantages compared to BTZ-043, like easier chemical synthesis, due to the absence of chiral centres, low cost of goods, and better pharmacodynamics. The drug has additive effects with many anti-TB agents, both marketed and in development, and has synergic effects with BDQ and clofazimine in preclinical models.[3]

Other Mechanisms

In addition to classes mentioned above there are novel compounds with alternative mechanisms of action:

- *Alpibectir:* Alpibectir is an amido piperidine compound being developed in combination with ethionamide. Ethionamide is a prodrug that must be bioactivated inside *M. tuberculosis* to exert its antitubercular activity. Alpibectir (also known as BVL-GSK098) increases the level of bioactivation of ethionamide. It has entered a Phase 2 EBA, safety, and tolerability study.[3]
- *Sanfetrinem cilexetil:* Sanfetrinem cilexetil is a β-lactam that was previously developed to treat otitis media in children and was identified in a screen as active against *M. tuberculosis*. It has entered a Phase 2 EBA, safety, and tolerability trial in 2022.[3,7]
- *Inhibitors of cholesterol catabolism: GSK2556286 (GSK-286) and CLB073*— GSK-286 is a new chemical entity with a novel mechanism of action related to cholesterol catabolism. Its intramacrophage activity in vitro is impressive and preclinical studies demonstrate that it penetrates into necrotic lesions. A Phase 1 safety, tolerability, and PK study began in 2020.[3,7] Similarly, CLB073 blocks *M. tuberculosis's* ability to metabolize cholesterol—essentially starving it. CLB073 is in development by Gates MRI and Scripps Research.

CONCLUSION

Compared to the year 2000, when the TB drug discovery and development pipeline was virtually dormant and the global community rallied to form a nonprofit organization, TB alliance to carry out research on new TB treatments, the situation has changed. The current pipeline of anti-TB candidates being tested globally is rich, has candidates in all stages of development, and is marked by several organizations and consortia who are working in this field, many with multiple candidates in Phase-1 and later. This unprecedented pipeline of anti-TB candidates may result in more novel, shorter, and possibly universal regimens for all forms of TB regardless of preexisting resistance.

It is important to mention that initial approvals of BDQ, delamanid, and pretomanid were based on limited data from pivotal clinical trials. However, while BDQ and delamanid were approved by regulatory authorities in 2012 and 2014 as add-ons to current and complex DR regimens without specific combination agents, pretomanid was the first drug developed and approved by regulatory authorities for use within a specific novel regimen (BPaL) in 2019/2020, representing a new approach to anti-TB regimens.[9]

In addition to safety and efficacy, new TB drugs and regimens should also be affordable, easy to adopt and implement, and suitable for coadministration with antiretroviral therapy in individuals coinfected with human immunodeficienchy virus (HIV), and suitable for use in elderly, pediatrics and other specific populations.

Figure 1 shows all new chemical entities being evaluated globally for TB treatment, also available on Working Group on New TB Drugs (WGND) https://www.newtbdrugs.org/

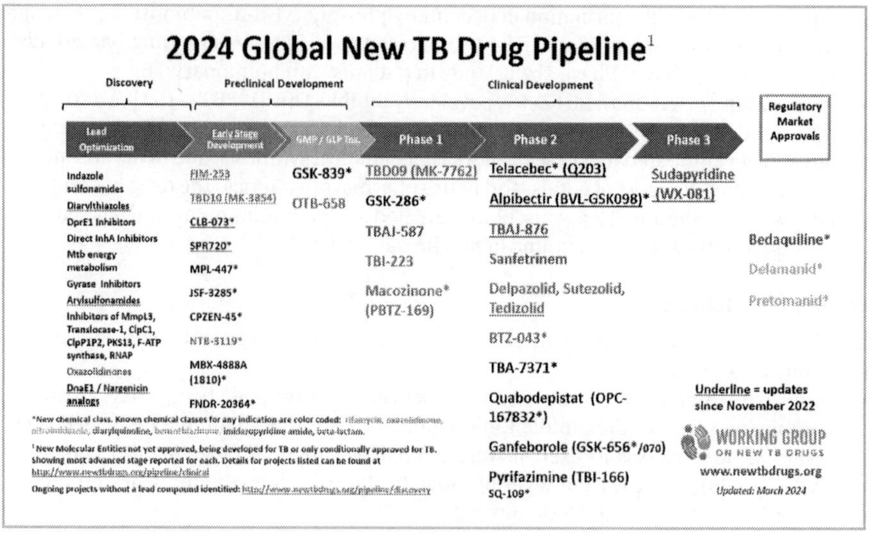

FIG. 1: New chemical entities being evaluated globally for TB treatment ***(For color version, see Plate 2)***.

REFERENCES

1. WHO. (2023). WHO global TB report 2023. [online] Available from https://www.who.int/teams/global-tuberculosis-programme/tb-reports/global-tuberculosis-report-2023 [Last accessed Sept., 2024].
2. Khan FA, Salim MAH, du Cros P, Casas EC, Khamraev A, Sikhondze W, et al. Effectiveness and safety of standardised shorter regimens for multidrug-resistant tuberculosis: individual patient data and aggregate data meta-analyses. Eur Respir Soc. 2017;50:1700061.
3. Working Group for New TB Drugs. (2016). Clinical Pipeline. [online] Available from https://www.newtbdrugs.org/pipeline/clinical [Last accessed Sept., 2024].
4. Chen RH, Burke A, Cho JG, Alffenaar JW, Davies Forsman L. New Oxazolidinones for Tuberculosis: Are Novel Treatments on the Horizon? Pharmaceutics. 2024;16(6):818.
5. Almeida D, Li SY, Lee J, Hafkin B, Mdluli K, Fotouhi N, et al. Contezolid can replace linezolid in a novel combination with bedaquiline and pretomanid in a murine model of tuberculosis. Antimicrob Agents Chemother. 2023;67(12):e0078923.
6. Wang J, Nie W, Ma L, Li Q, Geng R, Shi W, et al. Clinical Utility of Contezolid-Containing Regimens in 25 Cases of Linezolid-Intolerable Tuberculosis Patients. Infect Drug Resist. 2023;16:6237-45.
7. Hoelscher M, Barros-Aguirre D, Dara M, Heinrich N, Sun E, Lange C, et al. Candidate anti-tuberculosis medicines and regimens under clinical evaluation. Clin Microbiol Infect. 2024;30(9):1131-8.
8. Hoelscher M, De Jager V, Dreisbach J, Dawson R, Narunsky K, Svensson E, et al. BTZ-043 shows good safety and strong bactericidal activity in a seamless phase 1b/2a study in patients with pulmonary TB. [online] Available from https://amr-conference.com/wp-content/uploads/2024/01/Dreisbach.pdf [Last accessed Sept., 2024].
9. Black TA, Buchwald UK. The pipeline of new molecules and regimens against drug-resistant tuberculosis. J Clin Tuberc Other Mycobact Dis. 2021;25:100285.

CHAPTER

25

Current Regimens for Drug-resistant Tuberculosis

Kamal Chopra, Kranti Garg, VK Arora

Abstract

Management of drug-resistant tuberculosis (DR-TB) has always remained a challenge. Evidence-based policy recommendations issued from time to time guide the healthcare providers in the management of DR-TB. That is why the World Health Organization (WHO) and the National TB programs rapidly change DR-TB management guidelines as new evidence gathers in any part of the world.

This chapter briefly discusses the various regimens which are being currently administered to the patients with DR-TB, duration of treatment, eligibility and inclusion and exclusion criteria and replacement sequences.

Keywords: Tuberculosis, DR-TB, drug regimen

INTRODUCTION

Drug-resistant tuberculosis (DR-TB) strains present a major health challenge as they are difficult to treat.[1] Increase in incidence of DR-TB threatens global progress toward tuberculosis (TB) elimination. Evidence-based policy recommendations are in the ever continuum of development and have been issued from time to time to guide healthcare providers for providing treatment and care.

The various regimens currently recommended for patients with DR-TB are tabulated **(Table 1)** and summarized here.[2]

SHORTER ORAL BEDAQUILINE-CONTAINING MULTIDRUG-RESISTANT/RIFAMPICIN-RESISTANT TUBERCULOSIS REGIMEN

Regimen:

- *Initial intensive phase (IP)* of (4–6) bedaquiline (Bdq) (6 months), levofloxacin (Lfx), clofazimine (Cfz), pyrazinamide (Z), ethambutol (E), high-dose-isoniazid (H^h), and ethionamide (Eto)
- Followed by continuation phase (CP) of Lfx, Cfz, Z, and E for next 5 months

Duration: 9–11 months.

- *First 4 months*: Bdq, Lfx, Cfz, Z, E, H^h, and Eto.
- *From start of 5th month to end of 6th month – (If IP not extended)*: Bdq, Lfx, Cfz, Z, and E.

TABLE 1: Regimens used for DR-TB treatment.[2]

Regimen	Initial intensive phase	Continuation phase
Bedaquiline-containing shorter oral MDR/RR-TB regimen	(4–6) Bdq (6 months), Lfx, Cfz, Z, E, H^h, and Eto	(5) Lfx, Cfz, Z, and E
Injectable containing shorter regimen	(4–6) Mfx^h, Km/Am, Eto, Cfz, Z, H^h, and E	(5) Mfx^h, Cfz, Z, and E
All oral long M/XDR-TB regimen	(18–20) Lfx Bdq (6 months or longer) Lzd, Cfz, and Cs	
BPaL (bedaquiline, pretomanid, and linezolid) regimen	6–9 Bdq-Pa-Lzd	
H mono-/poly-DR-TB regimen	Lfx, R, E, and Z for 6 or 9 months	

(Bdq: bedaquiline; Cfz: clofazimine; Cs: cycloserine; DR-TB: drug-resistant tuberculosis; E: ethambutol; Eto: ethionamide; H^h: high-dose-isoniazid; Lfx: levofloxacin; Lzd: linezolid; Mfx^h: high-dose-moxifloxacin; MDR-TB: multidrug-resistant tuberculosis; Pa: pretomanid; RR-TB: rifampicin-resistant tuberculosis; XDR-TB: extensively-drug resistant tuberculosis; Z: pyrazinamide)

- Followed by Lfx, Cfz, Z, and E for next 3 months.
- If IP is extended up to 6 months, Bdq, H^h, and Eto are stopped at 6th month.
- This has been field tested as a packaged regimen so replacement of drug or extension of treatment duration not permitted. If any change is required, patient may be shifted on longer regimen.

Eligibility criteria:
- Rifampicin resistance detected/inferred.
- MDR/RR-TB with H-resistance detected/inferred based on *InhA* or *KatG* mutation only (not both).
- No resistance to fluoroquinolones.
- History of no exposure to medications used in this regimen (Bdq, Lfx, Eto, or Cfz) for >1 month, unless susceptibility to these medicines is confirmed.
- Adults and children 5–18 years of age, weighing at least 15 kg.
- Patients with controlled stable arrhythmia (after cardiac consultation)

Exclusion criteria:
- Multidrug-resistant/rifampicin-resistant tuberculosis (MDR/RR-TB) patients with resistance to both *KatG* and *InhA* mutation of H.
- Resistance to FQ.
- Intolerance to any drug or risk of toxicity from a drug in the regimen.
- Extensive parenchymal disease with bilateral cavities.
- Severe extrapulmonary tuberculosis (EP-TB) [presence of miliary TB or TB meningitis or central nervous system (CNS) TB]
- Pregnant and lactating women.
- Uncontrolled cardiac arrhythmia requiring regular drugs.
- *Having any of the following at screening*:
  - QTcF > 500 at baseline and normal electrolytes.
  - Any other risk factor for heart failure.

SHORTER INJECTABLE CONTAINING REGIMEN

Regimen:
- Initial intensive phase of Mfx^h, Km/Am, Eto, Cfz, Z, H^h, and E for 4–6 months
- Followed by CP of Mfx^h, Cfz, Z, and E for 5 months.

Duration: 9–11 months.

- If there is need to prolong IP, injectable agent three times/week.

Eligibility criteria:

- Confirmed MDR/RR-TB.
- No resistance to fluoroquinolones and SLIs.
- Use of second-line medications of this regimen for >1 month.

Exclusion criteria:

- Multidrug-resistant/rifampicin-resistant tuberculosis patients with both *KatG* and *InhA* mutation.
- Intolerance to any drug or risk of toxicity from a drug in the regimen (drug-drug interactions).
- Extensive parenchymal disease with bilateral cavities.
- Severe EP-TB (presence of miliary TB or TB meningitis or CNS TB)
- Pregnant and lactating women

Note: This is a packaged regimen and so replacement of drug or extension of treatment duration is not permitted.

LONGER ORAL MULTIDRUG-RESISTANT/EXTENSIVELY DRUG-RESISTANT-TB REGIMEN

Regimen: It consists of 18–20 months treatment with Lfx, Bdq (6 months), Lzd, Cfz, and Cs.

Duration:

- 18–20 months.
- In pre-XDR-TB and XDR-TB patients—the duration is of 20 months with appropriate modifications.

Eligibility criteria:

- Extensively-drug resistant (XDR)-TB patients.
- Multidrug-resistant/rifampicin-resistant tuberculosis patients who are not eligible for shorter regimen because of additional drug resistance, drug toxicity or nonavailability of drugs.

Replacement sequence:

- Drug replacement can be done according to efficacy, resistance pattern, prior use, side-effects profile and background resistance.
- *Preferably oral:* Injectables only if no effective drug is available.
- Replacement sequence recommended is delamanid (Dlm), amikacin, pyrazinamide, ethionamide, para-aminosalicylic acid (PAS), ethambutol, and penems.
- Bedaquiline and Dlm can be used in combination in such patients when regimen cannot be designed using all groups A and B drugs.
- Delamanid and Am should not to be used in the last 12 months phase of treatment.
- Imipenem-cilastatin (Imp-Cln) only to be used as the last resort as it is costly and difficult to administer.

BEDAQUILINE, PRETOMANID, AND LINEZOLID REGIMEN (BPAL REGIMEN)

Regimen:

- 6–9 Bdq-Pa-Lzd
- *Bedaquiline:* 400 mg once daily for 2 weeks, then 200 mg three times per week afterward, pretomanid: 200 mg once daily, linezolid: 1,200 mg once daily (after 1st month, dose

of linezolid can be reduced to 600 mg or 300 mg once daily in patients with linezolid-induced peripheral neuropathy or myelosuppression).

Duration: 6–9 months

Eligibility:
- Pulmonary MDR/RR-TB with resistance to fluoroquinolones, with or without resistance to injectable agents.
- At least 14 years, and ≥35 kg weight.
- No known allergy/demonstration of resistance to any of the bedaquiline, pretomanid, and linezolid (BPaL) component drugs.
- Patient has not been previously exposed to any of the component drugs for 2 weeks or longer.
- In extrapulmonary TB cases (including meningitis, other CNS TB, or TB osteomyelitis), it is not recommended.

Contraindications: No absolute contraindications.

Relative contraindications: Concurrent use of medications having toxicities similar to BPaL component drugs, high risk of cardiac arrhythmia, severe anemia, thrombocytopenia or leukopenia, severe hepatic failure, severe renal failure, severe neuropathy, as these are common side effects of drugs being used in BPaL regimen.

Note: This has also been tried as packaged regimen so replacement of drug or extension of treatment duration not permitted.

H MONO-/POLY-DRUG-RESISTANT-TUBERCULOSIS REGIMEN

Regimen: (6 or 9) Lfx R, E, and Z

Eligibility criteria: H mono-/poly-DR-TB where rifampicin resistance is ruled out.

Exclusion criteria: No specific exclusion criteria

In addition to the various regimens discussed above, adjuncts to DR-TB treatment such as surgery, use of oral corticosteroids, immunomodulators, etc., may need to be explored on a case-to-case basis.

Sometimes, patients remain persistently sputum-culture-positive despite standardized regimens, and disease is too advanced for resective surgery. In a final attempt to achieve sputum conversion and before declaring treatment to have failed, a regimen is designed combining new and previously used drugs. Such a regimen is referred as salvage regimen. Adjuvants such as N-acetylcysteine (NAC) are also given as a part of salvage therapy to minimize side-effects like ototoxicity. It is encouraged that salvage regimens are formulated under the program in patients encountering failure of standardized regimens.

It has also been noted that while administering standardized regimens, treatment access is improved at a reduced cost and complexity, however, potential risk of resistance amplification stays. Diagnostic adjuncts such as whole-genome predictions of susceptibility, targeted sequencing panels, and expanded phenotypic assays can help to individualize therapy and provide personalized care for patients with DR-TB. Documented susceptibility to the agents used in such individualized treatment regimens will prevent patients from receiving suboptimal treatment, and decrease the risk of DR-TB transmission.

CONCLUSION

Patient-centered approach should be prioritized while taking decision regarding the most suitable standard treatment regimen for a DR-TB patient. Proper selection of the therapy and regular monitoring of the patient during the course of treatment will help to maximize adherence and successful outcomes. Adjuncts, salvage therapy, and individualized treatment regimens should be used wherever needed and feasible. Periodic reviews of management of the supply chain and storage conditions for pharmaceuticals should also be undertaken. Collective efforts in a channelized manner will ensure our success in TB elimination.

REFERENCES

1. Guidelines for Programmatic management of Drug Resistant Tuberculosis in India. (2021). National Tuberculosis Elimination Programme, Central TB Division, Ministry of Health and Family Welfare, Government of India. [online] Available from https://tbcindia.mohfw.gov.in/wp-content/uploads/2023/05/8368587497Guidelines-for-PMDT-in-India-1.pdf [Last accessed Sept., 2024].
2. World Health Organization. (2022). WHO Operational Handbook on tuberculosis: Module 4: treatment: drug-resistant Tuberculosis Treatment, 2022 update. [online] Available from https://www.who.int/publications/i/item/9789240065116 [Last accessed Sept., 2024].

CHAPTER 26

Challenges in Early Detection, Management, and Prevention of Multidrug-resistant Tuberculosis in Geriatric Patients

Varsha Reddy J, Alex Anthony, VK Arora

Abstract

Multidrug-resistant tuberculosis (MDR-TB) significantly contributes to increasing the overall burden of tuberculosis. The management of MDR-TB is challenging, and the outcomes are worse in elderly patients. Aging is associated with changes in pharmacotherapy, pharmacokinetics, and pharmacodynamics, as well as a higher prevalence of comorbidities. These challenges are further complicated by the pre-existing tuberculosis-related challenges of diagnosis and management, as well as the unique features of MDR-TB. The review discusses these key points in a narrative manner and underlines the need for an integrated approach, which can tackle multiple aspects of the disease simultaneously.

Keywords: Geriatric, MDR-TB, atypical

INTRODUCTION

Tuberculosis (TB) remains the second leading cause of death from infectious diseases worldwide, with multidrug-resistant TB (MDR-TB) posing a significant challenge. Controlling TB in nursing homes is particularly challenging due to the high risk of MDR-TB transmission among elderly residents with compromised immune systems.

EPIDEMIOLOGY OF MULTIDRUG-RESISTANT TUBERCULOSIS IN GERIATRIC PATIENTS

Despite a recent increase in MDR-TB cases, the incidence of MDR-TB in elderly patients has only recently been documented. This paper aims to highlight the high incidence rate of MDR-TB in elderly patients and identify potential risk factors.[1] Studies have shown that elderly patients are more likely to develop MDR-TB, with increasing age being an independent risk factor.[2]

GLOBAL BURDEN

Multidrug-resistant tuberculosis is a major public health concern, with an estimated 3.4% of new TB cases and 18% of previously treated TB cases having MDR-TB in 2019.[3] The older generation accounts for one-third of the global TB population, with those aged 55–64 years having the highest TB burden. Managing MDR-TB in the geriatric population poses significant challenges, including diagnosis, treatment, and prevention.[4]

RISK FACTORS AND CHALLENGES IN DETECTING MULTIDRUG-RESISTANT TUBERCULOSIS IN GERIATRIC PATIENTS

Studies have examined risk factors for TB development, including demographic, social, economic, environmental, and other variables. One study found that older men are at a higher risk of TB than younger women, with disadvantaged positions contributing to this risk.[5] Another study identified associations between MDR-TB and younger age, tobacco use, diabetes, and human immunodeficiency virus (HIV) coinfection.

Early detection of MDR-TB in geriatric patients is crucial but challenging. Typical symptoms may not be present, leading to delayed diagnosis. Atypical presentations, comorbidities, and nonspecific radiological features further complicate diagnosis. Laboratory diagnostics, including bacteria culture and drug susceptibility testing, are essential. Histopathological studies may be necessary for accurate diagnosis.

Challenges in early detection include:

- Atypical presentations
- Comorbidities
- Nonspecific radiological features
- Delayed diagnosis
- Need for comprehensive surveillance

DIAGNOSTIC DELAYS

Delays in diagnosing MDR-TB occur in three areas: (1) patient's delay, (2) health service delay, and (3) diagnostic delay. These delays are experienced in both new and previously treated TB cases. Help-seeking behavior, diagnostics, and treatment approaches influence these delays. Structural barriers in healthcare facilities may contribute to patient's delay, while the orientation of the Revised National Tuberculosis Control Program (RNTCP) and unfriendly health services may also play a role.

STRATEGIES FOR MANAGEMENT OF MULTIDRUG-RESISTANT TUBERCULOSIS IN GERIATRIC PATIENTS

The World Health Organization (WHO) has approved bedaquiline, delamanid, and pretomanide for treating MDR-TB and rifampicin-resistant TB. However, antituberculosis drugs have limited penetration in granulomas, requiring prolonged treatment durations. Bedaquiline and delamanid are recommended for geriatric patients, but early diagnosis, assessment, and management of MDR-TB and TB disease are challenging in older adults.

PHARMACOLOGICAL TREATMENTS

The emergence of MDR-TB is a concern, and its dissemination is global. Patients with tuberculosis, especially older adults, require attention to improve identification, management, and prevention. This manuscript aims to provide useful advice on prophylaxis, directly observed therapy, postexposure treatment, awareness raising, and care of residence spaces.

SURGICAL INTERVENTIONS

Surgery may be considered for MDR-TB patients when clinical and bacteriological parameters worsen or fail to respond to optimized chemotherapy. Surgery should be performed in specialized centers with experienced surgeons and anesthetists. Meticulous preoperative patient's selection is crucial, and indications for surgical treatment include pulmonary MDR-TB with localized and progressive symptoms.

PREVENTIVE MEASURES AND PUBLIC HEALTH INTERVENTIONS

Delayed or inappropriate treatment of latent tuberculosis infection (LTBI) can have severe consequences, especially for geriatric patients and nursing home residents. These individuals are at a higher risk of *M. tuberculosis* infection and, once infected, are more likely to develop active TB. Atypical presentations of TB and delays in detection and diagnosis are common in this population.

To reduce the burden of TB in the elderly, improved TB control measures are necessary, including increased use of directly observed preventive therapy. Preventive measures such as stopping transmission, modifying patient's care, and managing risk factors are crucial. Health education and promotion campaigns can also help to promote good nutrition, alcohol-free living, and attending medical centers.

INFECTION CONTROL MEASURES

Robust TB infection control measures are essential in settings where TB patients congregate to reduce transmission risk. MDR-TB poses a particular risk due to delays in diagnosis and treatment. Effective infection control measures depend on identifying and addressing specific risk factors.

VACCINATION PROGRAMS

While Bacillus Calmette-Guérin (BCG) vaccination may protect against MDR-TB, its effectiveness in reducing MDR-TB burden is unclear. Developing a highly effective MDR-TB vaccine is challenging due to the variety of forms and components of vaccine preparations.

CONCLUSION

Ending MDR-TB transmission by 2035 and the MDR-TB epidemic by 2045 requires concrete actions aimed at early detection, management, and prevention. Advances in diagnostic assays, novel drugs, and treatment regimens are being made, but the association between population aging and MDR-TB risk is not well understood. Large-scale implementation of near-to-patient MDR-TB molecular rapid diagnostic assays is eagerly anticipated.

REFERENCES

1. Li JJ, Lu ZL, Kou WR, Chen Z, Wu YF, Yu XH, et al.; Chinese Coronary Secondary Prevention Study Group. Impact of Xuezhikang on coronary events in hypertensive patients with previous myocardial infarction from the China Coronary Secondary Prevention Study (CCSPS). Ann Med. 2010;42:231-40.
2. Lv H, Zhang X, Zhang X, Bai J, You S, Li X, et al. Global prevalence and burden of multidrug-resistant tuberculosis from 1990 to 2019. BMC Infect Dis. 2024;24:243.

3. Bu Q, Qiang R, Fang L, Peng X, Zhang H, Cheng H. Global trends in the incidence rates of MDR and XDR tuberculosis: Findings from the global burden of disease study 2019. Front Pharmacol. 2023;14:1156249.
4. Shadrach BJ, Kumar S, Deokar K, Singh GV, Hariharan, Goel R. A study of multidrug resistant tuberculosis among symptomatic household contacts of MDR-TB patients. Indian J Tuberc. 2021;68:25-31.
5. Xi Y, Zhang W, Qiao RJ, Tang J. Risk factors for multidrug-resistant tuberculosis: a worldwide systematic review and meta-analysis. PLoS One. 2022;17:e0270003.

Section 5: Associated Diseases

CHAPTER

27

Multidrug-resistant Tuberculosis during Pregnancy

Namita Chopra

Abstract

Multidrug-resistant tuberculosis (MDR-TB) is known since drugs for treatment of tuberculosis were discovered and are a challenge for healthcare providers in managing it among females of child-bearing age group. As limited experience of use of second-line drug is available, so MDR-TB management during pregnancies poses a challenge.

Keywords: Tuberculosis, multidrug resistant, pregnancy

INTRODUCTION

Multidrug-resistant tuberculosis (MDR-TB) is defined as *infection with M. tuberculosis* strain resistant to rifampicin and isoniazid. MDR-TB is found in nearly every country. In India, the incidence of MDR-TB is reported to be between 1 and 3% among previously untreated TB cases and between 12 and 17% among those undergoing next time treatment according to National Tuberculosis Elimination Program (NTEP).[1] Biological and immunological changes in pregnancy may cause subclinical infection to lead to active tuberculosis.[2] Also, teratogenic risk of reserve drugs is also not clear. Therefore, effective contraception is strongly advocated for all nonpregnant women receiving treatment with reserve drugs. But, MDR-TB, if left untreated or undiagnosed in pregnancy, can cause higher maternal morbidity, mortality, and increased risk of transmission of TB to fetus. There is increased risk of obstetrical complications such as spontaneous abortions, growth retardation, oligohydramnios, preterm labor, and increased neonatal mortality. Treatment with reserve drugs is required for managing these cases. Standard treatment regimens for drug-resistant tuberculosis (DR-TB) also require some replacement of drugs during pregnancy.

- Treatment of MDR-TB is as such very challenging but if associated with pregnancy, it is still a bigger challenge to manage. This is due to the fact that second-line drugs used for MDR-TB are very toxic and often causes vomiting, which is already a concern in pregnancy. So, it is better to counsel a presumptive MDR-TB to avoid pregnancy till MDR treatment is complete. But, if the patient is already pregnant, advise her to get medical termination of pregnancy (MTP) as permitted in law (up to 24 weeks' pregnancy).
- If the patient is not willing for MTP or the period of gestation is more than permissible limit for MTP, treatment should be started with adequate precautions (like streptomycin) to be avoided during first trimester and ethionamide up to 32 weeks because of suspected teratogenic effects. Newer drugs bedaquiline (Bdq) and delamanid (Dlm) are avoided as their safety profile in pregnancy is still not clear.

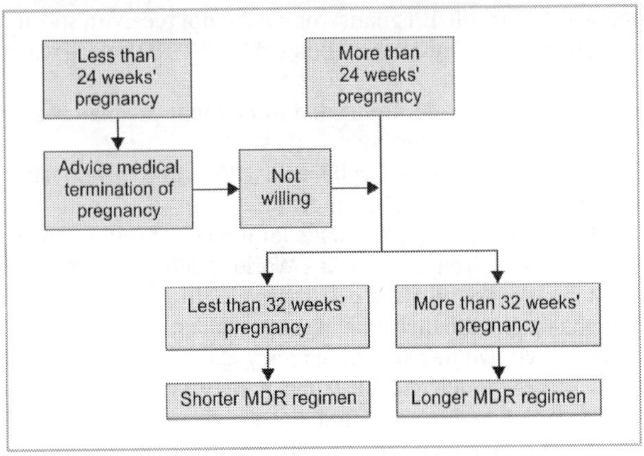

FLOWCHART 1: Management of MDR-TB case during pregnancy.

Notes:
- Ethionamide may be used after 32 weeks' pregnancy.
- Amikacin may be considered in postpartum period.

(MDR-TB: multidrug-resistant tuberculosis)

- The following **Flowchart 1** presents the management of MDR-TB case during pregnancy.
- Pregnant women initiated on Bdq must be encouraged to provide formula feed to their newborn child, till further evidence on the safety of this drug during lactation is available.

These are two-drug regimens used for such cases.

1. *Shorter regimen:* Consisting of 4 months intensive phase with seven drugs (Bdq, levofloxacin, clofazimine, pyrazinamide, and ethambutol followed by 5 months of levofloxacin, clofazimine, pyrazinamide, and ethambutol).

   (4–6) bedaquiline (Bdq) (6 months), levofloxacin (Lfx), clofazimine (Cfz), Z, E, H^h, Eto/(5) Lfx + cfz + Z + E
2. *Longer regimen:* (18–20) levofloxacin (Lfx), bedaquiline (Bdq) (6 months or longer) linezolid (LZD), clofazimine (Cfz), and cycloserine (Cs)

Pregnant patients with MDR-TB who receive effective treatment regimens can achieve a high success rate in treatment and positive pregnancy outcomes.

MULTIDRUG-RESISTANT TREATMENT OUTCOMES DURING PREGNANCY

- The use of treatment regimens recommended under the NTEP including newer drugs—including Bdq, Dlm, and linezolid—for the management of MDR-TB with pregnancy lead to enhance treatment success rate.
- In a study it was found that the treatment success rate was significantly higher among patients on linezolid-containing regimens (85.0%) as compared to patients without linezolid-containing regimens (65.6%). However, these results may be influenced or affected with the administration of additional drugs like Bdq and Dlm.
- Past review studies have indicated that linezolid has increased treatment success rates less number of adverse outcomes among patients taking MDR-treatment. These studies suggest that linezolid used to treat MDR-TB during pregnancy.
- Potential teratogenicity of ethionamide (Eto) in the first trimester and risk of hypothyroidism in the infant in second trimester precludes its use during the first 32

weeks' pregnancy. As a result, pregnant woman cannot receive a shorter oral regimen with Bdq for MDR/rifampin-resistant tuberculosis (RR-TB) before reaching 32 weeks' pregnancy.

- Second-line injectables are contraindicated throughout pregnancy as they affect the 8th cranial nerve (auditory) of the fetus.
- Hypothyroidism with p-amino salicylic acid (PAS) and myelo suppression with linezolid (Lzd) should also be kept in mind.
- A recent study has shown promising results for the use of Bdq in pregnancy (with an association with low birth weight only). The World Health Organization (WHO) hence recommends that a longer oral MDR or extensively-drug resistant (XDR) TB regimen should be individualized with inclusion of drugs with an established safety profile.
- In patients with DR-TB, women with pregnancy <24 weeks should be counseled for discontinuation of pregnancy (MTP). If the patient is unwilling, shorter oral Bdq containing MDR/RR-TB regimen should not be given in pregnancies <32 weeks' gestation. Either a shift to or continuation of longer oral Bdq containing MDR/XDR-TB regimen (as the case be) is necessary.[3]
- Well-being of the developing fetus should be monitored by the use of ultrasound sonography (USG) scans, particularly at 18 and 32 weeks' gestation.
- Breastfeeding should be encouraged if the patient is smear/culture negative. However, Bdq and Dlm are not recommended during lactation, and hence, formula feed may be given to the baby.

ADVERSE EVENTS

Adverse events are common among pregnant women with MDR-TB, with more than half of the patients experiencing at least one type of drug-related adverse event. With gastrointestinal disorders, ototoxicity, and psychiatric disorders being the most common. The high frequency of adverse events among pregnant women receiving MDR-TB drugs should be monitored closely and managed immediately for adverse effects.

PREGNANCY OUTCOMES

- Teratogenic effect of radiography and antitubercular drugs on the developing fetus needs to be considered. [Teratogenic potential of drugs in the drug-resistant TB (DR-TB) regimen needs to be strictly considered in decision making.]
- Women of child-bearing age, awaiting results of culture and drug-susceptibility tests receiving DR-TB drugs should be strongly counseled to use birth control measures (oral contraceptives should be avoided due to drug–drug interactions and chances of decreased efficacy as a result of vomiting). Testing for pregnancy should be done routinely during pretreatment evaluation and while on treatment. A decision regarding continuation/termination of pregnancy may be done in consultation with the gynecologist/obstetrician, after weighing potential risks to the fetus.
- Most frequently observed adverse pregnancy outcomes were preterm birth, low birth weight and pregnancy loss. The prevalence of preterm birth among patients with MDR-TB to 9.5–11% as compared to the prevalence of preterm birth among patients with drug-susceptible TB (8.0%).[4]
- The chances of still birth in the study (1.9%) were comparable to as reported for patients with other diseases such as coronavirus disease 2019 (COVID-19) (1.4%) and among nonpregnant females (1.8%).[5]
- Primary causes of pregnancy loss were miscarriage and therapeutic abortion.

BREASTFEEDING

It is concluded that although pregnancy possesses many challenges in the treatment of MDR-TB, the advantages of continuing treatment with modifications outweigh risks to both mother and fetus. Status of pregnant women and the period of gestation and severity of disease are deciding factors before start of the treatment and to achieve at least sputum conversion before delivery.[6]

- Breastfeeding should be continued if patient is sputum smear negative because only a meager fraction of therapeutic dose of drugs is excreted in milk and the impact on infants of such exposure throughout the entire course of MDR-TB treatment has not been determined.
- Nevertheless, if the mother is sputum smear-positive, infant care should be done by family members until she becomes sputum negative, if possible.
- Different countries have various recommended policies regarding whether child should be separated from the mother and the use of breast milk or top milk. In well-resourced settings, providing infant formula can be an alternative to breastfeeding. However, the evidence supporting this approach is limited.
- All efforts should be made to provide breastfeed to the child. Breast milk can be expressed in a mother who is MDR-TB.
- Congenital tuberculosis is very rare and the risk is the highest right after birth. According to the WHO guidelines, newborns should receive the Bacillus Calmette–Guérin (BCG) vaccine at birth. The importance of isoniazid (INH) prophylaxis for infant born with MDR-TB mother is not well established.[7]

CONCLUSION

To conclude, in pregnant women, strict counseling needs to be done for MTP, especially regarding the risk of delaying treatment, the potential effects of new drugs on the fetus including fetal abnormalities (if MTP is not opted) and the need for more intense maternal-fetal-neonatal follow-up. Appropriate counseling and an informed decision-making process for consent needs to be undertaken in each case.

REFERENCES

1. National Tuberculosis Elimination Programme, Central TB Division, Ministry of Health and Family Welfare, Government of India. (2021). Guidelines for Programmatic management of Drug Resistant Tuberculosis in India, 2021. [online] Available from https://tbcindia.mohfw.gov.in/wp-content/uploads/2023/05/8368587497 Guidelines-for-PMDT-in-India-1pdf [Last accessed Sept., 2024].
2. Shin S, Guerra D, Rich M, Seung KJ, Mukherjee J, Joseph K, et al. Treatment of multidrug-resistant tuberculosis during pregnancy: a report of 7 cases. Clin Infect Dis. 2003;36(8):996-1003.
3. World Health Organization. (2020). WHO Consolidated Guidelines on Tuberculosis: Module 4: Treatment: Drug-Resistant Tuberculosis Treatment. [online] Available from https://www.who.int/publications/i/item/9789240007048 [Last accessed Sept., 2024].
4. Tola HH, Khadoura KJ, Jimma W, Nedjat S, Majdzadeh R. Multidrug resistant tuberculosis treatment outcome in children in developing and developed countries: a systematic review and meta-analysis. Int J Infect Dis. 2020;96:12-8.
5. Turan O, Hakim A, Dashraath P, Jeslyn WJL, Wright A, Abdul-Kadir R. Clinical characteristics, prognostic factors, and maternal and neonatal outcomes of SARS-CoV-2 infection among hospitalized pregnant women: a systematic review. Int J Gynaecol Obstet. 2020;151(1):7-16.
6. Centers for Disease Control and Prevention. Guidelines for preventing the transmission of *Mycobacterium tuberculosis* in health-care facilities, 1994. MMWR Recommend Reports. 1994;43(RR13):1-132.
7. Schardein JL. Chemically Induced Birth Defects. New York, NY, USA: Marcel Dekker; 1993.

CHAPTER

28

Molecular Changes in Diabetes and Multidrug-resistant Tuberculosis

Sandeep Katiyar, SK Katiyar

Abstract

Tuberculosis (TB) remains a significant global health challenge, particularly in low- and middle-income countries, where the emergence of multidrug-resistant TB (MDR-TB) complicates efforts to control the disease. Individuals with latent TB face an increased risk of progressing to active TB if their immune system is compromised, especially those with diabetes mellitus (DM). The longstanding connection between DM and TB is further intensified by the rising global prevalence of diabetes, particularly in developing nations. Together, DM and TB weaken the immune system through various molecular changes and inflammatory responses, undermining the body's defense against TB and increasing the risk of both developing active disease and reactivating latent TB. Moreover, DM complicates TB treatment, contributing to poor outcomes, drug resistance through gene mutations, and higher mortality rates. The growing comorbidity of TB and DM underscores the need for integrated management strategies to address this pressing public health issue.

Keywords: Tuberculosis, MDR-TB, diabetes mellitus, comorbidity, cellular immunity

INTRODUCTION

Tuberculosis (TB), a highly prevalent disease in middle and low-income countries, is caused by *Mycobacterium tuberculosis* (MTB). Despite significant advancements in the field, TB remains one of the leading infectious killers worldwide. The World Health Organization (WHO) has made significant efforts to eradicate TB; however, the emergence of drug-resistant cases has stalled these efforts. Patients resistant to both rifampicin and isoniazid (INH) are classified as having multidrug-resistant TB (MDR-TB), which poses a major challenge to the prevention and treatment of TB.[1,2] A significant portion of the population is latently infected with TB, and they have the potential to develop active TB if their immune system becomes compromised. This risk is particularly heightened in individuals with diabetes mellitus (DM), who often experience subclinical inflammation.

The connection between DM and TB, as well as their combined impact on comorbidity, was first noted nearly a thousand years ago by Avicenna. Those with DM and latent DM are more susceptible to TB infection than nondiabetics. However, advancements in medical science have since enabled more effective treatments for both diseases, reducing the negative impact of diabetes on TB. Unfortunately, the rising prevalence of diabetes, driven by lifestyle changes, coupled with the ongoing spread of TB in developing countries, is causing the two diseases to re-emerge as a significant source of comorbidity and a serious public health concern.[3,4] Although the exact physiological mechanisms underlying the association between TB and DM are not fully understood, several hypotheses have been proposed, including decreased cellular immunity, reduced levels of interferon gamma (IFN-Y), and impaired function of alveolar macrophages.[5] In addition to its association with TB, diabetes has also been linked to drug resistance in TB cases.

BURDEN OF TUBERCULOSIS AND DIABETES AND THEIR INTER-RELATIONSHIP

Despite knowing the causative organism, having effective antituberculous chemotherapy, and implementing control measures, TB remains to be highly prevalent disease and one of the biggest killers, particularly in developing countries. According to the WHO, there were approximately 10.6 million new cases and 1.3 million deaths globally in 2022. India bears a significant portion of the global TB burden, accounting for nearly one-fourth of the world's new TB cases. In 2022, India saw approximately 0.32 million deaths due to this disease.[6]

In the recent past, there has been a rapid increase in the number of diabetes cases, from 285 million in 2010 to a projected 439 million by 2030, resulting in an estimated 3.5 million deaths.[7,8] According to another estimate approximately 537 million adults in 2021 were living with DM and if the current trend continues, it is estimated that by 2035, around 643 million adults will have DM.[9] This rise is more evident in south-Asian countries. A meta-analysis of studies from 31 countries found that the prevalence of DM among TB patients varied from 1.8 to 45% in developing countries, with the majority ranging between 10 and 30%.[5] Diabetes also impacts drug resistance in TB and in 2017, approximately 400 million new cases of diabetes were reported, among which 558,000 individuals also had MDR-TB.[10]

The epicenter of these overlapping epidemics is primarily in developing countries, with India playing a major role in the global burden of both diseases. In regions where TB is endemic, there is a notably high prevalence of diabetes, and similar patterns are observed in countries with a high burden of diabetes, as reported by the WHO.[11] Various studies have highlighted a significant association between the active phase of TB and diabetes, as opposed to the latent phase, underscoring the interplay between these two conditions.[12-14]

The relationship between DM and TB is complex and influenced by various factors such as the type and severity of DM, the age of the individual, and the prevalence of TB in the area. Studies have shown that this relationship is more evident in younger individuals, with a stronger association observed in those with poorly regulated glucose control or higher insulin intake. This suggests that individuals with type 1 diabetes (DM1) are more susceptible to TB compared to those with type 2 diabetes (DM2).[15-17]

However, clinical characteristics and radiological analyses of patients with both DM and TB do not consistently indicate a clear correlation between the two conditions.[18-20] While some studies have reported conflicting results, a few indicate that TB-DM patients may have higher glycated hemoglobin (HbA1c) levels compared to patients with only TB.[13,21,22] Additionally, there is evidence suggesting that in TB-DM patients, the lower lobes of the lungs are more likely to be involved compared to patients with TB alone.[23-25]

CHANGES AT CELLULAR LEVEL IN DIABETES MELLITUS

Type 1 Diabetes Mellitus

Type 1 diabetes mellitus (T1DM) is an autoimmune disorder characterized by the body's immune system attacking and destroying the insulin-producing beta (β) cells in the pancreas. This autoimmune response occurs when the β-cells' autoantigens are mistakenly identified as foreign, leading to the production of autoantibodies against these cells.

The destruction of insulin-producing β cells triggers the activation of T-helper cells, specifically Th1 and Th2. Th1 cells stimulate the production of interleukin 2 (IL-2), which plays a crucial role in activating cytotoxic T cells (Tc cells). These Tc cells then release perforins and granzymes, leading to the destruction of β cells in the islets of Langerhans. Additionally, the Th1 cells produce IFN-Y, which activates macrophages. These macrophages, in turn, produce proinflammatory cytokines such as IL-1β and tumor necrosis factor (TNF), further contributing to the destruction of β cells.

Type 2 Diabetes Mellitus

Type 2 diabetes mellitus (T2DM) is a chronic metabolic disorder characterized by insulin resistance, where the body's cells do not respond effectively to insulin. As a result, despite the presence of insulin, glucose uptake by the cells is impaired, leading to hyperglycemia.

Over time, this insulin resistance triggers a compensatory mechanism where the pancreas produces more insulin to lower blood glucose levels. However, this persistent demand for insulin eventually leads to β-cell exhaustion, reducing the effectiveness of insulin and worsening the hyperglycemic condition.[26]

CHANGES AT CELLULAR LEVEL IN TUBERCULOSIS

Tuberculosis is primarily acquired through the inhalation of aerosols containing MTB. Once inhaled, the bacilli are engulfed by alveolar macrophages, triggering an immune response. However, some of the bacilli survive this initial defense by secreting early secreted antigenic target 6 (ESAT-6), which inhibits the phagosome-lysosome fusion mechanism that typically leads to the destruction of the bacteria. Additionally, ESAT-6 inhibits apoptosis of the infected macrophages.

As a result, the bacteria evade destruction, undergo cytosolic translocation, and begin to multiply within the macrophages, leading to necrosis of these cells. The release of bacilli into the extracellular space further stimulates an immune response, including the activation of polymorphonuclear cells (PMNs) and monocytes. These cells enhance the phagocytic activity and transport the bacteria to the lymph nodes.

Activated dendritic cells (DCs) play a critical role in this process by presenting bacterial antigens (epitopes) to T cells, leading to the activation of CD4+ and CD8+ T cells and other immune cells. This immune response attempts to contain the infection through the formation of granulomas, which are clusters of immune cells that encase the bacteria, restricting its replication.

However, in immunocompromised individuals, such as those with human immunodeficiency virus (HIV) or diabetes, the immune response may be insufficient to control the bacteria. In these cases, the granulomas fail to contain the bacilli, leading to active TB disease. Conversely, individuals with a robust immune response may develop a latent TB infection, where the bacteria remain dormant and nonreplicating. This latent infection can become active if the individual's immune system becomes compromised.

Type 2 diabetes mellitus has been shown to increases the risk of latent TB infection progressing to active disease, highlighting the interplay between TB and metabolic disorders.[26]

Genomic analysis of patients with T2DM has revealed an increase in cases of MDR-TB. This is due to mutations in genes that confer resistance to drugs such as ethionamide, fluoroquinolones, and INH. The hyperglycemic condition in T2DM patients also contributes to the overproduction of reactive species, such as polyols and hexosamine flux, leading to increased levels of protein kinase C (PKC), receptor for advanced glycation end-products (RAGEs), and advanced glycation end-products (AGEs). The activation of these pathways triggers oxidative stress, resulting in inflammation and cellular damage.

IMPACT OF DIABETES MELLITUS ON TUBERCULOSIS

Diabetes mellitus is known to impair the host's immune system through various mechanisms. Additionally, MTB infection can further weaken innate immunity, intensifying the effects in DM patients. In individuals with diabetes, key immune cells such as macrophages, neutrophils, monocytes, and lymphocytes may have altered functions. These changes not only impair the immune response but also contribute to complications such as vitamin deficiencies, renal dysfunction, and pulmonary microangiopathy, further exacerbating the condition. The interaction between the metabolic and genetic mechanisms of these two diseases is complex and not yet fully understood. However, diabetes hinders the body's ability to fight TB, leading to poorer patient outcomes.[27-29] The influence of DM with TB on the immune system involves several molecular changes, which are described below:

- *Alterations in the immune system*: Coexisting DM and TB result in decreased cellular immunity, primarily due to the impaired function of crucial immune cells such as macrophages, neutrophils, and T cells. Additionally, there is a reduction in the production of key cytokines such as IFN-γ, TNF-α, and IL-2. These cytokines are critical in mounting an effective defense against MTB during various phases of infection.
- *Increased inflammatory response*: Uncontrolled DM causes chronic subclinical inflammation throughout the body, which can significantly contribute to the pathogenesis of TB. The oxidative stress induced by hyperglycemia further weakens the immune system, making it more susceptible to infection and less effective in combating MTB.
- *Other mechanisms*: Impaired phagocytosis reduces the body's ability to effectively destroy MTB. Additionally, the formation of AGEs and the activation of PKC interfere with normal immune responses, further compromising the body's defense against TB in individuals with diabetes.
- *Drug resistance occurrence*: Gene mutations are more likely to occur in MTB among DM patients, increasing the risk of drug resistance. Additionally, the impaired response to anti-TB drugs in these patients further contributes to the development of drug-resistant strains.

Thus, patients with DM, including those with latent DM, exhibit several changes at the molecular level and are at a higher risk of developing TB, and find it difficult to eliminate MTB. Various studies have demonstrated a greater prevalence of TB in individuals with DM, which can occur through the reactivation of previously dormant bacilli from a latent infection or due to recent exposure to the bacteria.[30,31] The latter is frequently linked to nosocomial (hospital-acquired) infections.[32]

The hyperglycemic condition in T2DM patients also contributes to the overproduction of reactive species, such as polyols and hexosamine flux, leading to increased levels of PKC, RAGE, and AGEs. The activation of these pathways triggers oxidative stress, resulting in inflammation and cellular damage.

Additionally, the rise in glycated proteins in T2DM patients impairs the mechanisms of phagocytosis and complement activation, leading to the spread of microbial infections.

The gut microbiota in T2DM patients shows an increase in *Lactobacillus* and *Firmicutes taxa*. This shift in gut bacteria composition makes individuals more prone to T2DM and results in the upregulation of butyrate production. Butyrate has been reported to reduce MTB-induced activation, cytokine production, and antigen presentation by DCs, thereby increasing susceptibility to TB.

Furthermore, blood transcriptome analysis in T2DM and TB patients has shown either upregulation or downregulation of various genes, leading to alterations in pathways that regulate immune responses. These changes contribute to increased susceptibility to TB **(Fig. 1)**. A detailed discussion of all these genetic and metabolic alterations is beyond the scope of this chapter.[26]

Chest X-rays and computed tomography (CT) scans of patients with uncontrolled T2DM often reveal more severe forms of TB, characterized by increased lesions and cavities. Furthermore, T2DM has been associated with a higher early mortality rate among TB patients.[33,34]

Furthermore, individuals with uncontrolled blood sugar levels are more susceptible to TB infection compared to those with well-regulated glucose levels which have also been shown by the studies. This underscores the importance of managing diabetes effectively to reduce the risk and severity of TB in these patients.[7,35] Research has also shown that DM negatively impacts the treatment outcomes of TB patients compared to nondiabetic individuals.

Diabetes can also potentially lead to higher drug toxicity, as the condition predisposes individuals to drug-induced liver injury, which may exacerbate the adverse effects of TB treatment. The increased mortality rate and treatment failure observed in some DM patients with TB may be attributed to several factors, including a decline in cellular immunity, delayed sputum conversion, and increased drug resistance.[36,37]

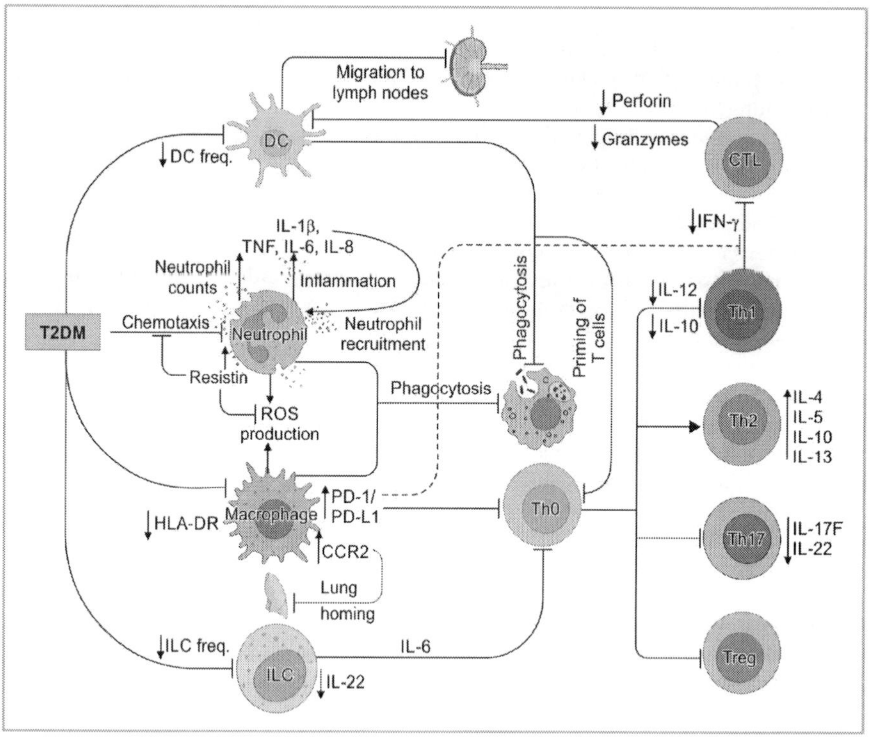

FIG. 1: TB and T2DM immunological dysregulation. Effects of T2DM on the various innate (DC, neutrophil, macrophage, and ILC) and adaptive (CTL, Th1, Th2, Th17, and Tregs) immune cells ***(For color version, see Plate 2)***.

(DC: dendritic cell; ILC: innate lymphoid cell; TB: tuberculosis; T2DM: type 2 diabetes mellitus)

Prevalence of drug resistance is also higher in patients with DM. Rifampin (RIF) and INH are commonly used drugs for treating TB. Patients of TB with DM experience a 1.7 times higher rate of treatment failure compared to those without diabetes,[38] often manifesting as MDR-TB. Studies have reported that 16% of TB-DM patients exhibit three times higher MDR-TB compared to the 5.9% found in TB patients without DM.[39] Genomic analysis of patients with T2D has revealed mutations in the MTB isolates, leading to resistance to anti TB-drugs such as INH, ethionamide, and fluoroquinolones.[40,41] This resistance is primarily attributed to lowered immunity and diabetes-related changes.[11]

Furthermore, a gender bias has been observed, with middle-aged and elderly men being more prone to TB-DM coinfection than women. In women, elevated levels of uric acid appear to play a significant role in this increased susceptibility.[42]

CONCLUSION

The statistics presented indicate a concerning correlation between TB and DM, highlighting how DM can worsen the clinical course of TB. The altered physiological state caused by DM appears to significantly impact TB outcomes. However, a more comprehensive approach is needed, considering physical, genetic, and physiological factors in both control and experimental studies. Addressing these variables will lead to more accurate and reproducible results, ultimately improving our understanding of the interplay between TB and DM.

REFERENCES

1. Uplekar M, Weil D, Lonnroth K, Yi Y, Dou X, Zhou L. WHO's new end TB strategy. Lancet. 2015;385(9979):1799-801.
2. Pan Y, Yu Y, Lu J, Yi Y, Dou X, Zhou L. Drug resistance patterns and Trends in patients with suspected drug-resistant tuberculosis in Dalian, China: a retrospective study. Infect Drug Resist. 2022;15:4137-47.
3. Chang JT, Dou HY, Yen CL, Wu YH, Huang RM, Lin HJ, et al. Effect of type 2 diabetes mellitus on the clinical severity and treatment outcome in patients with pulmonary tuberculosis: a potential role in the emergence of multidrug-resistance. J Formos Med Assoc. 2011;110(6):372-81.
4. Restrepo BI. Convergence of the tuberculosis and diabetes epidemics: Renewal of old acquaintances. Clin Infect Dis. 2007;45(4):436-8.
5. Baghaei P, Marjani M, Javanmard P, Tabarsi P, Masjedi MR. Diabetes mellitus and tuberculosis facts and controversies. J Diabetes Metab Disord. 2013;12:58.
6. World Health Organization. Global Tuberculosis Report. Geneva: World Health Organization; 2023.
7. Harries AD, Lin Y, Satyanarayana S, Lönnroth K, Li L, Wilson N, et al. The looming epidemic of diabetes-associated tuberculosis: Learning lessons from HIV-associated tuberculosis. Int J Tuberc Lung Dis. 2011;15(11):1436-44.
8. International Diabetes Federation. IDF diabetes atlas, 4th edition. Brussels, Belgium: International Diabetes Federation; 2009.
9. Pan Y, Yu Y, Yi Y, Dou X, Lu J, Zhou L. The differences in drug resistance between drug-resistant tuberculosis patients with and without diabetes mellitus in northeast China: a retrospective study. BMC Infect Dis. 2023;23:162.
10. World Health Organization. Global tuberculosis report. Geneva: World Health Organization; 2018.
11. Carey IM, Critchley JA, DeWilde S, Harris T, Hosking FJ, Cook DG. Risk of infection in type 1 and type 2 diabetes compared with the general population: a matched cohort study. Diabetes Care. 2018;41(3):513-21.
12. Deshmukh PA, Shaw T. Pulmonary tuberculosis and diabetes mellitus. Ind J Tub. 1984;31:114-7.
13. Alisjahbana B, Sahiratmadja E, Nelwan EJ, Purwa AM, Ahmad Y, Ottenhoff TH, et al. The effect of type 2 diabetes mellitus on the presentation and treatment response of pulmonary tuberculosis. Clin Infect Dis. 2007;45(4):428-35.

14. Tatar D, Senol G, Alptekin S, Karakurum C, Aydin M, Coskunol I. Tuberculosis in diabetics: Features in an endemic area. Jpn J Infect Dis. 2009;62(6):423-7.
15. Dobler CC, Flack JR, Marks GB. Risk of tuberculosis among people with diabetes mellitus: An Australian nationwide cohort study. BMJ Open. 2012;2(1):e000666.
16. Jeon CY, Harries AD, Baker MA, Hart JE, Kapur A, Lönnroth K, et al. Bi-directional screening for tuberculosis and diabetes: a systematic review. Trop Med Int Health. 2010;15(11):1300-14.
17. Boucot KR, Dillon ES, Cooper DA, Meier P, Richardson R. Tuberculosis among diabetics: The Philadelphia survey. Am Rev Tuberc. 1952;65(1:2):1-50.
18. Bashar M, Alcabes P, Rom WN, Condos R. Increased incidence of multidrug-resistant tuberculosis in diabetic patients on the Bellevuem chest service, 1987 to 1997. Chest. 2001;120(5):1514-9.
19. Ocal S, Saka D, Ogretensoy M. Mild and severe forms of tuberculosis in diabetic and non-diabetic patients. J Diabetes. 2009;1(2):107-11.
20. Al-Tawfiq JA, Saadeh BM. Radiographic manifestations of culture-positive pulmonary tuberculosis: Cavitary or non-cavitary? Int J Tuberc Lung Dis. 2009;13(3):367-70.
21. Webb EA, Hesseling AC, Schaaf HS, Gie RP, Lombard CJ, Spitaels A, et al. High prevalence of mycobacterium tuberculosis infection and disease in children and adolescents with type 1 diabetes mellitus. Int J Tuberc Lung Dis. 2009;13(7):868-74.
22. Wang JY, Lee LN, Hsueh PR. Factors changing the manifestation of pulmonary tuberculosis. Int J Tuberc Lung Dis. 2005;9(7):777-83.
23. Perez-Guzman C, Torres-Cruz A, Villarreal-Velarde H, Salazar-Lezama MA, Vargas MH. Atypical radiological images of pulmonary tuberculosis in 192 diabetic patients: a comparative study. Int J Tuberc Lung Dis. 2001;5(5):455-61.
24. Umut S, Tosun GA, Yildirim N. Radiographic location of pulmonary tuberculosis in diabetic patients. Chest 1994;106(1):326.
25. Ruslami R, Nijland HM, Adhiarta IG, Kariadi SH, Alisjahbana B, Aarnoutse RE, et al. Pharmacokinetics of antituberculosis drugs in pulmonary tuberculosis patients with type 2 diabetes. Antimicrob Agents Chemother. 2010;54(3):1068-74.
26. Ssekamatte P, Sande OJ, van Crevel R, Biraro IA. Immunologic, metabolic and genetic impact of diabetes on tuberculosis susceptibility. Front Immunol. 2023;14:1122255.
27. Restrepo BI, Schlesinger LS. Impact of diabetes on the natural history of tuberculosis. Diabetes Res Clin Pract. 2014;106(2):191-9.
28. Ruslami R, Aarnoutse RE, Alisjahbana B, van der Ven AJ, van Crevel R. Implications of the global increase of diabetes for tuberculosis control and patient care. Trop Med Int Health. 2010;15(11):1289-99.
29. Martinez N, Kornfeld H. Diabetes and immunity to tuberculosis. Euro J Immunol. 2014;44(3):617-26.
30. Ponce-De-Leon A, Garcia-Garcia Md Mde L, Garcia-Sancho MC, Gomez-Perez FJ, Valdespino-Gomez JL, Olaiz-Fernandez G, et al. Tuberculosis and diabetes in southern Mexico. Diabetes Care. 2004;27(7):1584-90.
31. Jimenez-Corona ME, Cruz-Hervert LP, Garcia-Garcia L, Ferreyra-Reyes L, Delgado-Sánchez G, Bobadilla-Del-Valle M, et al. Association of diabetes and tuberculosis: impact on treatment and posttreatment outcomes. Thorax. 2013;68(3):214-20.
32. Bock NN, Jensen PA, Miller B, Nardell E. Tuberculosis infection control in resource-limited settings in the era of expanding HIV care and treatment. J Infect Dis. 2007;196 Suppl 1:S108-13.
33. Mave V, Gaikwad S, Barthwal M, Chandanwale A, Lokhande R, Kadam D, et al. Diabetes mellitus and tuberculosis treatment outcomes in Pune, India. Open Forum Infect Dis. 2021;8(4):ofab097.
34. Arriaga MB, Araújo-Pereira M, Barreto-Duarte B, Nogueira B, Freire MVCNS, Queiroz ATL, et al. The effect of diabetes and prediabetes on antituberculosis treatment outcomes: A multicenter prospective cohort study. J Infect Dis. 2021;225(4):617-26.
35. Chiang CY, Bai KJ, Lin HH, Chien ST, Lee JJ, Enarson DA, et al. The influence of diabetes, glycemic control, and diabetes-related comorbidities on pulmonary tuberculosis. PloS One. 2015;10(3):e0121698.
36. Chalasani N, Fontana RJ, Bonkovsky HL, Watkins PB, Davern T, Serrano J, et al. Causes, clinical features, and outcomes from a prospective study of drug-induced liver injury in the United States. Gastroenterology. 2008;135(6):1924-34.

37. Baghaei P, Tabarsi P, Chitsaz E, Saleh M, Marjani M, Shemirani S, et al. Incidence, clinical and epidemiological risk factors, and outcome of drug-induced hepatitis due to antituberculous agents in new tuberculosis cases. Am J Ther. 2010;17(1):17-22.
38. Degner NR, Wang JY, Golub JE, Karakousis PC. Metformin use reverses the increased mortality associated with diabetes mellitus during tuberculosis treatment. Clin Infect Dis. 2018;66:198-205.
39. Munir MK, Adnan M, Shabbir I, Rahat T, Rehman S. Therapeutic outcome of pulmonary tuberculosis in type-2 diabetes patients. APMC. 2018;12(2):93-7.
40. Ruesen C, Chaidir L, Ugarte-Gil C, van Ingen J, Critchley JA, Hill PC, et al. Diabetes is associated with genotypically drug-resistant tuberculosis. Eur Respir J. 2020;55(3):1901891.
41. Viswanathan V, Vigneswari A, Selvan K, Satyavani K, Rajeswari R, Kapur A. Effect of diabetes on treatment outcome of smear-positive pulmonary tuberculosis—a report from South India. J Diabetes Complications. 2014;28:162-5.
42. Lin M, Liao J, Gong Y, Han X, Chen Y, Tang Z, et al. Diabetes and multidrug-resistance gene mutation: Tuberculosis in Zunyi, Southwest China. Ann Palliat Med. 2020;9(5):3152-61.

CHAPTER

29

Psychiatric Disorders in Drug-resistant Tuberculosis

Mina Chandra, Kalpana Chandra

Abstract

Drug-resistant tuberculosis (DR-TB) is an emerging public health emergency. India has one of the highest rates of DR-TB and multidrug-resistant (MDR) TB in the world. The common psychiatric comorbidities in DR-TB are depressive, anxiety, psychotic, and medication-induced psychiatric disorders. Psychiatric disorders share a bidirectional relationship with DR-TB with DR-TB having with higher rates of psychiatric morbidity while the prevalence of MDR-TB is higher in individuals with severe mental illness like psychosis. The etiopathogenic mechanisms of psychiatric comorbidity in DR-TB include frailty, incapacity, nutritional impairment, inflammatory cascade, hypothalamus-pituitary axis (HPA) axis dysregulation, immune suppression, along with the long duration of treatment with toxic drugs with high rates of adverse events and psychiatric side effects such as cycloserine, fluoroquinolones, and isoniazid. The psychosocial contributory factors for psychiatric comorbidity in DR-TB include stigma, discrimination, unemployment, financial challenges, higher costs of treatment, poorly ventilated housing, lack of safer occupational options, and social support.

Psychiatric comorbidity worsens prognosis in DR-TB due to its symptomology, drug-drug interaction, poor treatment adherence, psychosocial distress, poor social support, and stigma. Early diagnosis and appropriate pharmacological and nonpharmacological treatment (counseling, social support, and supportive psychotherapy) of psychiatric comorbidity in DR-TB, as part of routine care platforms improve physical and mental health outcomes.

Concerted public health approaches for management of psychiatric comorbidity in DR-TB should focus on mental health literacy, capacity building of healthcare providers, defined referral pathways, financial support/social security, nutritional support, and supported employment options. Linkages between National Mental Health Program and Indian National Strategic Plan for Tuberculosis Elimination at policy and at ground level are essential for success of such initiatives.

While DR-TB is a global public health challenge and a national priority for India, early diagnosis and management of psychiatric comorbidity can help to improve outcomes.

Keywords: Tuberculosis, MDR-TB, psychiatric disorders, depression, anxiety, psychosis

INTRODUCTION

Tuberculosis (TB) control is a part of United Nations Sustainable Development Goal on Communicable Diseases (SDG 3.3). The major challenge for TB control is drug resistance. Drug-resistant TB (DR-TB) is an emerging public health emergency which threatens the progress made by TB programs worldwide.[1]

With global public health efforts against TB and DR-TB, the proportion of new cases of multidrug-resistant (MDR) TB/rifampicin-resistant TB (RR-TB) declined from 4.0% [95% uncertainty interval (UI): 3.1–4.9%] to 3.3% (95% UI: 2.6–4.0%) between 2015 and 2022. In addition, the proportion of previously treated cases with MDR/RR-TB reduced from 25% (95% UI: 15–36%) to 17% (95% UI: 11–23%) in the same period.[2] Despite such concerted efforts, India still has one of the highest rates of DR-TB and MDR-TB in the world.[3]

Drug resistance in TB is a heterogenous construct based on the resistance to different anti-TB drugs. Drug resistance in TB can be classified as:

- *RR-TB*: Resistance to rifampicin
- *Polydrug-resistant TB (PDR-TB)*: Resistance to more than one anti-TB drug, other than isoniazid and rifampicin
- *MDR-TB*: Resistance to at least isoniazid and rifampicin
- *Pre-extensively drug-resistant TB (PreXDR-TB)*: MDR-TB plus resistance to either a fluoroquinolone or a second-line injectable agent
- *XDR-TB*: MDR-TB plus resistance to fluoroquinolone and second-line injectable agents

These definitions are important as the original research work on psychiatric morbidity in DR-TB has been done on TB populations with different drug resistance profiles.[4]

Despite these limitations in the existing literature, it can be stated with confidence that DR-TB and psychiatric illnesses share a bidirectional relationship. DR-TB is associated with higher rates of psychiatric morbidity[5] while the prevalence of MDR-TB is significantly higher in individuals with severe mental illness such as psychosis (18.3–33%) as compared to controls (2.7%).[6]

Psychiatric comorbidities in turn are associated with poorer treatment outcomes with higher morbidity and mortality in patients with DR-TB.

EPIDEMIOLOGY OF PSYCHIATRIC COMORBIDITY IN DR-TB

There is a similarity in prevalence rates of psychiatric disorders in patients with different types of DR-TB living in different settings in different countries.

The prevalence of psychiatric disorders in patients with MDR-TB was determined to be 32.8% in an Indonesian study, of which 14.1% of patients had multiple psychiatric diagnoses.[7]

Similar rates were reported from an Indian study from Mumbai wherein one-third of the patients with DR-TB were diagnosed to have a psychiatric disorder and of which half the patients developed psychiatric disorder during the course of treatment.[4]

The common psychiatric disorders include depressive disorders, anxiety disorders, psychotic disorders (including schizoaffective disorder, bipolar I disorder current episode severe manic with psychotic features) and medication-induced psychiatric disorders **(Box 1)**.[7]

A brief summary of various psychiatric comorbidities in DR-TB is given here.

Depressive Disorders

The pooled prevalence of depression in DR-TB was reported to be 25% [95% confidence interval (CI) 14–39] in a recent meta-analysis.[1]

BOX 1 Psychiatric comorbidity in drug-resistant tuberculosis (DR-TB).

- Depressive disorders
- Anxiety disorders
- Psychotic disorders
- Medication-induced disorders

Depressive disorders were diagnosed in 48.0% patients while mixed anxiety depression additionally was diagnosed in 23.5% patients of DR-TB in a Mumbai-based study.[4]

A recent Indonesian study also reported that more than two-thirds of the patients with MDR-TB had depression with rates of mild-to-severe depression ranging between 31.4 and 9.8%, respectively.[8]

Depression in DR-TB is associated with older age, female gender, poverty, smoking, and immunocompromised states such as diabetes and HIV coinfection. Depression in DR-TB is also mediated by psychosocial factors such as limitation of familial, social and occupational roles, perceived and actual social isolation, reduced self-esteem, mental distress, feelings of shame, social stigma, fear of rejection, fear of infecting others, and fear of death.[9]

Anxiety Disorders

The pooled prevalence of anxiety in DR-TB was reported to be 24% (95% CI 2–57) in a recent meta-analysis.[1]

In an Indian study on DR-TB patient in Mumbai, mixed anxiety depression was diagnosed in 23.5% patients while anxiety with neurocognitive disorders was diagnosed on 4.9% patients.[4]

However, exponentially high rates of anxiety were reported from an Indonesian study on MDR-TB wherein <14% patients of MDR-TB found to be free from anxiety. The rates of moderate-to-severe anxiety varied between 46.1% and 6.9% respectively in this study.[8]

Psychosis

The pooled prevalence of psychosis in DR-TB was reported to be 10% (95% CI 7–14) in a recent meta-analysis.[1] Psychotic symptoms include delusions, hallucinations disorganized speech, disorganized behaviors, and catatonic symptoms.

Psychotic symptoms have been reported to be significantly associated with male sex and lower level of educational attainment in an Indonesian study on MDR-TB.[7]

Medication-induced Psychiatric Disorders

Antituberculosis treatment (ATT) medications such as isoniazid, ethambutol, and cycloserine have been documented to be associated with psychosis (including symptoms of delusions, hallucinations, and behavioral disturbances), manic symptoms, depression, suicidal ideation/attempts, and insomnia.[10]

The most commonly implicated agent for medication-induced psychiatric disorders in patients with DR TB is cycloserine. In an Indonesian study on MDR-TB, psychiatric disorders were found to be significantly associated with increasing dose of cycloserine.[7] Cycloserine has been implicated for both depression and psychosis in a Mumbai-based study on DR-TB, though cycloserine has been reported to have antidepressant property due to its effect on gamma-aminobutyric acid (GABA) and N-methyl-D-aspartate (NMDA) receptor.

Cycloserine is a GABA transaminase inhibitor resulting in increased levels of GABA. Cycloserine is also NMDA receptor partial agonist which enhances receptor activation in the presence of glutamate.[8]

However, the rate of medication-induced psychosis in the aforesaid Mumbai study was just 2.0%.[4]

Such ATT-related psychiatric morbidity may require modification of ATT regimen.

Other drugs used to treat DR-TB, such as bedaquiline, delamanid, and imipenem, were not significantly associated with treatment emergent psychiatric comorbidities in the aforesaid Mumbai study.[4]

ETIOPATHOGENIC MECHANISMS OF PSYCHIATRIC COMORBIDITY IN DR-TB

Psychiatric comorbidity in DR-TB can be attributed to a spectrum of biopsychosocial factors. The biological factors include frailty, incapacity, nutritional impairment, and immune mechanisms such as inflammatory cascade, HPA axis dysregulation, immune suppression, and probable reduced vaccine response. Suppression of cellular immunity due to poor mental health can result in reactivation of latent TB infection (LTBI) or progression from subclinical to clinical disease.[6,9,11]

Additional contributory factors are the long duration of treatment with toxic regimens comprising of drugs having high rates of adverse events and psychiatric side effects such as cycloserine, fluoroquinolones, and isoniazid.

The psychosocial contributory factors include stigma, discrimination, unemployment, financial challenges, higher costs of treatment, poorly ventilated housing, lack of safer occupational options, lack of social support, social isolation, and abandonment **(Table 1)**.[1,4,6,9,11]

TREATMENT OF PSYCHIATRIC COMORBIDITY IN DR-TB

There is a pressing need to identify and manage psychiatric comorbidities in persons with DR-TB as part of routine care platforms to improve physical and mental health outcomes.[9]

Psychiatric comorbidity might disturb MDR-TB treatment due to its symptomology, drug-drug interactions, and poor treatment adherence resulting in adverse outcomes.

A person with TB is in repeated contact with some healthcare facility including directly observed therapy (DOT) centers throughout the course of his treatment. Defined screening protocols especially for patients with DR-TB can help identify possible cases of psychiatric disorders which can be referred for psychiatric treatment in time.[11]

TABLE 1: Biopsychosocial factors for psychiatric comorbidity in drug-resistant tuberculosis (DR-TB).

Biological contributory factors	Psychosocial contributory factors
Frailty, incapacity, and nutritional impairment	Stigma and discrimination
Treatment with toxic regimens with high rates of adverse events and psychiatric side effects	Unemployment, financial challenges, and high costs of treatment
Hypothalamus-pituitary axis (HPA) axis dysregulation	Poorly ventilated housing
Inflammatory cascade	Lack of safer occupational options
Immune suppression and reduced vaccine response	Lack of social support, social isolation, and abandonment

Treatment of psychiatric disorders requires appropriate pharmacological management with comprehensive knowledge of both anti-TB drugs and psychotropic medications including pharmacokinetics and pharmacodynamic (PK/PD) parameters, changes in absorption and distribution, possible side effects, and drug-drug interactions.[12]

If any antitubercular drugs is suspected to cause psychiatric disorder, it must be removed from the treatment regimen and another antitubercular introduced in its place.

Early diagnosis and appropriate psychiatric treatment require affordable, accessible, and culturally acceptable interventions by trained mental health professionals such as psychiatrists and clinical psychologists in collaborative care settings.[8]

PROGNOSTIC IMPLICATIONS OF PSYCHIATRIC COMORBIDITY IN DR-TB

The presence of psychiatric comorbidity has prognostic implications in DR-TB. Comorbid psychiatric disorders such as depression and anxiety adversely impact prognosis and treatment outcomes on account of treatment nonadherence,[10] psychosocial distress, poor social support and stigma irrespective of age, race, demographic characteristics, geographical location, and social status.[13]

Of all psychiatric comorbidities, depression is independently associated with higher rates of morbidity, mortality, drug resistance, risk of TB reactivation, and community TB transmission.[11]

At the same time, appropriate treatment of psychiatric comorbidity results in better treatment outcomes for patients with MDR-TB. There was significantly better treatment outcomes for patients of DR-TB with psychiatric comorbidity, who received comprehensive psychiatric care integrated into DR-TB care delivery, in a Mumbai-based study ($p = 0.014$).[4]

PUBLIC HEALTH APPROACHES FOR PSYCHIATRIC COMORBIDITY IN DR-TB

Public health approaches for management of psychiatric comorbidity in DR-TB should focus on mental health literacy, capacity building of healthcare providers, defined referral pathways, and provision of pharmacological and nonpharmacological interventions such as counseling, social support, and supportive psychotherapy.[11] Patient support measures for DR-TB should include financial support/social security, nutritional support and supported employment options.[14]

The public health models for management of psychiatric comorbidity in DR-TB include integrated care model, collaborative care model, patient-centered care model and defined referral pathways to care model, and linkages between programs addressing mental health and TB like National Mental Health Program and National Strategic Plan for Tuberculosis Elimination both at policy and ground level are essential for success of such initiatives.

RESEARCH ON PSYCHIATRIC COMORBIDITY IN DR-TB

Multidisciplinary research is also required to address the issue of psychiatric morbidity in DR-TB. Epidemiological studies are needed to define the burden of psychiatric comorbidity in DR-TB in diverse population, in urban, rural, and tribal settings across all age groups and in all genders. Further, research on etiopathogenic mechanisms of comorbid psychiatric disorders in TB is required to understand biopsychosocial underpinnings for optimal therapeutic interventions.

CONCLUSION

The DR-TB is a global public health challenge and a national priority for India. Early diagnosis and management of psychiatric comorbidity are important steps for improving outcomes in DR-TB. To implement successful psychiatric management in DR-TB, capacity building and evidence-based integrated care models must be incorporated in public health strategy for addressing DR-TB.

REFERENCES

1. Alene KA, Clements ACA, McBryde ES, Jaramillo E, Lönnroth K, Shaweno D, et al. Mental health disorders, social stressors, and health-related quality of life in patients with multidrug-resistant tuberculosis: A systematic review and meta-analysis. J Infect. 2018;77:357-67.
2. World Health Organization. (2023). Global Tuberculosis Report 2023. [online] Available from https://www.who.int/teams/global-tuberculosis-programme/tb-reports/global-tuberculosis-report-2023/tb-disease-burden/1-3-drug-resistant-tb [Last accessed September, 2024].
3. Vishwakarma D, Gaidhane A, Sahu S, Rathod AS. Multi-Drug Resistance Tuberculosis (MDR-TB) Challenges in India: A Review. Cureus. 2023;15(12):e50222.
4. Laxmeshwar C, Das M, Mathur T, Israni T, Jha S, Iyer A, et al. Psychiatric comorbidities among patients with complex drug-resistant tuberculosis in Mumbai, India. PLoS One. 2022;17(2):e0263759.
5. Espinosa JV, Hernández-Pando R. Psychiatric Problems in Pulmonary Tuberculosis: Depression and Anxiety. J Tuberculosis Res. 2021;9:31-50.
6. Hayward SE, Deal A, Rustage K, Nellums LB, Sweetland AC, Boccia D, et al. The relationship between mental health and risk of active tuberculosis: A systematic review. BMJ Open. 2022;12(1):e048945.
7. Supriyanto I, Liung S, Suprihatini, Ismanto SH. Psychiatric disorders in patients with multidrug resistant tuberculosis (MDR-TB) in Sardjito Hospital, Yogyakarta, Indonesia. J Anal ResClin Med. 2017;5(3):91-6.
8. Susanto TD, Widysanto A, Cipta DA, Tanar A, Wirawan GR, Kosim AB, et al. Anxiety and depression level of patients with multidrug-resistant tuberculosis (MDR-TB) in two hospitals in Banten province, Indonesia. Dialogues Health. 2023;2:100115.
9. Janse Van Rensburg A, Dube A, Curran R, Ambaw F, Murdoch M, Bachmann M, et al. Comorbidities between tuberculosis and common mental disorders: a scoping review of epidemiological patterns and person-centred care interventions from low-to-middle income and BRICS countries. Infect Dis Poverty. 2020;9:4.
10. Pachi A, Bratis D, Moussas G, Tselebis A. Psychiatric morbidity and other factors affecting treatment adherence in pulmonary tuberculosis patients. Tuberc Res Treat. 2013;2013:489865.
11. Chandra M, Rana P, Chandra K, Arora VK. Tuberculosis—depression syndemic: A public health challenge. Indian J Tuberc. 2019;66(1):197-202.
12. Riccardi N, Canetti D, Rodari P, Besozzi G, Saderi L, Dettori M, et al. Tuberculosis and pharmacological interactions: A narrative review. Curr Res Pharmacol Drug Discov. 2020;2:100007.
13. Agbeko CK, Mallah MA, He B, Liu Q, Song H, Wang J. Mental Health Status and its Impact on TB Treatment and its Outcomes: A Scoping Literature Review. Front Public Health. 2022;10:855515.
14. Todowede O, Afaq S, Adhikary A, Kanan S, Shree V, Jennings HM, et al. Barriers and facilitators to integrating depression care in tuberculosis services in South Asia: A multi-country qualitative study. BMC Health Serv Res. 2023;23:818.

CHAPTER

30

Antimicrobial Resistance Fight: Preventing Drug Resistance

Ankita Anand, Kamal Chopra, Sanjay Rajpal

Abstract

Tuberculosis (TB) is a disease that can be prevented, treated, and cured. In 2022, the global tally of newly diagnosed TB cases was reported to be 7.5 million.[1] However, Drug-resistant tuberculosis (DR-TB) remains a significant public health challenge. Among all recorded TB cases, approximately 410,000 individuals were diagnosed with multidrug-resistant or rifampicin-resistant TB (MDR/RR-TB).[1] Given the rise of antimicrobial resistance and the emergence of DR-TB, traditional methods of preventions are increasingly proving inadequate. Preventing the spread of MDR-TB and extensively drug-resistant TB (XDR-TB) is a global health imperative and requires enhanced efforts to strengthen the TB control in resource-limited settings. Repurposing existing drugs, developing analogs of current anti-TB medications, and exploring novel compounds with different mechanisms will be critical in the future success of DR-TB treatment strategies. By implementing these strategies, the spread and emergence of DR-TB can be controlled, and overall TB management can be improved.

Keywords: Tuberculosis, drug resistance, MDR-TB, XDR-TB, DR-TB, repurposed drugs, genotypic DST

INTRODUCTION

The COVID-19 pandemic significantly impacted tuberculosis (TB) by causing a notable global decline in the number of new TB diagnoses and official notifications. After a substantial increase from 2017 to 2019, there was an 18% drop from 7.1 million in 2019 to 5.8 million in 2020, with a partial rebound to 6.4 million in 2021. By 2022, the number of new TB cases diagnosed and officially reported worldwide had increased to 7.5 million and ~410,000 of these were patients with MDR/RR-TB.[1]

World Health Organization (WHO) in 2023 published 50 interventions for antimicrobial resistance, approximately 10 of the priority areas were dedicated to drug-resistant (DR) TB.[2] Primary resistance along with poor patient compliance and poor treatment adherence due to longer duration of treatment with combination of drugs raises the threat of the emergence of multidrug-resistant TB (MDR-TB) and extensively drug-resistant TB (XDR-TB).

Emergence of drug resistance *Mycobacterium tuberculosis* (MTB) accentuates the need of early diagnosis of resistant strains, the search for potential targets of drug resistance, shorter treatment options, and effective medical interventions.

Social determinants such as poverty and factors such as undernutrition, overcrowding, and smoking and DR-TB go hand in hand. TB incidence and mortality decrease with improvements in living conditions and nutrition. Another major risk factors for TB progression and severity are comorbidities like human immunodeficiency virus (HIV), diabetes mellitus, malignancies, and silicosis. It has been observed that among people living with HIV, and in diabetics the risk of MDR/rifampicin-resistant (RR)-TB was 1.42-fold and twofold higher respectively than for those not living with HIV and in nondiabetics.[3] Addressing these social determinants, can help to reduce the risk of TB and its progression to MDR-TB.

In the early 90s, DR-TB transmission and its epidemic was illustrated mainly by acquired resistance but later by the end of the decade, most of the new cases of DR-TB were infected by already resistant strains, i.e., primary resistance. Preventing MDR-TB involves a combination of strategies to minimize the spread of the disease and ensure effective treatment.

EARLY DIAGNOSIS AND PROMPT TREATMENT

Initial clinical assessment along with rapid identification of TB cases, and diagnosis of drug-resistant strains with help of different advanced molecular tests, allows for timely and appropriate treatment.

The WHO now requires drug susceptibility testing (DST) for all TB patients to better inform treatment decisions and enhance treatment results. However, in countries with a high burden of TB, the availability of resources is still a major obstacle. Traditionally, phenotypic DST is the first choice for the diagnosis of MDR/XDR-TB; however, it has drawbacks such as long turnaround time, highly complex, and labor-intensive process and also requires specialized infrastructure which limits its accessibility and directly affects effective treatment.

In recent times, new automated rapid molecular diagnostic assays for genotypic DST have developed including whole genome sequencing and targeted genomic sequencing. These tests can simultaneously detect resistance through detection of specific genetic markers. This rapid point of care test will optimize the TB diagnosis and facilitate a precision DR-TB treatment and thus will prevent the amplification of resistance.

PROMPT AND APPROPRIATE TREATMENT

Individualized treatment regimens, based on the drug susceptibility profile, involving healthcare workers under DOT therapy to ensure adherence which helps in preventing development of further resistance. Avoiding misuse, incomplete or inappropriate, and overuse of TB drugs can prevent the development of resistance. Medical adherence and treatment outcome can be improved with supportive care such as addressing side effects and complications of treatment and ensuring nutritional support will reduce emergence of drug resistance strains. Adverse effects of the drug subvert treatment adherence resulting in treatment interruption, life-threatening complications, and death. Reducing the adverse effects of TB drugs is crucial for improving patient adherence and treatment outcomes. These can be minimized by regular clinical monitoring, early detection, educating the patient about symptoms, and reporting these events.

INTEGRATED APPROACHES

Integrated approaches such as public health surveillance to robustly monitor TB incidence, pattern of resistance their treatment outcomes at the community and national levels. Training healthcare professionals in the use of advanced diagnostic tools for accurate diagnosis and to use effective treatment protocols which will further add in capacity building and reduce the emergence and spread of drug resistance TB. Screening of close contacts of infectious patients with early detection of DR-TB will be useful in stopping the spread of DR-TB.

PATIENT EDUCATION AND SUPPORT

Educating patients about TB, its transmission, and the importance of completing the full course of treatment helps in reducing transmission and preventing the development of drug-resistant strains.

INFECTION CONTROL MEASURE

It plays an important role in reducing the transmission. It includes improving ventilation in healthcare settings with proper air changes, using masks, and ensuring good hygiene practices.

STRENGTHENING HEALTH SYSTEMS

Investing in upgrading the laboratory and diagnostic facility along with robust quality control measures for reliable and accurate diagnostic results.

MAINTAINING A PROPER DRUG SUPPLY CHAIN MECHANISM

Ensuring a consistent supply of all TB drugs and its storage to maintain its efficacy for the uninterrupted treatment.

CURRENT CONVENTIONAL DRUG DELIVERY APPROACHES

These approaches contribute to the emergence of drug resistance due to higher pill burden, extended duration of treatment, and increased toxicity of drugs which increase the probability of rise of drug resistance, coupled with poor patient adherence and exacerbate the problem. Various types of *nanocarriers' systems* can be designed to release drugs slowly and steadily over extended periods, reducing the need for multiple doses which can lower the pill burden and simplify treatment regimens. These carriers can encapsulate multiple drugs, enabling combination therapy in a single delivery system which can help to simplify the dosing schedules and enhance patient adherence. It will help in improving the bioavailability and stability of drugs, leading to more effective treatment and decreasing the emergence of DR-TB.[4]

THE DEVELOPMENT AND USE OF NOVEL ANTI-TB DRUGS

The development and use of novel anti-TB drugs that target different aspects of MTB bacilli will be crucial and important for overcoming current resistance. Use of repurposed drugs for combination therapy with other agents to improve the efficacy and improving the treatment outcome. Exploring host-directed therapeutics such as interferon gamma, vitamin D, and immune modulators to improve DR-TB treatment efficacy and reduce disease severity.[5]

CONCLUSION

Understanding the transmission of DR strains, followed by effective monitoring, is crucial. This can be achieved by identifying specific genetic markers and ensuring timely diagnosis of drug resistance and usage of rapid genotypic DST tools for newer drugs. Prompt and accurate detection is essential to prevent MTB from evolving into highly resistant strains. Implementing antibiotic stewardship measures to rationalize antibiotic use is essential to preserve the efficacy of new drugs and extend the lifespan of existing treatments, thus prolonging the utility of existing regimens, minimizing the development of resistance, ongoing promotion of new drugs. To enhance TB management and control the spread of MDR-TB, alternative strategies should be considered such as pathogen-centric, host-centric and nano-based drug delivery systems, use of novel drugs, and repurposed drugs.

REFERENCES

1. WHO. (2023). Global Tuberculosis Report 2023. World Health Organization. [online] Available from https://www.who.int/teams/global-tuberculosis-programme/tb-reports/global-tuberculosis-report-2023 [Last accessed September, 2024].
2. WHO. (2024). Global Research Agenda for Antimicrobial Resistance in Human Health. [online] Available from https://www.who.int/publications/m/item/global-research-agenda-for-antimicrobial-resistance-in-human-health [Last accessed September, 2024].
3. Sultana ZZ, Hoque FU, Beyene J, Akhlak-Ul-Islam M, Khan MHR, Ahmed S, et al. HIV infection and multidrug resistant tuberculosis: a systematic review and meta-analysis. BMC Infect Dis. 2021;21:51.
4. Alshawwa SZ, Kassem AA, Farid RM, Mostafa SK, Labib GS. Nanocarrier Drug Delivery Systems: Characterization, Limitations, Future Perspectives and Implementation of Artificial Intelligence. Pharmaceutics. 2022;14(4):883.
5. Young C, Walzl G, Du Plessis N. Therapeutic host-directed strategies to improve outcome in tuberculosis. Mucosal Immunol. 2020;13:190-204.

CHAPTER

31

Mitigating Strategies to Prevent Drug Resistance

Niti Singh, Sarman Singh

Abstract

Mycobacterium tuberculosis (MTB) is the causative agent of tuberculosis (TB). Resistance to standard anti-TB drugs has become a major challenge in the treatment and control of TB around the globe and in India. The resistance to mycobactericidal drug rifampicin (RIF) with or without isoniazid (INH) resistance is known as multidrug-resistant TB (MDR-TB), even though as per new WHO definition, the RIF resistance alone has been considered as surrogate of MDR. The risk of developing MDR-TB (resistance to both INH and RIF) is the product of cumulative individual chances (10^{14}) in the bacterial population, and it is exaggerated by the suboptimal treatment or noncompliance to drug regimens. The understanding of the mechanisms of drug resistance helps in the development of newer drugs with novel targets to treat drug-resistant TB. Resistance to INH is a complex process that generates mutations in numerous genes, including *katG, inhA, ahpC, kasA*, and *ndh* which have all been associated with INH resistance while resistance to RIF is mainly associated with the mutations in the *rpoB* gene of MTB. Several strategies need to be adopted to mitigate emergence of drug resistance that include active case detection and early detection of drug resistance patterns in the isolates. Counseling for treatment compliance and social, nutritional, financial, and psychological support to the effected patient and the family is of paramount importance.

Keywords: MDR-TB, *rpoB* gene, mutations, MGIT-960

INTRODUCTION

Mycobacterium tuberculosis (MTB) is the causative agent of tuberculosis (TB). Resistance to standard anti-TB drugs has become a major challenge in the treatment and control of TB around the globe. The resistance to mycobactericidal drug rifampicin (RIF) with or without isoniazid (INH) resistance is known as multidrug-resistant TB (MDR-TB).[1] MDR-TB threatens the progress made so far by the TB elimination programs. Patients infected with MDR-TB are practically refractory to standard first-line treatment. The number of primary DR-TB decreased from 3.90% in 2015 to 3.10% in 2020 but again started increasing in 2021 and reached to 3.60%.[2] India notified 24.20 lakh MDR cases in the year 2022; an increase of 13.0% in comparison to 2021 and reported a total number of 63,801 MDR cases. In 2017, India launched its revised National Strategic Plan (NSP) (2017–2025) with the ambitious and challenging goal of eliminating TB by 2025, 5 years before the 2030 target set by the United Nation's-Sustainable Developmental Goal (UN-SDG) and WHO End Tuberculosis Strategy. To achieve the objectives of the NSP, India must reduce TB cases by at least 10% every year, compared to the global target of 2%. The revised NSP includes several new recommendations including scaling up of rapid molecular diagnostic services to reduce the burden of drug-resistant TB (DR-TB).

MECHANISM OF DRUG RESISTANCE

The current therapeutic management of MTB is inadequate due to the comparatively prolonged course of treatment, associated side effects of drugs, unorganized treatment regimens prescribed by individual doctors, and nonadherence to the prescribed regimen. These aspects can lead to therapeutic failure and development of DR-TB. Drug resistance to the anti-TB drugs has existed and been reported within few years of discovering these drugs. The understanding of the entire mechanisms of drug resistance helps in the development of newer rapid diagnostic tools and newer drug(s) with novel targets for selectively killing the DR-MTB. It is a matter of consolation that drug resistance in MTB is genetically controlled **(Table 1)** and not plasmid mediated like other bacteria.[3]

Resistance to INH is a complex process that generate mutations in numerous genes, including *katG, inhA, ahpC, kasA*, and *ndh* that have been associated with INH resistance. The INH is a prodrug necessitating stimulation by the catalase/peroxidase enzyme encoded by *katG* gene. A reduction in catalase/peroxidase activity as a result of nutation in the *katG* gene (S315T) is the most common mechanism associated with INH resistance. Other such mechanisms involve mutations in the *inhA* promoter (15C-T) that result in overexpression of inhA, which confers low-level resistance to INH. Mutations in these two genes account for resistance in approximately 90–95% isolates and mutations in *ahpC, kasA*, and *ndh* genes account for resistance in about 5–10% isolates.[3]

Even though MDR-TB is defined as resistance to RIF with or without INH, resistance to RIF is considered surrogate for MDR. RIF acts against actively growing and slowly metabolizing (nongrowing) bacilli. Resistance to RIF is mainly associated with the mutations in the *rpoB* gene of MTB. Furthermore, >95% of MTB clinical isolates that are resistant to RIF have a mutation in an 81bp "hot spot" region of *rpoB* known as the rifampicin resistance-determining region (RRDR) between codons 507 and 533 **(Fig. 1)**. Position of these mutations within the *rpoB* gene is associated with different levels of phenotypic resistance to RIF.[4,5] Some mutations are associated with a high level of resistance to RIF while others are known to confer only low-level resistance.[4]

TABLE 1: Mechanisms of drug resistance to primary anti-mycobacterial drugs.

Agent	Mode of action	Target	Gene	Most prevalent mutation
Isoniazid	Inhibition of mycolic acid synthesis	Mycolic acids	*katG*	Ser-315-Thr
Rifampicin	Inhibition of RNA polymerase	RNA polymerase	*rpoB*	Ser-450-Leu
Pyrazinamide	Inhibition of energy production and trans-translation	Fatty acid synthase-I, ribosomal protein S1	*pncA*	Asp-12-Ala/Asn, Leu-85-Pro
Ethambutol	Inhibition of arabinogalactan synthesis	Arabinosyl transferases	*embCAB*	Met-306-Val/Ile/Leu

The mutations are dominated by single nucleotide changes, resulting in substitutions of a single amino acid (especially mutations at codons 531, 526, and 516). However, in-frame deletion and insertion mutations also occur at lower frequencies at codons 511, 516, 518, and 522. In RRDR region of *rpoB* gene 16 single base changes, two insertions, one deletion and five multiple mutations (with two or three codons implicated) are most frequently reported. However, the mechanism of resistance in about 5% of MTB RIF-resistant isolates is unknown, suggesting alternative mechanisms, such as lowered cell wall permeability or efflux pump activity. Mutations that confer or are associated with INH and RIF resistance are independent of each other, with frequency rates of 106 and 108 of the bacterial population, respectively.

PREDICTORS OF DRUG RESISTANCE

Defaulting to prescribed drug regimen is one of the biggest reason for treatment failure and development of drug resistance. Most treatment defaulters are in the 20–39 years age group, which is probably due to the fact that individuals of this age group are more likely to migrate for business and other job opportunities and to have erratic working hours, making them more likely to miss taking medication. Nevertheless, the largest number of treatment failures are among patients aged > 60 years. Most likely due to their lowered immune status. Therefore, adherence to prescribed regimen and good nutritional supplementation are most helpful in the success of treatment.

The risk of developing MDR-TB (resistance to both INH and RIF) is the product of cumulative individual chances (10^{14}) in the bacterial population. MDR-TB is thus less likely to occur in new cases and those having paucibacillary disease. However, in the case of nonadherence to treatment, the use of poor-quality drugs or malabsorption, "functional monotherapy" may lead to resistance. These reasons may predispose patients receiving first-line anti-TB drugs for longer durations to develop MDR-TB. Most of the RIF resistance strains (45.4%) showed mutations at codon S531L of the *rpoB* gene. Mutations involving D516V and H526Y (MUT1 and 2A in *rpoB*) in the *rpoB* gene were infrequent in our study

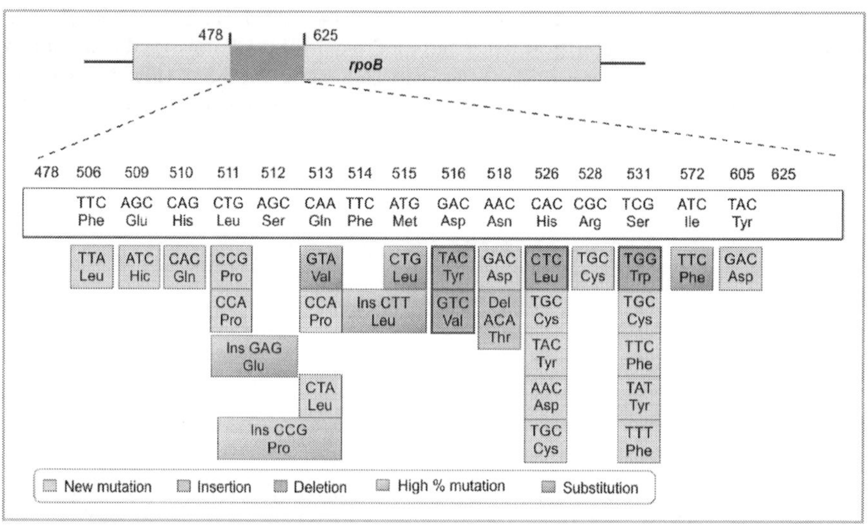

FIG. 1: The hotspot region (HSR) (red) of the *rpoB* gene which depicts that any mutation in this area is likely to confer high level RIF resistance. The flanking blue regions indicates mutation in these areas are associated with low-level resistance.[4] ***(For color version, see Plate 3)***

(data not shown here). However, it sharply contrasts with the higher rates reported from studies in the West. Mutations involving codon 315 of *katG* were most commonly seen among INH-resistant strains in our study, similar to other studies from the Indian subcontinent.

NEW PIPELINE OF NOVEL DRUGS

The clinical development and regulatory approvals of bedaquiline, delamanid, and pretomanid in last few years have made a significant progress in the management of DR-TB, providing all-oral regimens. The Nix-TB and ZeNix trials of a bedaquiline–pretomanid–linezolid regimen demonstrated for the first time that certain forms of DR-TB can be cured in the majority of patients within 6 months. However, as more and more clinical use of these drugs and regimens is being undertaken globally, resistance to these drugs is also being reported from various parts of India and globally. Therefore, there is urgent need to search for novel molecules for the treatment of MDR-TB. The investigational drugs in clinical development, such as second-generation oxazolidinones (sutezolid, delpazolid, and TBI-223) and diarylquinolines (TBAJ-876 and TBAJ-587) promise improved potency and safety. Compounds with novel targets involved in diverse bacterial functions such as cell wall synthesis (DrpE1 and MmpL3), electron transport, DNA synthesis (GyrB), cholesterol metabolism, and transcriptional regulation of ethionamide bioactivation pathways also provide hope with early clinical efficacy studies and the potential to enhance antibacterial activity when added to new or established anti-TB drug regimens.[4,6]

Amongst others, the highly optimistic and with potent antimycobacterial activity, agents such as BTZ-043, PBTZ 169, and OPC-167832 are also being studied. New and exciting prospective agents with novel mechanisms of impact against TB include 3-aminomethyl benzoxaboroles and telacebec. Recent studies have found that addition of molecule GSK2556286 increases the bactericidal and sterilizing activity of BPa-containing regimens in a well-established BALB/c mouse model of TB. The investigators used this model to evaluate the potential of new regimens combining bedaquiline or the more potent diarylquinoline TBAJ-587 with GSK2556286 and the DprE1 inhibitor TBA-7371, all of which are currently in early-phase clinical trials. They found the combination of bedaquiline, GSK2556286, and TBA-7371 to be more active than the first-line regimen and nearly as effective as BPaL in terms of bactericidal and sterilizing activity. The authors concluded that GSK2556286 and TBA-7371 have the potential to replace pretomanid, an oxazolidinone, or both components, in combination with bedaquiline or TBAJ-587.[6]

STRATEGIES TO MITIGATE EMERGENCE OF DRUG RESISTANCE

Even though in last two decades a lot of progress has been made in field of TB diagnosis and management, including the endorsement of liquid culture for culture isolation, and drug susceptibility testing (DST), rolling out of molecular tests that include GeneXpert MTB/Rif, the Line Probe Assay, and indigenous Truenat test. However, this progress has remained hampered by the vastness of the country, remote and difficult terrains of the infected population, leading to missing a large number if infected population to report to health centers for diagnoses and treatment of TB. On top of that, increasing rates of MDR-TB, comorbidities such as diabetes and human immunodeficiency virus (HIV) are other challenges. The following are some known reasons for not being able to combat the drug resistance, and our suggested strategies to handle these challenges:

- More than half number of TB patients remain unreported, and an even higher percentage of MDR-TB patients cannot have timely second-line DST done due to nonavailability of facility in the rural parts of India and in public sector. Therefore, self-testing triage algorithms should be developed and adopted by the national TB elimination program for active case finding.[7]

- RIF is an important constituent of not only first-line treatment but also for MDR-TB (second line) treatment. However, prior to start of MDR-TB treatment, it is necessary to carry out rapid DST to avoid the misuse of ineffective drugs. Therefore, as mentioned above, not only for active case detection, but network for molecular DST laboratories must be strengthened by government of India.
- Frequency of emergence of MDR-TB is more in those patients who are carrying a higher bacillary load suggesting impaired clearance of bacilli due to ineffective anti-TB treatment. In the light of this finding, it might be beneficial to offer baseline DST to individuals with high bacillary load in sputum samples, particularly in resource-limited settings. Hence conventional microscopy with acid-fast bacilli (AFB) load and/or with cycle threshold (Ct) value in the molecular tests should be reported to help treating physicians a considered view for dose and regimen prescription with frequent follow-up of such cases.

CONCLUSION

Whenever, possible multiple tests should be applied, as no single test is Gospel's truth. In low-level drug resistance (using minimum inhibitory concentration of >0.5 μg/mL), the conventional phenotypic culture-based DST methods can miss drug resistance. Similarly, the molecular assays also may not be carrying the probes for these rare but clinically relevant low-level resistance conferring mutations such as *Ile572Phe, Leu533Pro,* and *His526Leu.* This aspect has to be looked at and newer molecular tools to detect these mutations should be developed.

The Government must also rethink the adult immunization with standard Bacillus Calmette–Guérin (BCG) or its newer versions, because there is sufficient evidence that by the adulthood the efficacy of the BCG vaccination given at birth wanes off giving hardly any protection.[8]

REFERENCES

1. WHO. (2022). Global Tuberculosis Report 2022. [online] Available from https://www.who.int/teams/global-tuberculosis-programme/tb-reports/global-tuberculosis-report-2022 [Last accessed September, 2024].
2. WHO. (2022). WHO consolidated guidelines on tuberculosis. Module 4: treatment - drug-resistant tuberculosis treatment, 2022 update. [online] Available from https://www.who.int/publications/i/item/9789240063129 [Last accessed September, 2024].
3. Wang W, Liu R, Yao C, Huo F, Shang Y, Zhang X, et al. Reevaluating Rifampicin Breakpoint Concentrations for *Mycobacterium tuberculosis* Isolates with Disputed rpoB Mutations and Discordant Susceptibility Phenotypes. Microbiol Spectr. 2022;10(1):e02087-21.
4. Black TA, Buchwald UK. The pipeline of new molecules and regimens against drug-resistant tuberculosis. J Clin Tuberc Other Mycobact Dis. 2021;25:100285.
5. Rufai SB, Singh J, Kumar P, Mathur P, Singh S. Association of *gyrA* and *rrs* gene mutations detected by MTBDRsl V1 on *Mycobacterium tuberculosis* strains of diverse genetic background from India. Sci Rep. 2018;8(1):9295.
6. Li S-Y, Tyagi S, Soni H, Betoudji F, Converse PJ, Mdluli K, et al. Bactericidal and sterilizing activity of novel regimens combining bedaquiline or TBAJ-587 with GSK2556286 and TBA-7371 in a mouse model of tuberculosis. Antimicrob Agents Chemother. 2024;68(4):e0156223.
7. Singh S. End tuberculosis: Challenges and opportunities. Tuberc Res Treat. 2024;2024:2307742.
8. Martinez L, Cords O, Liu Q, Acuna-Villaorduna C, Bonnet M, Fox GJ, et al. Infant BCG vaccination and risk of pulmonary and extrapulmonary tuberculosis throughout the life course: a systematic review and individual participant data meta-analysis. Lancet Glob Health. 2022;10(9):e1307-16.

CHAPTER

32

Airborne Transmission of Drug-resistant Tuberculosis

Rajnish Gupta, Ashish Ranjan, Ajantha Panneerselvam

Abstract

Tuberculosis (TB), including drug-resistant TB (DRTB), is transmitted by air from an infectious TB patient. An individual with active and untreated TB typically spreads the infection to around 10–15 people annually. Close contacts or household contacts of a person with active TB are particularly at risk of contracting the disease from the case. HIV infection is the greatest risk factor for progression from latent TB infection (LTBI) to TB disease. Infectiousness is increased in presence of cough, cavitation on chest X-ray, positive acid-fast bacilli (AFB) in sputum smear and failure to cover the mouth and nose when coughing. Further, environmental factors may increase the risk of TB transmission.

Over half of new cases of multidrug resistant (MDR)-TB arise in individuals who have not previously received treatment. This highlights the urgent need to prevent TB transmission. Administrative controls are crucial in mitigating the risk by identifying and isolating individuals who exhibit respiratory symptoms or signs of TB. Effective ventilation may be achieved by natural ventilation, mechanical ventilation, ultraviolet germicidal irradiation (UVGI) devices or filtration and other methods. Basic precautions such as hand hygiene, cough hygiene, cleaning and disinfection, waste management, and use of personal protective equipment (PPE) can minimize TB transmission. Whenever possible, effort should be done to treat MDR-TB cases at home. An initial period of isolation and treatment in a hospital is desirable in selected cases like extensive drug-resistant (XDR)-TB to reduce transmission. Rapid diagnosis of TB, MDR-TB, and XDR-TB with a clinical suspicion and rapid molecular and liquid culture tests is important to prevent the spread of TB from an index case into the community or family. Appropriate and effective treatment regimens devised for DRTB cases should be accordingly administered for the specific therapy duration.

This chapter discusses the mechanism of TB transmission, factors increasing the infectiousness of TB and progression to disease, comparison between drug-sensitive TB (DSTB) and DRTB transmission, prevention of transmission of TB and recommendations for specific healthcare settings such as airborne precaution room, MDR-TB ward, bronchoscopy room, and intensive care unit (ICU).

Keywords: Tuberculosis, transmission, prevention, TB, DRTB, air change per hour

INTRODUCTION

Airborne transmission of tuberculosis (TB) and drug-resistant TB (DRTB) is a significant health problem that not only tends to spread TB infection in the community and increases the TB burden, but also throws greater challenges to TB control especially with regard to DRTB cases. Hence, it is important to understand the mechanism of TB transmission, the propagating factors and the ways to prevent TB transmission in community including the specific healthcare settings which face greater likelihood of TB transmission.

MECHANISM OF TUBERCULOSIS TRANSMISSION

Tuberculosis (TB) is caused by the bacterium *Mycobacterium tuberculosis (M. tuberculosis).* The disease is infectious when it affects the lungs or larynx. Individuals with such infections can release numerous tiny particles called droplet nuclei into the air through coughing or sneezing, though smaller amounts can be released during normal activities like talking or breathing. These droplet nuclei, which are too small to be seen by the naked eye and measure approximately 1–5 μ,[1] can remain suspended in the air for extended periods. Anyone who shares air with an infectious person is at risk of contracting TB. About 2–12 weeks after being infected with *M. tuberculosis,* the immune system usually controls further bacterial growth, leading to a positive immunologic test result for *M. tuberculosis* infection. Some bacteria can persist in the body for many years, resulting in latent tuberculosis infection (LTBI). People with LTBI do not show symptoms and are not infectious. However, around 5–10% of those with LTBI who do not receive treatment may develop active TB disease during their lifetime,[2] with the highest risk of progression occurring in the first few years after infection.

Mycobacterium tuberculosis could be either susceptible to anti-TB treatment (ATT) or resistant to at least one or more of the drugs resulting in the development of DRTB. As compared to the drug susceptible TB, those with DRTB require more number of effective drugs tolerated by the patient for a specific-treatment duration.

RISK FACTORS OF TUBERCULOSIS INFECTION

An individual with active and untreated TB typically spreads the infection to around 10–15 people annually.[3] The likelihood of an individual becoming infected after exposure to *M. tuberculosis* is mainly determined by the concentration of infectious droplet nuclei present in the air and the length of time spent in contact with someone who has active TB disease. Increased proximity and extended exposure duration significantly elevate the risk of infection.

Close contacts or household contacts of a person with active TB are particularly at risk of contracting the disease from the case. Others, such as residents and employees in congregate settings like correctional facilities, long-term care facilities, and homeless shelters, as well as healthcare workers (HCWs) who are exposed to patients without protection, are also at high risk.[4]

RISK FOR PROGRESSION FROM LATENT TUBERCULOSIS INFECTION TO TUBERCULOSIS DISEASE

Individuals at higher risk of progressing from LTBI to active TB disease include those with HIV infection, infants, and children under 4 years old, and people with various immunocompromising conditions such as silicosis, diabetes mellitus, chronic renal failure, specific hematologic disorders (such as leukemia and lymphomas), certain malignancies (such as cancers of the head, neck, or lung), body weight that is 10% or more below the ideal weight, prolonged use of corticosteroids, immunosuppressive treatments [including tumor necrosis factor-α (TNF-α) antagonists], organ transplants, end-stage renal disease (ESRD), and individuals who have undergone intestinal bypass or gastrectomy.[4]

Individuals who use tobacco or alcohol or illicit drugs may also be at increased risk for infection and disease. HIV infection is the greatest risk factor for progression from latent TB to TB disease. Individuals with HIV who are severely immunocompromised and then become newly infected with *M. tuberculosis* face a higher risk of developing TB disease compared to those who are newly infected but do not have human immunodeficiency virus (HIV).[5]

CHARACTERISTICS OF TB PATIENTS THAT INCREASE THE RISK FOR INFECTIOUSNESS

The following characteristics increase the risk for infectiousness in TB patients:[4]

- Presence of a cough
- Cavitary lesions on a chest X-ray
- Positive acid-fast bacilli (AFB) in sputum smear
- Lung disease with involvement of the larynx
- Failure to cover the mouth and nose while coughing
- Incorrect use, lack of, or insufficient duration of antituberculosis treatment (ATT)
- Undergoing procedures that induce coughing or generate aerosols (such as bronchoscopy, sputum induction, or administration of aerosolized medications)

ENVIRONMENTAL FACTORS THAT INCREASE THE RISK OF TB TRANSMISSION

The risk of *M. tuberculosis* transmission is heightened by several environmental factors, including:[4]

- Exposure to TB in small and enclosed spaces
- Inadequate ventilation, either local or general, leading to insufficient dilution or removal of infectious droplet nuclei
- Recirculation of air that contains infectious droplet nuclei
- Insufficient cleaning and disinfection of medical equipment
- Improper handling of specimens

COMPARISON BETWEEN DRUG-SENSITIVE TUBERCULOSIS AND DRUG-RESISTANT TUBERCULOSIS TRANSMISSION

There is limited evidence for determining the mechanism and the risk factors of the spread of drug-sensitive (DS)-TB or drug-resistant (DR)-TB as well as of the differences in the rates of transmission between them. While untreated, both DS-TB and DR-TB appear to progress in the same manner.

Rapid diagnosis of TB, MDR-TB, and XDR-TB is important to prevent the spread of TB from an index case into the community or family. Delay in carrying out drug-susceptibility test (DST) in TB patients may result in transmission for months before they are identified as drug-resistant.[6]

In the 1950s, Richard Riley conducted classic experiments in Baltimore where patients with strongly positive smears and cavitary tuberculosis were connected via a ventilation system to 100s of sentinel guinea pigs housed in cages in the penthouse above the clinical ward. Out of 77 patients, only 3 were responsible for 35 of the 48 (73%) guinea pig infections observed. These infections occurred when patients with DRTB who were on inadequate therapy were admitted. In contrast, no guinea pig infections were recorded when drug-susceptible patients were admitted and started on treatment the same day. This demonstrated that starting treatment immediately upon admission was highly effective in preventing transmission, compared to the significant infectiousness observed in patients who were left untreated for a period to measure their infectivity.[7]

A DNA fingerprinting analysis of 55 MDR/XDR *M. tuberculosis* strains collected from TB patients across Japan in 2002 revealed that 21 (38%) of these strains were grouped into nine clusters with geographic connections, indicating ongoing community transmission of MDR/XDR-TB. Additionally, XDR *M. tuberculosis* strains were more likely to be clustered compared to non-XDR MDR strains (71% vs. 24%; $p = 0.003$), highlighting that transmission is a key factor in the rise of XDR-TB cases. These results underscore the urgent need for more effective strategies to control the spread of highly drug-resistant TB.[8]

Experiments have demonstrated that the development of drug resistance often results in a reduction in the fitness of disease-causing organisms. Fitness, which is determined by both virulence and transmissibility, has traditionally been thought by biologists to be lower in drug-resistant strains of *M. tuberculosis* compared to drug-susceptible strains. However, less fit bacteria can acquire additional mutations over time that may compensate for their initial fitness disadvantage. Furthermore, not all mutations that lead to drug-resistance impact fitness; some mutations can confer resistance without affecting the organism's overall fitness.[6]

Middlebrook and Cohn reported that isoniazid-resistant strains of tubercle bacilli were less pathogenic or avirulent in guinea pigs compared to the parent isoniazid-sensitive strains.[9] Similarly, Gagneux and colleagues found that laboratory strains of *M. tuberculosis* with mutations exhibited statistically significant fitness defects, although the impact varied by strain and mutation. In contrast, when drug-resistant strains from TB patients were compared to drug-susceptible strains from the same patients, some drug-resistant strains showed no loss in fitness. The authors suggested that these clinical strains might have acquired additional mutations over time that compensated for the initial fitness cost.[10]

Another study indicated that the prevalence of active TB among contacts of MDR or XDR-TB cases (3.4%) was similar to the overall prevalence of active TB among contacts of all TB cases (3.1%) in low- and middle-income countries.[11] However, a 3-year prospective cohort study conducted from 2010 to 2013 in South Lima and Callao, Peru, found that 35 out of 1,055 (3.3%) household contacts of 213 MDR-TB index cases developed TB, compared to 114 out of 2,362 (4.8%) household contacts of 487 drug-susceptible index cases. The hazard ratio for developing TB among MDR-TB contacts was half that for drug-susceptible contacts (hazard ratio: 0.56; 95% CI 0.34–0.90; $p = 0.017$). This study's findings suggest that the lower relative fitness of MDR-TB may facilitate control efforts, though the emergence of fitter MDR strains over time could complicate these efforts.[12] Further research is needed to clarify the fitness and transmissibility of drug-resistant and drug-susceptible TB strains.

PREVENTION OF DRUG-RESISTANT TUBERCULOSIS TRANSMISSION

Reports suggest that more than half of new MDR-TB cases occur in people who have not been treated previously.[13] Therefore, many new cases result from transmission, though some may result from poor management. Hence, there is a clear need to prevent transmission of DRTB.

Administrative controls: Administrative controls are crucial for minimizing the risk of TB transmission. They involve identifying individuals with respiratory or TB symptoms, isolating them in suitable environments (such as triage or well-ventilated screening areas), expediting their passage through the healthcare facility to limit exposure to others, and promptly diagnosing and treating them. Hospitalization should be minimized or avoided when possible. These administrative measures are fundamental for the effective implementation of other controls, including environmental controls and personal protective equipment.[1]

Environmental controls:[1] Choice of environmental control is variable. The basic principle is dilution of infectious particles through real or "effective" air exchange. Effective ventilation may be achieved by natural ventilation, mechanical ventilation, ultraviolet germicidal irradiation (UVGI) devices or filtration and other methods.

- *Natural ventilation:* It is created by the use of external natural forces such as wind and temperature and is the preferred method in most circumstances.

  Natural ventilation is "controlled" when openings are fixed and unrestricted (i.e., those that cannot be closed) on opposite sides of a room to maintain air flow at all times. It provides the most effective natural ventilation.
- *Mechanical ventilation:* Mechanical ventilation is achieved by using a supply (HVAC) or exhaust fan to facilitate air exchange and drive airflow. It operates by creating either negative or positive pressure within the room to promote air changes. For optimal performance, it is crucial that all doors and windows remain closed, allowing only controlled air leakage into or out of the space.

  Air conditioners should be avoided or used with great caution in patient's care areas. However, rooms equipped with air conditioning or heating can still achieve proper ventilation. **Figure 1** illustrates an air conditioner positioned away from the exhaust fan and near the door, allowing cooled air to circulate across the room. An exhaust fan, capable of providing the necessary air exchange, is installed on the opposite side. Adequate air intake is ensured by maintaining a few inches of clearance under the door to allow free movement of air into the room.

  Mechanical ventilation also encompasses "Mixed Mode ventilation," where exhaust and/or supply fans are combined with natural ventilation to ensure adequate air dilution when natural ventilation alone is insufficient.

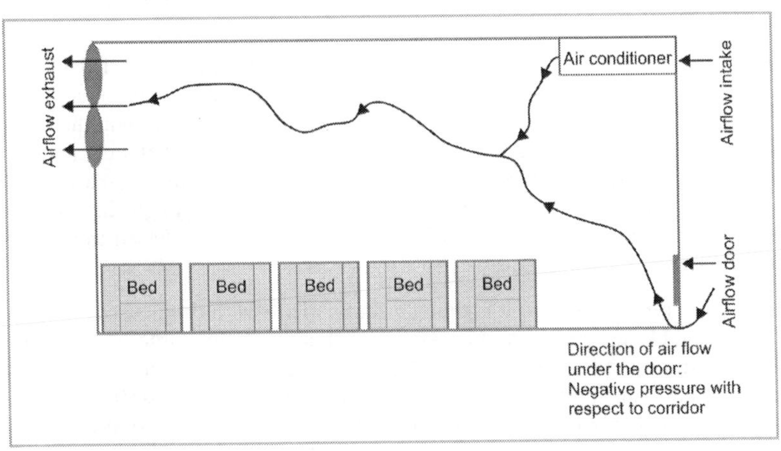

FIG. 1: Shows adequate air exchange in a room with air conditioning/heating.

In specific high-risk environments, such as airborne precaution rooms, MDR-TB wards and clinics, and bronchoscopy suites, it is advisable to implement directional control of airflow. This is particularly important for managing infectious patients with diseases like drug-resistant tuberculosis (DRTB) or other acute respiratory illnesses.

- *Ultraviolet germicidal irradiation (UVGI)[1]/GUV[14] devices:* The UVGI fixtures are properly designed, mounted on the wall or ceiling and create an upper room air disinfection zone. They eliminate the ability of microbes to replicate by inactivating both bacterial and viral DNA. UVGI is maximally germicidal at a wavelength of 254 nm. Good room air mixing between the upper and lower room allows effective disinfection of air in the lower breathing zone. Without proper air mixing, UVGI will continuously sterilize the same volume of air without mixing contaminated air with the sterilized air. To ensure safety, staff, and patients should be exposed to <6.0 mg/cm^2 of UVGI over an 8-hour period.[1]

  GUV is a contemporary term for UVGI, with the word "irradiation" omitted from the abbreviation to reduce concerns about ionizing radiation, which GUV does not involve. Upper-room GUV systems are engineered to produce high levels of ultraviolet-C (UVC) irradiance above the heads of room occupants, while minimizing UVC exposure in the lower, occupied areas of the room. These systems are appropriate for any environment with a high risk of *M. tuberculosis* transmission, especially in settings with a substantial burden of drug-resistant TB (DR-TB).[14]
- *Filtration with HEPA filters:* These systems are suitable for environments where natural ventilation is not feasible and where there is a high risk of TB transmission and morbidity, such as small spaces like bronchoscopy suites, laboratories, or individual TB patient's rooms. Only true-HEPA filters, which are rated to remove 99.97% of particles as small as 1 µ, should be utilized.

Standard precautions and personal protective equipment (PPE): Basic precautions such as hand hygiene (washing with soap or rubbing with alcohol-based formulation), cough hygiene (covering the mouth and nose during coughing with a tissue, or cloth, or a medical mask), cleaning and disinfection, waste management, and use of PPE (e.g., particulate respirators certified as N95 or FFP2, gloves, facial protection, and gowns) based on infection control assessment can minimize TB transmission.[1] Adequate infection control supplies, i.e., PPE, etc., should be available in high-risk situations, e.g., when dealing with DRTB, and during high-risk aerosol-generating procedures such as bronchoscopy or sputum induction.

Community-based MDR-TB treatment programs: Since treatment of MDR-TB cases in hospitals can be a risk factor for transmission, it is desirable that the time patients are in hospitals is minimized. Whenever possible, effort should be done to treat these cases at home, though hospital admission may be required in the initial part of their management or in the presence of complications or drug side-effects. Community-based MDR-TB treatment programs exist in different regions of the world, although they have raised concern about transmission. But, well-implemented community-based treatments can minimize the risk of transmission.

Isolation and initial treatment: It is thought that patients with drug-susceptible TB may be isolated for 14 days after commencement of treatment. This timeframe is informed by multiple studies dating back to the 1960s that examined the impact of chemotherapy on transmission. Smear and culture positivity are indicators of transmission risk before therapy starts but do not reflect transmission risk once treatment has commenced.[5] There is evidence that patient's infectiousness is abolished probably after less than 2 weeks of treatment. This abolition of infectiousness is different from "cure," which may take months, and from negative results of bacteriological examinations, direct and culture, which may take weeks.[15] Thus, based on these assumptions, a time period of 14 days may suffice for the abolition of infectiousness in drug-susceptible TB. However, the same may not be true in DRTB case management especially with regard to XDR-TB, which may take a longer time to abolish the infectiousness. Research can throw more light, however, an initial period of isolation and treatment in a hospital is desirable in selected cases like XDR-TB to reduce transmission.

Prompt diagnosis: Patients with unsuspected TB, whether drug-susceptible or drug-resistant, are the most likely to spread the infection to others. This is because they are not receiving treatment and may remain undiagnosed for days or weeks. It is essential that every TB case is diagnosed promptly followed by appropriate therapy so that transmission whether at home or in the hospital is reduced at earliest. It is even more important for DRTB cases, who require greater number of drugs for a longer duration and are at an increased risk of development of drug side-effects and disease complications. Therefore, clinical suspicion, bacteriological and radiological confirmation, and the use of rapid molecular tests such as CBNAAT/TRUNAAT, line probe assay (LPA) and *Mycobacterium* growth indicator tube (MGIT) culture can greatly help in a prompt DRTB diagnosis including the MDR or XDR-TB. The conventional solid culture and DST, which took 3–4 months in DRTB diagnosis, have been largely replaced with the rapid molecular and liquid culture tests for a prompt diagnosis, thus, paving the way for institution of a prompt and effective drug treatment.

Prompt treatment: Theoretically, if all drug-susceptible TB patients take their first-line drugs regularly till the completion of their treatments with good tolerance and no adverse effects, acquired drug resistance should not arise. However, that is not the usual case. Acquired drug resistance can arise due to improper prescriptions by the health providers or by drug intolerance or inadequate drug intake for the specified duration by the patient.

It is extremely important that a treatment regimen most likely to be effective, based on the past history of drug intake and the results of rapid tests (molecular or MGIT culture), is commenced at the earliest to halt further DRTB transmission. The initial period of treatment may be carried out during the isolation specially in cases of XDR-TB, while most other DRTB cases including MDR-TB can be treated within community. Appropriate addressal of drug side-effects and disease complications helps in the treatment adherence and its completion thereby ensuring no further transmission to the contacts.

Availability of diagnostics and drugs: In order to prevent transmission on account of a diagnostic delay or a treatment interruption due to want of any drug, the healthcare provider and the government must ensure a ready availability of the diagnostics and the drugs for a prompt diagnosis and treatment of DRTB cases in their areas. The supplies and the supply chain should be maintained.

Tuberculosis preventive treatment (TPT): All household contacts and close contacts of active cases of TB whether drug-susceptible or -resistant should be given TPT as per national guidelines to prevent transmission and development of any form of TB in them.

Training, health education, and counseling: There is a need to train the health workers, patients, and visitors in observation of infection control measures to decrease DRTB transmission. Health educators and counselors need to stress upon the patients to complete the course of treatment, ways to identify and address the adverse effects, observe cough hygiene and sputum disposal, use of masks, sputum testing at intervals, need for TPT to household and close contacts, etc.

Regular assessment of TB in healthcare workers (HCWs): All HCWs involved in management of TB patients including DRTB should be regularly assessed for development of TB in them

TABLE 1: Minimum air-change per hour (ACH) required for various healthcare settings.[1]

Healthcare setting	ACH
Registration areas	>6 ACH*
Outpatient departments and their waiting areas	>6 ACH
Inpatients departments	>6 ACH
• High-risk settings and their waiting areas • ART centers • TB/Chest departments (outpatient and inpatient) • Bronchoscopy procedure rooms • MDR-TB wards and clinics • Airborne precaution rooms	>12 ACH**

*Equivalent to >40 (L/s) for a 4 × 2 × 3 m (24 m^3) room.

**Equivalent to >80 (L/s) for a 4 × 2 × 3 m (24 m^3) room.

(MDR-TB: multidrug-resistant tuberculosis)

as they are at risk despite observing precautions. Timely TB detection can decrease further transmission.

SPECIFIC HEALTHCARE SETTINGS

National standards recommend following minimum air change per hour (ACH) according to the specific healthcare setting **(Table 1)**.

AIRBORNE PRECAUTION ROOM

Following recommendations should be followed for "airborne precaution rooms."[1]

- Put signage on the door.
- Ensure appropriate hand-washing facilities.
- Personal protective equipment (PPE) and other supplies should be available outside the room (i.e., in the change room).
- Room should be cleaned daily.
- Ensure appropriate room ventilation (>12 ACH).
- Ensure directional control of airflow, with air flow only entering the room when the door is open, and exhausted outside safely.
- Negative pressure "Ventilation," i.e., the pressure of the room should be maintained slightly less than the pressure of the entry area, so that air flows into the room when doors are open.
  - A negative pressure differential of >2.5 Pa (0.01-inch water gauge).
  - An airflow differential with exhaust exceeding supply by >125 ft^3/min (56 L/second).
  - Room sealing should permit no more than approximately 0.5 ft^2 (0.046 m^2) of leakage.
  - Air should be exhausted to the outside, or a HEPA filter should be used if the room air is being recirculated.

MULTIDRUG-RESISTANT TUBERCULOSIS WARD

Following are the recommendations for the MDR-TB Ward:[1]

- The MDR ward should be situated away from other wards and equipped with sufficient hand-washing facilities, along with rigorous maintenance and cleaning protocols.
- The ventilation system should ensure a minimum of 12 air changes per hour (ACH), ideally achieving >15 ACH.
- If these ventilation standards cannot be consistently met due to varying times of day or seasons, the use of UVGI can be considered as an alternative.
- There should be a minimum of 6 ft of space between adjacent beds to ensure adequate separation.
- Promote cough hygiene through visible signage and ensure adherence by training both patients and staff, with ongoing reinforcement from staff members.
- Sputum should be disposed of properly using individual containers with lids, filled with 5% phenol, for collection.
- All staff members must receive training on standard precautions, airborne infection control (AIC), and the correct use of personal respiratory protection.

BRONCHOSCOPY ROOM

Following are the recommendations for the bronchoscopy room:[1]

- Generally, bronchoscopy should be avoided unless essential clinical information cannot be obtained through less invasive methods.
- Steps should be taken to minimize the risk of exposure to healthcare personnel and other patients within or near the bronchoscopy room.
- The ventilation must be >15 ACH/hour. Air flow should be directional from room entrance to the back and outside. The room should have local exhaust ventilation that vents room air to the outside. Specific air cleaning methods such as UVGI or HEPA filtration may be installed.
- Judicious use of PPE and N5 respirator is needed by healthcare personnel involved in bronchoscopy and specimen handling.

INTENSIVE CARE UNIT

Following are the recommendations for ICU:[1]

- The ICU should establish airborne precaution rooms or areas, with air flowing into these areas and being exhausted out without recirculation. If air is recirculated back into the ICU, it must be decontaminated using HEPA filters.
- A minimum of 12 air changes/hour is recommended for ICU ventilation, though a higher rate may be preferable. Alternatively, a ventilation rate of 80 L/sec/patient should be achieved. Ventilation should be controlled (e.g., mixed-mode or mechanical) and may include air conditioning and/or special filtration.
- Ideally, each patient should have an individual cubicle with adequate space for the patient's bed and necessary equipment for critical and respiratory care. This setup helps to prevent nosocomial infections among other patients and staff in the ICU and simplifies disinfection after patient's discharge.
- Bacterial/viral filters should be installed on the exhalation valves of intubated patients and replaced regularly according to manufacturer's guidelines. Used filters should be disposed off properly, and ventilator tubing should be disinfected as recommended by the manufacturer.

- Proper disposal of respiratory secretions from suctioning mechanically ventilated patients, as well as used PPE, is essential.
- Visitor access should be limited.
- Healthcare workers should follow stringent precautions, including general hygiene practices like hand disinfection, while caring for ICU patients.
- For aerosol-generating procedures (e.g., nebulization, cardiopulmonary resuscitation, endotracheal intubation, manual ventilation, oral/airway suctioning, or bronchoscopy), N95 respirators should be used along with other PPE such as gloves, gowns, and goggles.
- Adequate supplies should be available for general hygiene (e.g., soap, running water, alcohol-based hand rubs, and disposable towels) and for cleaning and disinfecting patient beds and equipment at regular intervals. Sufficient personal protective equipment should also be ensured.

AIRBORNE INFECTION CONTROL SYSTEM IN COUNTRY[1]

National Guidelines on Airborne Infection Control have been formulated by the National Airborne Infection Control Committee (NAICC) which is a multilateral national level coordinating body and provides technical guidance to states. During regular meetings, the Committee monitors the implementation of these guidelines within the country.

The State Airborne Infection Control Committee (SAICC) acts as a coordinating body at the level of state and supervises the activities of the District Airborne Infection Control Committee (DAICC). The infection control activities at district level are undertaken by the Sub-committee of Biomedical Waste Management/Infection Control (SC-BWMIC) under guidance of District Health Society (DHS) and in coordination with the SAICC, State Health Society and the TB subcommittee under DHS.

Key functions of the committee in airborne infection control at district level are:
- *Dissemination and implementation:* Promote and execute the National Guidelines on Airborne Infection Control across healthcare and other relevant settings in the district. Advocate for and evaluate AIC practices at the facility level within the district.
- *Training and status review:* Provide training and conduct status reviews for facility administrators, supervisors, and healthcare providers on AIC modules.
- *Planning and evaluation:* Oversee the planning, preparation, implementation, supervision, monitoring, review, and evaluation of infection control measures at all facilities in accordance with national guidelines.
- *Risk assessment and recommendations:* Conduct risk assessments at facilities and develop technical recommendations for administrative, engineering, and architectural measures aimed at reducing the risk of respiratory infection transmission.
- *Effective tool utilization:* Ensure the effective use of tools to assess risk, identify straightforward solutions, and monitor the effectiveness of interventions designed to reduce airborne disease transmission in healthcare facilities.

CONCLUSION

In short, airborne transmission of TB and DRTB can be prevented by institution of administrative controls, placement of environmental controls, observation of personal precautions, use of rapid diagnostics and appropriate drugs in TB management and counseling of health staff and patients.

REFERENCES

1. Directorate General of Health Services, Ministry of Health and Family Welfare, Govt of India, New Delhi. (2010). Guidelines on Airborne Infection Control in Healthcare and Other Settings. [online] Available from chrome-extension://efaidnbmnnnibpcajpcglclefindmkaj/https://naco.gov.in/sites/default/files/Guidelines_on_Airborne_Infection_Control_April2010Provisional.pdf [Last accessed Sept., 2024].
2. CDC. Guidelines for preventing the transmission of *Mycobacterium tuberculosis* in healthcare facilities, 1994. MMWR. 1994;43(No. RR-13).
3. WHO. (2024). Tuberculosis. [online] Available from https://www.who.int/westernpacific/health-topics/detail/tuberculosis [Last accessed Sept., 2024].
4. Centers for Disease Control and Prevention. Guidelines for preventing the transmission of *Mycobacterium tuberculosis* in Health-Care Settings, 2005. MMWR. 2005;54(No. RR-17).
5. American Thoracic Society, CDC. Targeted tuberculin testing and treatment of latent tuberculosis infection. MMWR. 2000;49(No. RR-6).
6. National Academies of Sciences, Engineering, and Medicine. Preventing transmission of drug-resistant tuberculosis. In: National Academies of Sciences, Engineering, and Medicine. Facing the Reality of Drug-Resistant Tuberculosis in India: Challenges and Potential Solutions: Summary of a Joint Workshop by the Institute of Medicine, the Indian National Science Academy, and the Indian Council of Medical Research. Washington, DC: The National Academies Press; 2012. pp. 49-58.
7. Riley RL, Mills CC, Nyka W, Weinstock N, Storey PB, Sultan LU, et al. Aerial dissemination of pulmonary tuberculosis. A two-year study of contagion in a tuberculosis ward. Am J Epidemiol. 1959;142(1):3-14.
8. Murase Y, Kato S, Yamada H, Maeda S, Ohkado A, Mitarai S, et al. Clonal expansion of multidrug-resistant and extensively drug-resistant tuberculosis, Japan. Emerg Infect Dis. 2010;16(6):948-54.
9. Middlebrook G, Cohn ML. Some observations on the pathogenicity of isoniazid-resistant variants of tubercle bacilli. Science. 1953;118:297-9.
10. Gagneux S, Long CD, Small PM, Van T, Schoolnik GK, Bohannan BJ. The competitive cost of antibiotic resistance in *Mycobacterium tuberculosis*. Science. 2006;312(5782):1944-6.
11. Fox GJ, Barry SE, Britton WJ, Marks GB. Contact investigation for tuberculosis: a systematic review and meta-analysis. Eur Respir J. 2013;41:140-56.
12. Grandjean L, Gilman RH, Martin L, Soto E, Castro B, Lopez S, et al. Transmission of Multidrug-Resistant and Drug-Susceptible Tuberculosis within Households: A Prospective Cohort Study. PLoS Med. 2015;12(6):e1001843.
13. Nardell E, Dharmadhikari A. Turning off the spigot: Reducing drug-resistant tuberculosis transmission in resource-limited settings. Int J Tubercul Lung Dis. 2010;14(10):1233-43.
14. WHO. WHO Guidelines on tuberculosis infection prevention and control, 2019 update. Geneva: World Health Organization; 2019.
15. Rouillon A, Perdrizet S, Parrot R. Transmission of tubercle bacilli: The effects of chemotherapy. Tubercle. 1976;57(4):275-99.

CHAPTER

33

Problematic Issues in Implementation of Drug-resistant Tuberculosis Case Management

Shivani Pawar, Sanjay Rajpal, Kamal Chopra

Abstract

India grapples with a formidable public health crisis in the form of multidrug-resistant tuberculosis (MDR-TB). This drug-resistant variant poses a substantial threat to the nation's health infrastructure, necessitating urgent and comprehensive interventions. This chapter delves into the core challenges impeding effective MDR-TB management in India.

Keywords: Tuberculosis, multidrug resistance, challenges

HIGH PREVALENCE AND DIAGNOSTIC SHORTFALLS

India bears a disproportionate burden of multidrug-resistant tuberculosis (MDR-TB), with an estimated 119,000 cases, constituting approximately a quarter of the global incidence.[1-3] A significant impediment to effective control lies in the challenges faced at various levels.

The first challenge lies at the patient's end. Patient awareness of their symptoms and willingness to seek medical advice is the primary step required for early diagnosis. Lack of education, poor socioeconomic status, and stigma attached to TB are some of the common barriers to seeking health advice.[4]

Even when patients seek medical advice, they go to primary healthcare services or local private practitioners. There are issues at the level of healthcare providers in identifying presumptive drug-resistant TB suspects.

The scarcity of adequate diagnostic infrastructure, particularly the lack of widespread access to drug-susceptibility testing (DST), results in underdiagnosis. There is a lack of diagnostic facility in the private sector and a significant proportion of private practitioners are not aware of the free diagnostics under the National Tuberculosis Elimination Program (NTEP). In addition, there is a lack of knowledge about the interpretation of results of the various molecular results. All these factors lead to delays in crucial treatment initiation and thereby, contributing to the spread of the disease.

TREATMENT ADVERSITIES

The treatment regimen for MDR-TB is arduous, prolonged, and often associated with significant adverse effects. Patients endure a treatment course of at least 9 months in case of shorter oral regimen and 18–20 months in case of all oral longer regimen, of expensive drugs that frequently induce severe side effects. Ensuring continuous availability of these multiple drugs for all registered patients under the NTEP can face roadblocks.

The WHO regimen for MDR and extensively drug-resistant tuberculosis (XDR-TB) is only for the National TB programs and not for private practitioners. The newer antitubercular drugs such as bedaquiline, pretomanid, and delaminid are not available in the private sector. Hence, any patient started under the NTEP cannot be transferred to the private sector.

All these factors collectively contribute to poor treatment adherence, ultimately compromising treatment outcomes. Moreover, there is a likelihood that healthcare providers in the private sector are not well-versed or updated with the current regimen of drug-resistant tuberculosis (DR-TB) management.

HEALTHCARE SYSTEM DEFICIENCIES

The National Tuberculosis Elimination Program, while striving for universal access to TB care, encounters substantial challenges in its efforts to address MDR-TB. The scarcity of skilled healthcare professionals, specialized diagnostic laboratories, and essential second-line antituberculosis drugs severely hampers the capacity to deliver effective MDR-TB management.

Recording and reporting of drug-resistant cases is a challenge. As per the TB notification policy, all patients with TB are to be notified through Nikshay portal. However, integrating the private sector into this system is yet to be fully achieved.

CASCADING IMPACT OF POOR TUBERCULOSIS CONTROL

A substantial proportion of MDR-TB cases originate from the mismanagement of regular TB, underscoring the critical need for comprehensive improvements in overall TB care.

Strengthening primary TB prevention and treatment programs is essential for mitigating the emergence of drug resistance.

SOCIOECONOMIC AND BEHAVIORAL DETERMINANTS

Socioeconomic disparities, including poverty, malnutrition, and limited access to healthcare, exacerbate the vulnerability of populations to TB, including MDR-TB. Addressing these underlying social determinants is crucial for achieving sustained progress in TB control.

CONCLUSION

A multifaceted approach is imperative to effectively address the challenges posed by MDR-TB in India. Key strategies include:

- *Diagnostic enhancement:* Expanding access to rapid, accurate diagnostic tools, and ensuring widespread availability of DST services are fundamental for early case detection.
- *Therapeutic advancements:* Developing shorter, more tolerable, and effective treatment regimens is crucial for improving patient's outcomes and adherence.
- *Healthcare system strengthening:* Investing in the training of healthcare professionals, establishing well-equipped diagnostic laboratories, and ensuring a consistent supply of essential anti-TB drugs are essential for strengthening the healthcare response to MDR-TB.
- *Community engagement:* Empowering communities through health education, social support, and patient-centered care can significantly improve treatment outcomes and prevent the spread of MDR-TB.

- *Research and innovation:* Continued research and development are vital for discovering novel diagnostic tools, drugs, and vaccines, as well as optimizing treatment strategies.

By implementing these strategies, India can make significant strides in combating MDR-TB, reducing its devastating impact on public health, and ultimately achieving the goal of eliminating TB as a public health threat.

REFERENCES

1. Vishwakarma D, Gaidhane A, Sahu S, Rathod AS. Multi-Drug Resistant Tuberculosis (MDR-TB) Challenges in India: A Review. Cureus. 2023;15(12):e50222. National Center for Biotechnology Information. (2024). National Center for Biotechnology Information (NCBI) databases and resources on tuberculosis. [online] Available from https://www.ncbi.nlm.nih.gov/ [Last accessed Sept., 2024].
2. Mancuso G, Midiri A, De Gaetano S, Ponzo E, Biondo C. Tackling Drug-Resistant Tuberculosis: New Challenges from the Old Pathogen *Mycobacterium tuberculosis*. Microorganisms. 2023;11:2277.
3. Masini T, Furin J, Udwadia Z, Guglielmetti L. Optimal management of drug-resistant tuberculosis: Can India lead the way? Indian J Med Res. 2023;157(2-3):220-2.

CHAPTER 34

Multidrug Resistance in Tuberculosis: Contact Tracing and Isolation of Infected Individuals

Surya Kant, Ankit Kumar

Abstract

Contact tracing is crucial for the elimination of MDR-TB. It involves identifying and screening individuals who have been in close contact with an MDR-TB patient. This early detection helps to prevent latent TB from progressing to active disease and breaks transmission chains. Contact tracing significantly reduces TB transmission rates.

Isolation is another critical component in managing MDR-TB to prevent transmission. Effective isolation requires infection control measures, environmental controls like adequate ventilation, and healthcare worker protection.

Challenges in both contact tracing and isolation are resource constraints, associated stigma, logistical issues, adherence to protocols, and the psychosocial impact of prolonged isolation. Success stories, such as Mumbai's robust MDR-TB management strategy and Chennai's use of digital tools, highlight the effectiveness of these measures.

Strengthening of health systems, engaging communities, integrating digital technologies, addressing stigma, and providing support services for MDR-TB patients can reduce incidence of MDR-TB. By investing in health infrastructure, using technology, and addressing social determinants can significantly reduce the spread of MDR-TB.

Keywords: Multidrug resistant tuberculosis, contact tracing, isolation

INTRODUCTION

Multidrug-resistant tuberculosis (MDR-TB) is still a significant public health challenge of India and it poses greater threat due to its complex treatment regimens and higher mortality rates. The treatment for MDR-TB is lengthy with a combination of second-line drugs that are more toxic and less effective than first-line drugs. The emergence of MDR-TB is primarily due to incomplete, inappropriate, or irregular treatment of drug-susceptible TB. India has the highest burdens of tuberculosis (TB) and MDR-TB. According to the World Health Organization (WHO), there were an estimated 410,000 new cases of MDR-TB globally in 2022.[1] India targeted this goal to achieve by year 2025. The End-TB Strategy aims to reduce TB incidence by 80% and TB deaths by 90% for TB-affected households by 2030 that needs rigorous strategies for effective control and management.[2] Contact tracing and isolation in managing MDR-TB patients have shown their importance in preventing the spread of MDR-TB.[3]

IMPORTANCE OF CONTACT TRACING IN MULTIDRUG-RESISTANT TUBERCULOSIS

Contact tracing involves identifying and screening individuals who have been in close contact with an MDR-TB patient to detect and treat latent or active TB infection early. This strategy is crucial for following reasons:

- *Early detection and treatment:* Early identification of secondary cases prevents the progression of latent TB infection (LTBI) to active disease, thereby reducing the transmission risk.
- *Breaking the chain of transmission:* By identifying and treating contacts, the chain of transmission can be interrupted, preventing the spread of MDR-TB within communities.
- *Public health surveillance:* Contact tracing contributes to understanding the epidemiology of MDR-TB. It also helps public health authorities to implement targeted interventions.

STEPS IN CONTACT TRACING FOR MULTIDRUG-RESISTANT TUBERCULOSIS

1. *Index case identification:* The process begins with identifying the index case, which is the diagnosed MDR-TB patient. Detailed information about their contacts is gathered.
2. *Risk assessment:* Contacts are assessed based on their exposure level. Close contacts, such as household members, are prioritized.
3. *Screening and testing:* Contacts undergo screening using tuberculin skin tests (TST), interferon-γ-release assays (IGRAS), and chest radiographs. Symptomatic individuals are further evaluated with sputum smear microscopy, culture, and drug-susceptibility testing (DST).
4. *Follow-up and monitoring:* Contacts are followed up regularly to check for the development of TB symptoms and to ensure adherence to preventive therapy if needed.

Contact tracing has been reduced TB transmission rates significantly. The WHO End-TB Strategy emphasizes contact tracing as a key intervention for TB control, recommending that all close contacts of MDR-TB patients be systematically screened and managed accordingly.[2]

The National TB Elimination Program (NTEP) in India, formerly known as the Revised National TB Control Program (RNTCP), has integrated contact tracing into its strategy for managing TB and MDR-TB. This program has successfully traced and screened over 90% of household contacts of MDR-TB patients, leading to early detection and treatment of secondary cases.[4]

CHALLENGES IN CONTACT TRACING

- *Resource constraints:* Contact tracing is resource-intensive, requiring trained personnel, diagnostic tools, and follow-up mechanisms, which can be challenging in resource-limited settings.
- *Stigma and privacy concerns:* TB-related stigma may deter individuals from taking part in contact tracing efforts. Ensuring confidentiality and addressing stigma are crucial for effective contact tracing.
- *Logistical issues:* Tracking and monitoring contacts over extended periods can be logistically challenging, especially in high-burden settings.

ISOLATION OF MULTIDRUG-RESISTANT TUBERCULOSIS PATIENTS

Isolation is a critical part in the management of MDR-TB to prevent transmission to others. It involves separating individuals with active MDR-TB from those who are uninfected or susceptible.[5]

Types of Isolation

- *Home isolation:* When feasible, patients can be isolated at home with proper education on infection control measures such as ventilation, respiratory hygiene, and limiting close contact.
- *Hospital isolation:* In cases where home isolation is not possible, or patients need intensive care, hospital isolation in specialized wards with negative pressure rooms is recommended.
- *Community isolation centres:* These are designated facilities for isolating patients who cannot be managed at home or in hospitals, providing a controlled environment for treatment and infection control.

Implementation of Isolation Measures

- *Infection control measures:* Patients should be educated about infection control measures, including wearing masks, covering their mouth when coughing, and keeping personal hygiene.
- *Environmental controls:* Adequate ventilation, ultraviolet germicidal irradiation (UVGI), and high-efficiency particulate air (HEPA) filters should be used in isolation facilities to reduce the risk of airborne transmission.
- *Healthcare worker protection:* Healthcare workers should use personal protective equipment (PPE), including N95 respirators, and follow strict infection control protocols to prevent occupational exposure.

CHALLENGES IN ISOLATION

- *Adherence to isolation:* Ensuring patient adherence to isolation protocols can be challenging, particularly in socioeconomically disadvantaged settings.
- *Resource availability:* Establishing and keeping isolation facilities require significant resources, including infrastructure, equipment, and trained personnel.
- *Psychosocial impact:* Prolonged isolation can have a significant psychosocial impact on patients, needing support services to address mental health and social needs.
- Case studies and success stories.

THE MUMBAI MODEL

Mumbai implemented an aggressive MDR-TB management strategy that included robust contact tracing and isolation protocols. The Brihanmumbai Municipal Corporation (BMC) employed a multidisciplinary approach involving healthcare workers, community volunteers, and public health officials. The strategy resulted in improved detection rates and better treatment outcomes, highlighting the effectiveness of rigorous contact tracing and isolation measures.[6]

THE CHENNAI INITIATIVE

Chennai's TB control program incorporated digital tools for contact tracing and monitoring. Using a mobile application, healthcare workers could efficiently track contacts, schedule follow-ups, and update patient's records in real-time. This technological integration enhanced the accuracy and efficiency of contact tracing, contributing to the program's success in managing MDR-TB.[7]

CONCLUSION

Contact tracing and isolation are indispensable components in the fight against MDR-TB, especially in high-burden countries like India. The successful implementation of these measures is vital for controlling the spread of MDR-TB and ensuring better health outcomes for affected populations. The spread of MDR-TB can be significantly control by identifying and ensuring the effective isolation of infected individuals. However, these efforts require a coordinated approach involving healthcare systems and communities. Investing in robust health infrastructure, using technology, and addressing social determinants are crucial for the success of MDR-TB control programs. These collaborated efforts pave the way for a healthier and TB-free future.

REFERENCES

1. WHO. (2023). Global tuberculosis report 2023. [online] Available from https://iris.who.int/ [Last accessed Sept., 2024].
2. WHO. (2014). Global Tuberculosis Programme. [online] Available from https://www.who.int/teams/global-tuberculosis-programme/the-end-tb-strategy [Last accessed Sept., 2024].
3. Kant S, Maurya AK, Kushwaha RAS, Nag VL, Prasad R. Multi-drug resistant tuberculosis: An iatrogenic problem. Biosci Trends. 2010;4(2):48-55.
4. Ministry of Health and Family Welfare, Govt. of India. (2023). India Tb report 2023. [online] Available from https://tbcindia.mohfw.gov.in/ [Last accessed Sept., 2024].
5. WHO. WHO guidelines on tuberculosis infection prevention and control: 2019 update. [online] Available from https://www.ncbi.nlm.nih.gov/books/NBK539291/ [Last accessed Sept., 2024].
6. Arinaminpathy N, Deo S, Singh S, Khaparde S, Rao R, Vadera B, et al. Modelling the impact of effective private provider engagement on tuberculosis control in urban India. Sci Rep. 2019;9(1):1-9.
7. WHO. Chennai accelerates multi-pronged action to end TB. [online] Available from https://www.who.int/india/news/feature-stories/detail/chennai-accelerates-multi-pronged-action-to-end-tb [Last accessed Sept., 2024].

CHAPTER

35

Multidrug-resistant Tuberculosis: Infection Prevention and Control Measures in Healthcare Settings

Pratibha Narang

Abstract

The world has committed to the United Nation and World Health Organization (WHO) goals of ending tuberculosis (TB) epidemic by 2030. However, the same is not possible without strict institution of infection prevention and control (IPC) strategies across all approaches, especially in healthcare settings where the risk of transmission of *Mycobacterium tuberculosis* is high. Since TB is an airborne disease and patients with multidrug resistant TB (MDR-TB) remain infectious for much longer time even after initiation of treatment and carry high mortality rate with them, understanding the importance and implementation of these strategies by all concerned becomes all the more imperative. This chapter very briefly sums up the latest national and WHO IPC guidelines as advocated under the three hierarchy levels for TB and Programmatic Management of Drug-resistant TB (PMDT). The guidelines for drug sensitive TB (DS-TB) form the baseline for prevention of MDR-TB and the same have to be followed more stringently especially in special situations such as the MDR-TB wards and directly observed treatment short course (DOTS)-plus centers.

Keywords: MDR-TB, transmission, prevention, strategies, hierarchy levels

INTRODUCTION

Tuberculosis (TB) has always remained a major public health problem and today next to COVID-19 it is the leading cause of death from a single infectious agent despite being preventable and usually curable.[1] Like COVID, TB is an airborne disease and the causative agent *Mycobacterium tuberculosis* is carried in the airborne particles called droplet nuclei that are generated from a person with active pulmonary or laryngeal TB diseases while talking, coughing, sneezing, shouting, or singing. These particles are approximately between 1 and 5 μm in size and can remain suspended in the air for prolonged period. Inhalation of these particles can lead to disease in uninfected persons in the room. Droplets bigger than 5 μm settle down faster near the infected person and are less likely to reach the alveoli and infect others. This basic knowledge forms the principal understanding behind the institution of infection prevention and control (IPC) measures in healthcare settings, i.e., across any establishment that is engaged in direct patient care on site including home care where the risk of transmission is high.[2] It also include home setting. The purpose of

IPC practices is vital toward reduction in concentration of infectious droplet nuclei in the air and minimizing the exposure time of the aerosols to susceptible individuals. TB patients are most infectious when they are untreated or inadequately treated like undiagnosed drug-resistant (DR) cases.

PURPOSE AND SCOPE OF THE CHAPTER

An increasing challenge to public health is to prevent and control the transmission of drug resistant strains of *M. tuberculosis* which cause higher mortality compared to drug sensitive (DS) *M. tuberculosis* strains and are more difficult to treat. According to World Health Organization (WHO) estimates, in 2022 globally, there were 410,000 people [95% uncertainty interval (UI): 370,000–450,000] who developed multidrug resistant TB (MDR-TB) or rifampicin-resistant TB (RR-TB) and only two out of five who needed could actually be put on treatment.[1] This chapter is being written to give an update on IPC of MDR-TB in healthcare settings. However, evidence suggests that transmission of DR-TB is no different from DS-TB. Earlier it was thought that the resistant strains have lower transmissibility; however, it is now clear that globally DR-TB is sustained not through acquired resistance but through transmission of primary-resistant strains. Thus, infection control policies and strategies in both the cases are not much different and all facilities dealing with DR-TB must strictly and vigilantly follow and implement the standard airborne infection control measures set for DS-TB;[2-4] in fact, all symptomatic for TB, for the purpose of IPC, should be considered as MDR-TB suspects till the investigations prove otherwise.

Initial WHO global recommendations on the implementation of IPC for TB were published between 1999[5] and 2009.[6] After 10 years, in 2019,[2] these guidelines were updated and are still relevant in practice though in 2022 they were formatted into a module with no change.[7]

The Indian guidelines for IPC in TB were published in 2010[3] which hold good for MDR-TB as well and passing reference to them is made in Programmatic Management of Drug-resistant TB (PMDT) guidelines of 2017.[8] The PMDT guidelines of 2021[4] give the protocol in more detail for special areas such as the TB laboratory and MDR-TB wards. These guidelines apply to all healthcare facilities and high-risk areas which include outpatient departments (OPDs) and in patient departments where TB patients are hosted and seen, directly observed treatment short course (DOTS)-plus sites, microscopic centers, antiretroviral treatment (ART) centers, bronchoscopy suites, TB culture laboratories, intensive care unit (ICU) and operation theatres. This chapter gives an overview of the present ongoing accepted recommendations (readers are advised to refer to the above references for details). Since TB is an airborne disease these IPC measures should be implemented along with the national guidelines on standard precautions which also include universals precautions, body substance isolation, and airborne precautions for transmission of pathogens in health facilities.[9]

MEASURES FOR INFECTION PREVENTION AND CONTROL

The WHO guidelines on IPC in all healthcare settings[2,7] and national guidelines including DR-TB[3,4] recommend having an integrated implementation control plans at three levels of hierarchy. If these are implemented systematically and objectively in that order, it can minimize the risk of *M. tuberculosis* transmission by reducing the concentration of infectious droplet nuclei in the air and the exposure of such aerosols to susceptible individuals.

The hierarchy comprises of *administrative controls, environmental controls, and respiratory protection with personal protective equipment (PPE).*

Administrative Controls

These are the first and most important level in the hierarchy. They consist of management measures that are intended to reduce the risk of exposure from persons with infectious TB and are essential for the implementation of other two controls, i.e., (1) environmental controls and (2) PPE. However, IPC is complete only after all three are implemented as a package.

Policies and Protocols

First and foremost, administrators at all levels must show political commitment and leadership. Managerial activities should be taken up by national, state, hospital, and local authorities. The major responsibility of those in administrative control of the facility is to protect their healthcare workers (HCWs) and the patients attending the facility from acquiring TB. The HCWs are defined as all people in the health sector and other sectors, public or private, whose main activities are patient-care oriented such as doctors, nurses, pharmacists, laboratory technicians, and the support staff such as cleaners. Risk assessment should be made regarding TB transmission to both HCWs and patients, including those who are human immunodeficiency virus (HIV) positive, by identifying the number of TB patients attending the facility and time spent by them in different areas. Based on the assessment comprehensive budgeted infection control policies should be formulated, and within the existing hospital infection control team that takes care of infections for all purposes[9] a strong infection control officer, well trained in TB control, should be assigned the responsibility for implementation, enforcement, and evaluation of the policies including those for MDR-TB.

The main stress of IPC should be to identify persons with respiratory symptoms, separate them into appropriate environment, fast-track them through the healthcare facility to reduce exposure time to others, and diagnose/treat them with minimal delay. Hospitalization should be reduced or avoided to the greatest extent possible.

Training and Education

Educational programs regarding TB disease, its signs and symptoms, transmission, interaction between HIV and TB, should be organized for HCWs at regular intervals. The HCWs should also be trained for standard universal precautions, air borne infection control, use of PPE, and importance of educating the patients to follow the same including respiratory hygiene and cough etiquettes. HCWs should follow the standard policies regarding disinfection, linen management, and disposal of waste.[4,9]

Surveillance

Administrative control must consider performing site surveillance of HCWs for active TB disease and screening for latent TB infection (LTBI). Those with LTBI should be offered TB prophylaxis treatment (TPT) depending on the exposure whether DS-TB or DR-TB.[4] They should also provide HIV screening and regulate the posting of HIV-positive workers in areas with less exposure. Both HIV and LTBI positive persons should be kept on follow-up and treated appropriately when detected with latent or active infection.

Maintenance

It is also the responsibility of the administrators to evaluate the use of current facilities and institute renovation or development of new spaces as required.

Patient Care and Support Measures

Administrative control measures also include triaging of people with signs and symptoms of TB, or with TB disease. Such patients should be separated and taken up for sputum testing preferably with rapid molecular methods such as cartridge-based nucleic acid amplification test (CBNAAT) or Truenat and line probe assay (LPA). Those found to be MDR cases should be separated from other patients, including from DS patients, as transmission can occur between groups.

Patients with suspected or confirmed TB should be educated about respiratory hygiene and cough etiquette at the time of triage. They should be instructed to turn their heads and cover their mouths and nose during breathing, coughing, or sneezing. They can be provided with surgical masks, tissues, or cloths and if nothing is available they should use their sleeve, fixed elbow, or hand to reduce the dispersal of respiratory secretions.

The MDR-TB patients remain infectious for a long time even when put on treatment, and therefore they need frequent counseling to ensure adherence to treatment, cough etiquettes, and mask. The HCWs or family members have to be more cautious, HIV-positive persons should avoid attending to these patients and children, if in the household, should be asked to stay away. They should be followed up regularly for TB screening.

Environmental Controls

This *second level* of the hierarchy in control is to prevent the spread of infectious droplet nuclei by reducing their concentration in the air. The choice of method for the purpose is largely determined by local factors and resources. Effective ventilation may be achieved by natural ventilation where possible. In high-risk settings where optimal ventilation cannot be achieved through natural or mechanically aided means, properly designed, placed, and maintained shielded ultraviolet (UV) germicidal irradiation devices should be considered as a complementary control.

Types of ventilations used may be natural, mixed-mode, or mechanical ventilation with recirculated air through high-efficiency particulate air (HEPA) filters. Regardless of the type of ventilation system, design should seek to achieve airflow from the source of potential contamination to air exhaust points or to areas away from other patients that allows for sufficient air dilution. Particular attention should be paid to high-risk transmission areas such as TB chest OPD and TB wards, ART unit, bronchoscopy and procedure areas, sputum collection areas, and MDR-TB wards where the air changes per hour (ACH) should be >12.

Natural ventilation systems are used in resource-limited situations and where the climatic conditions permit opening of large windows and doors for cross ventilation. The direction of air flow should be kept in mind to avoid contamination of surrounding areas. Natural ventilation should be "controlled", with fixed, unrestricted openings (i.e., those that cannot be closed) that are insensitive to climactic conditions. Openings should constitute >20% of floor area and should be on two sides, preferably opposite sides. If constructed properly natural ventilation may provide better ventilation than rooms with mechanical ventilation. Using skylights or vents just under the ceilings also improve cross ventilation.

Mixed mode ventilation systems including exhaust fans on the windows may be used. If these fans are well-designed, scientifically fitted, maintained, and operated, they can improve ventilation and air mixing.

Closed mechanical ventilation uses equipment that manages the air flow so that the contaminated air is exhausted outside away through the HEPA filters before it is recirculated. HEPA filters remove 99.9% of particles ≥ 0.3 μm in size. *M. tuberculosis* droplet nuclei are between 1 μm and 5 μm in size and therefore are removed by filtration.

If feasible airborne infection isolation (AII) rooms can be designed with negative pressure so that air flows from the corridor into the room where TB patients are stationed and not in the reverse direction. Such rooms should be mechanically ventilated to a minimum of 12 ACH.

The use of germicidal ultraviolet (GUV) systems to reduce *M. tuberculosis* transmission to health workers in high-risk settings such as DR-TB wards, if affordable, has also been recommended.[2,4] This system inactivates airborne droplet nuclei and kills the surface organisms by irradiation. The two most common forms of GUV system are (1) the upper room irradiation and (2) duct irradiation. In upper room air irradiation, UV lights are shielded and directed toward the ceiling away from patients to reduce the risk of skin and eye toxicity while providing germicidal benefit. Well-designed GUV upper room systems can disinfect mycobacteria or surrogate organisms in a test room equivalent to 10–20 ACH. Duct irradiation is used to disinfect air exhausted from TB isolation rooms. These systems are potentially hazardous if not installed correctly, so need to be designed and installed by well-qualified engineers and technicians.

RESPIRATORY PROTECTION WITH PERSONAL PROTECTIVE EQUIPMENT

It is the *third level* of the hierarchy. It consists of the use of PPE in situations that pose a high risk of exposure to *M. tuberculosis*. PPE (e.g., particulate respirators certified as N95 or FFP2) should be available to HCWs as is required in high-risk situation especially when dealing with drug-resistant TB, during high-risk aerosol-generating procedures such as bronchoscopy or sputum induction and in the mycobacteriology laboratories and DR-TB wards. The N95 respirator has filter efficiency level of 95% or greater against particulate aerosols free of oil when tested against a 0.3 μm particles. The "N" means "Not resistant to oil". The FFP2 respirator has filter efficiency level of 94% or greater against 0.4 μm particles and is tested against oil and nonoil aerosol. These respirators when worn should be properly fitted with tight facial seal.

Surgical masks should be worn by the TB patients to reduce the number of infectious particles in the air, but they have only 50% filter efficiency and lack tight facial seal. They, therefore, should not be used by HCWs in place of N95 masks.

RECOMMENDATIONS FOR MDR-TB WARDS

The MDR-TB wards should be located away from other wards with proper hygiene facilities[4] and should have adequate ventilation (natural and/or assisted ventilation) to ensure >12 ACH, preferably 15 ACH, at all times. GUV should be used whenever feasible. Space between two adjacent beds should be at least 6 feet. All the staff of the MDR-TB ward should be trained in Universal Workplace Precaution, Waste segregation and disposal and Air borne Infection Control Practices, with special reference to TB and in the use of N95 particulate respirators. Avoid posting immunosuppressed staff. Cough hygiene and wearing of surgical masks by the patients should be promoted through trained HCWs and practice ensured through signage. For sputum disposal, the patients should be educated to spit directly into the container provided with lid containing 5% phenol. The sputum should then be disposed of as per the infection control guidelines. Visitors should be restricted to the greatest extent practical.

CONCLUSION

Tuberculosis still remains a major cause of morbidity and mortality amongst all the preventable infectious diseases and MDR-TB has added fuel to the fire. Elimination of this disease is not possible unless IPC measures are instituted to prevent its transmission from an infected person to a susceptible individual, and efforts more stringent than otherwise are needed in healthcare settings where the HCWs are constantly exposed to such patients; and in facilities where individuals in immunocompromised state are readily available. There are studies that have demonstrated distinct positive effect of IPC measures in curtailing the transmission of infection to HCWs in their facilities.[10,11] Institution of IPC norms as advocated in the order of hierarchy can surely achieve this goal. Though MDR-TB presents significant challenges, IPC practices for MDR-TB do not differ much from DS-TB but the advocated precautions should be followed more strictly. Committed adherence to infection prevention and control measures offers a tangible path toward reducing transmission and potentiating elimination of TB in healthcare settings. Worldwide allegiance toward implementing these protocols would certainly be critical in achieving this target.

REFERENCES

1. WHO. (2023). Global tuberculosis report 2023. [online] Available from https://www.who.int/teams/global-tuberculosis-programme/tb-reports/global-tuberculosis-report-2023 [Last accessed September, 2024].
2. World Health Organization. (2019). WHO Guidelines on Tuberculosis Infection Prevention and Control: 2019 Update. [online] Available from https://iris.who.int/handle/10665/311259 [Last accessed September 2024].
3. Directorate General of Health Services, Ministry of Health & Family Welfare. (2010). Airborne infection control healthcare and other settings: in the context of tuberculosis and other airborne infections. [online] Available from https://naco.gov.in/sites/default/files/Guidelines_on_Airborne_Infection_Control_April2010Provisional.pdf [Last accessed September, 2024].
4. National TB Elimination Program, Central TB Division, Ministry of Health & Family Welfare, Govt. of India. (2021). Guidelines for Programmatic Management of Drug Resistant Tuberculosis in India-2021. [online] Available from https://tbcindia.mohfw.gov.in/wp-content/uploads/2023/05/8368587497Guidelines-for-PMDT-in-India-1.pdf [Last accessed September, 2024].
5. WHO. (1999). Guidelines for the prevention of tuberculosis in health care facilities in resource-limited settings. [online] Available from https://www.who.int/publications/i/item/WHO-TB-99.269 [Last accessed September, 2024].
6. WHO. (2009). WHO policy on TB infection control in health-care facilities, congregate settings and households. [online] Available from https://www.who.int/publications/i/item/9789241598323 [Last accessed September, 2024].
7. WHO. (2022). WHO consolidated guidelines on tuberculosis: Module 1: Prevention - infection prevention and control. [online] Available from https://www.who.int/publications/i/item/9789240055889 [Last accessed September, 2024].
8. WHO. Guidelines for Programmatic Management of Tuberculosis Preventive Treatment in India. India: Ministry of Health & Family Welfare, Govt. of India; 2017.
9. Ministry of Health & Family Welfare, Govt. of India. (2020). National Guidelines for Infection Prevention Control in Healthcare Facilities. [online] Available from https://cdn.who.int/media/docs/default-source/searo/india/antimicrobial-resistance/ipcguidelines-web-sep2020.pdf?sfvrsn=9e77fcb0_2 [Last accessed September, 2024].
10. Azeredo ACV, Holler SR, de Almeida EGC, Cionek OAGD, Loureiro MM, Freitas AA, et al. Tuberculosis in Health Care Workers and the Impact of Implementation of Hospital Infection-Control Measures. Workplace health & safety. 2020;68(11):519-25.
11. Maloney SA, Pearson ML, Gordon MT, Del Castillo R, Boyle JF, Jarvis WR. Efficacy of control measures in preventing nosocomial transmission of multidrug-resistant tuberculosis to patients and health care workers. Annals of internal medicine, 1995;122(2):90-5.

CHAPTER

36

Importance of Prevention, Early Diagnosis, and Adherence to Treatment: Latent and Subclinical TB

Kranti Garg, Kamal Chopra

Abstract

The spectrum of tuberculosis (TB) is shifting from a binomial model of latent TB and TB disease, to a multistaged process. With advances in the understanding of the disease trajectory, it is important to identify the different stages of the disease and treat accordingly.

Efforts should be made to identify and treat latent TB infection/TB infection (TBI) in the high-risk groups as per Programmatic Management of TB Preventive Treatment in India. TB preventive treatment (TPT) acts as a barrier preventing progression of infection to disease, and shall help in achieving the goal to eliminate TB. At the same time, active TB disease should be diagnosed by passive and active case finding, and treated as per recommendations. The National TB Prevalence Survey in India (2019–2021) has highlighted the importance of diagnosing subclinical TB (scTB) as well, and prioritizing chest X-rays in asymptomatic individuals.

Early diagnosis and adherence to treatment in patients remain a challenge for the healthcare workers (HCWs). The acceptance for treatment is deemed to be even poorer in patients with TBI/scTB, as they are "otherwise well", and difficult to be motivated for long duration of treatment. Such roadblocks need to be taken care of, under the program, at the community level, with sensitization of the HCWs and general public. Reallocation of resources may be needed, as newer diagnostics and treatment strategies are being developed to prevent, identify, and treat TB at different stages.

Keywords: Latent TB, subclinical TB, TB preventive treatment

INTRODUCTION

Latent tuberculosis infection (LTBI) is a state of persistent immune response to stimulation by *Mycobacterium tuberculosis* antigens with no evidence of clinically manifest TB disease. "LTBI" term has been replaced nowadays with TB infection (TBI).[1] Individuals are asymptomatic, but at risk of developing TB disease.

Subclinical TB (scTB) is the presence of TB disease due to viable *M. tuberculosis* bacteria that does not cause clinical TB-related symptoms but causes other abnormalities that can be detected using existing radiologic or microbiologic assays.[2] The patients, being asymptomatic do not approach healthcare facilities for evaluation or treatment. They are negative on 4S (cough, night sweats, fever, and weight loss) screening, act as a reservoir, and are highly unlikely to be tested for TB.

Thus, TBI and scTB represent two of the four proposed states of TB including TBI, incipient infection, scTB, and active disease, the model which has replaced the binary paradigm of TB. TBI and scTB represent a potential barrier to TB elimination efforts.

India has the highest estimated burden of TBI globally, with nearly 35–40 crores individuals having TBI. It has been found that 5–10% of those infected develop TB disease during their lifetime, majority developing within first 2 years of initial infection.[1] The National TB Prevalence Survey in India (2019–2021) has found the prevalence of TBI in population aged ≥ 15 years as 21.7%. It has also provided rough estimates of scTB and revealed that 42.6% the TB cases diagnosed in the survey were asymptomatic and would have been missed if chest radiographs were not included.[3]

It is assumed that the traditional TB control measures may reduce the prevalence of symptomatic TB disease, but not TBI or scTB. As a part of TB preventive efforts, besides a focus on infection control measures, Government of India has come up with Programmatic Management of TB Preventive Treatment in India, and has centered its attention on preventing the TB "infected" individuals from progressing to TB disease. Before any patient is administered TB preventive treatment (TPT), active TB is ruled out, and TBI is recognized. Strengthening of the existing healthcare system is required to identify and rule out scTB as well, before any patient is started on TPT. The National TB Prevalence Survey in India (2019–2021) has also suggested that National TB Elimination Program (NTEP) should prioritize the use of chest X-rays in the program wherever possible.[3]

DIAGNOSTIC MODALITIES AND ADHERENCE TO TREATMENT

Programmatic Management of TB Preventive Treatment in India has listed the need for identifying TBI in high-risk groups (HRGs), and includes household contacts (HHCs), close contacts (CCs), people living with human immunodeficiency virus (HIV) (PLHIV), and patients on immunosuppressive therapy, having silicosis, on antitumor necrosis factor (TNF) treatment, on dialysis or preparing for organ or hematologic transplantation. Mapping out of high TB transmission settings (healthcare workers, prisons, mines, slums, tribal, migrant laborer's, etc.), has also been suggested. There has been a focus on integrating screening for TBI into various entry points for care such as antiretroviral therapy (ART) centers; maternal and child health, immunization, well baby, and nutrition clinics; cancer clinics and radiotherapy units; dialysis units; and transplant set-ups. Every effort is made to investigate for active TB, if the individual has any of the symptoms suggestive of TB disease. After ruling out active TB disease, and in those individuals who are asymptomatic, testing for TBI by interferon gamma release assay/tuberculin skin test (IGRA/TST) is done.[1,4,5] TPT is initiated in TBI "positive". In cases of nonavailability of TBI tests (IGRA/TST) or chest radiographs, TPT is still offered.[1]

The National TB Prevalence Survey has already advocated prioritizing the use of chest X-rays under the program wherever possible.[3] There is a need to escalate the availability of mobile X-ray units for population at large, for helping screen for scTB. Advanced radiological and microbiological assays at specialized settings should be made available, along-with a robust mechanism of obtaining and transporting the samples from the "asymptomatic" with scTB, for early diagnosis and management. scTB should also be considered as a differential while screening for TBI in HRGs and at various entry points for care. **Table 1** enumerates some of the diagnostic tools which aid in identifying TBI and scTB. A combination of two or more tools may be required to reach at a final diagnosis.[4,5]

Diagnosis and differentiation between TBI, scTB, and active TB disease at an early stage will help in administration of appropriate treatment. **Table 2** summarizes the differences in TBI, scTB, and active TB disease.

TABLE 1: Diagnostic tools which aid in identifying TB infection and subclinical TB.

TB infection	Subclinical TB

Skin tests:
• TST (RT23 PPD or PPD-S)
• ESAT 6 and CFP-10 based:
  ○ Cy-Tb (Serum Institute of India)
  ○ Diaskin test
  ○ C-TST (EC Skin test)
	Chest X-ray:
	• AI CAD (computer-aided detection using artificial intelligence) interpretation of chest radiography

IGRAs: • QuantiFERON®-TB GIT • QuantiFERON®-TB Gold Plus • T-SPOT®-TB • Beijing Wantai's TB-IGRA	Sputum smear microscopy
Novel approaches: • Host derived biomarkers • MTB derived biomarkers • Clinical and epidemiological scoring • Face mask sampling	Mycobacterial culture
	Xpert MTB/RIF
	Xpert MTB/RIF ultra
	MTB nucleic acid detection in oral mucosa and stool
	MTB proteins and metabolites in urine: • Urinary lipoarabinomannan (LAM) • FDG PET combined with CT imaging (PET/CT)

(FDG: fludeoxyglucose-18; IGRA: interferon gamma release assay; MTB: *Mycobacterium tuberculosis*; PET: positron emission tomography; PPD: purified protein derivative; RIF: rifampicin; TB: tuberculosis; TST: tuberculin skin test)

TABLE 2: Differences in TB infection, subclinical TB and active TB disease.

	TB infection	Subclinical TB	TB disease
TST	Positive	Positive	Usually positive
IGRA	Positive	Positive	Usually positive
Culture	Negative	Intermittently positive	Positive
Sputum smear	Negative	Usually negative	Positive/Negative
Infectious	No	Sporadically	Yes
Symptoms	None	None	Mild-to-severe
Preferred treatment	Preventive treatment	Multidrug therapy	Multidrug therapy

(IGRA: interferon gamma release assay; TB: tuberculosis; TST: tuberculin skin test)

Many a times, with the available diagnostics, it may not be possible to differentiate between the three different entities, and between recently acquired and old infections. Diagnostic tests lack reference standards and validity, and risks of false positives and negatives cannot be eliminated. Above all, progression to TB disease at any particular stage cannot be predicted.

The TPT can take care of TBI, however, it can turn hazardous for scTB and TB disease in the long run. It is unconfirmed whether scTB is a precursor of full-blown active TB disease, and can be treated differently with lesser number of drugs than the standard regimens. Till then, scTB and TB disease need to be treated with multidrug therapy in a similar manner. Infectiousness of TB from asymptomatic "scTB" patients is also not very clear, however, early diagnosis and adequate treatment are necessary to break the chain of transmission and eliminate the reservoir of infection and disease.

Preferences for treatment in "otherwise well" individuals need to be noted. A lot of counseling and motivation is required to convince patients for taking TPT or antitubercular treatment for a period of 6 months, as they are asymptomatic (TBI and scTB). Emphasis on adherence to the prescribed treatment is a must, lest the patients leave the medications in between, leading on to development of drug-resistant strains. Sensitization and training of healthcare workers, as they gradually move away from a "one size fits all" strategy to individualized patient-centered approaches is also of paramount importance. Various digital advances, particularly in patients with comorbidities, can be of immense help in monitoring adherence on a large scale, and easing the already overburdened healthcare system.

CONCLUSION

We need to differentiate between TBI, scTB, and TB disease early, at the point of diagnosis itself as far as possible, administer appropriate treatment regimens and ensure compliance. Infection control practices should be followed stringently.

Despite advances in medicine and years of fighting with a disease like TB, we are still too naïve in our understanding regarding the development of the disease and its transmission. In high burden countries, there is no consensus regarding the screening frequency. Extensive research is needed to elucidate the complete spectrum of the disease and predict progression, discover newer diagnostic modalities for early stages, and formulate shorter and optimal treatment regimens and host-directed therapies appropriate to a particular stage in the disease trajectory. While developing more nuanced algorithms for such a management strategy through stages, need for resource reallocation and subsequent economic consequences should be kept in mind.

REFERENCES

1. National Tuberculosis Elimination Programme, Central TB Division, Ministry of Health and Family Welfare, Government of India. (2021). Guidelines for Programmatic Management of TB Preventive Treatment in India 2021.[online] Available from https://tbcindia.mohfw.gov.in/wp-content/uploads/2023/05/Guidelines-for-Programmatic-Management-of-Tuberculosis-Preventive-Treatment-in-India.pdf [Last accessed September, 2024].
2. Stuck L, van Haaster AC, Kapata-Chanda P, Klinkenberg E, Kapata N, Cobelens F. How "Subclinical" is Subclinical Tuberculosis? An Analysis of National Prevalence Survey Data from Zambia. Clin Infect Dis. 2022;75(5):842-8.
3. Indian Council of Medical Research (ICMR), New Delhi. (2021). The National TB Prevalence Survey in India (2019-2021) Summary. [online] Available from https://tbcindia.mohfw.gov.in/wp-content/uploads/2023/05/25032022161020NATBPSReport.pdf [Last accessed September, 2024].
4. Chin KL, Anibarro L, Sarmiento ME, Acosta A. Challenges and the Way forward in Diagnosis and Treatment of Tuberculosis Infection. Trop Med Infect Dis. 2023;8(2):89.
5. Zellweger JP, Sotgiu G, Corradi M, Durando P. The diagnosis of latent tuberculosis infection (LTBI): currently available tests, future developments, and perspectives to eliminate tuberculosis (TB). Med Lav. 2020;111(3):170-83.

CHAPTER

37

Novel Tuberculosis Vaccines: A Promising Approach for Multidrug-resistant Tuberculosis Elimination

Thomas Vadakkan Devassy

Abstract

The rise of multidrug-resistant tuberculosis (MDR-TB) poses a significant challenge to global TB elimination efforts. To combat this, innovative preventive strategies are necessary. Recent advancements in TB vaccine development offer new hope. Multiple novel vaccines are in various stages of clinical trials, targeting different stages of TB infection. These vaccines employ diverse formulations, including live attenuated, killed, subunit, and viral-vectored approaches. India's latest contribution is the phase 3 clinical trial of *Mycobacterium tuberculosis* vaccine (MTBVAC), launched in March 2024. Future vaccines are anticipated to surpass the efficacy of the existing bacille Calmette–Guerin (BCG) vaccine, potentially accelerating TB elimination by 2035.

Keywords: MDR-TB, TB vaccine, MTBVAC, BCG

INTRODUCTION

The rise of multidrug-resistant (MDR) and rifampicin-resistant (RR) tuberculosis (TB) poses a significant global health threat, with an estimated 410,000 new cases in 2022.[1] Despite progress in treatment outcomes, the success rate remains suboptimal at 63%. The ongoing transmission of MDR-TB, coupled with the challenging side effect profile of treatment regimens, contributes to poor adherence and hinders efforts to control the spread of the disease. With a significant pool of latently infected individuals at risk of reactivation, innovative prevention strategies are crucial.[2] Building on the success of vaccines in combating infectious diseases, the development of a novel mycobacterial vaccine offers a promising avenue for preventing MDR-TB.

NOVEL TUBERCULOSIS VACCINES

The bacille Calmette–Guerin (BCG) vaccine, a live attenuated formulation, has been the sole globally approved TB vaccine for over a century. While BCG vaccination offers protection to children against severe extrapulmonary TB, its efficacy in preventing pulmonary or extrapulmonary TB in adults is limited. To address this gap, novel vaccines are being developed to provide protection against both drug-sensitive and drug-resistant mycobacterial infections. Several promising mycobacterial vaccine candidates have entered the clinical trial pipeline, aiming to improve upon the limitations of BCG and offer enhanced protection against TB.

TYPES OF TB VACCINES

The TB vaccines can be categorized in two ways—(1) by target population and (2) by vaccine composition.

By Target Population

- *Preventive/pre-exposure vaccines (POI)*: Aim to prevent infection
- *Preventive postexposure vaccines/prevention of disease (POD)*: Aim to prevent disease in already infected individuals
- *Therapeutic vaccines/prevention of recurrence (POR)*: Aim to prevent recurrence in treated individuals

By Vaccine Composition

- Live-attenuated whole cell vaccines
- Inactivated whole cell vaccines
- Adjuvanted protein subunit vaccines
- Viral-vectored vaccines

The TB vaccine initiative (TBVI) has provided an updated overview of current TB vaccines in the pipeline, summarized in **Table 1**.[3]

VACCINES FOR PREVENTION OF INFECTION

These vaccines are administered to individuals without prior exposure to mycobacteria, primarily newborns, and infants. The most promising candidates in this category are VPM1002 and *Mycobacterium tuberculosis* vaccine (MTBVAC). VPM1002 has demonstrated superior safety and efficacy compared to BCG. MTB VAC, a live-attenuated vaccine with deleted virulence genes *PhoP* and *fadD26*, is being developed in collaboration with Bharath Biotech in India. A phase 3 clinical trial for MTB VAC commenced in India on March 24, 2024, to evaluate its safety, immunogenicity, and efficacy in a region with high prevalence of drug-sensitive and resistant TB.

VACCINES FOR PREVENTION OF DISEASE

These vaccines target adolescents and adults who have already been exposed to mycobacteria. They typically contain antigens expressed during latent infection, such as fusion proteins combining antigens from both active and latent stages. Examples of these fusion vaccines include H56, M72, and ID93, designed to boost immunity in individuals with prior exposure to mycobacteria.

VACCINES FOR TB THERAPY

The TB vaccines are being explored to enhance treatment outcomes in active TB, particularly in cases of MDR and extensively drug-resistant (XDR)-TB, where pharmacological treatment has limited success. Research is ongoing, with completed phase 2 trials using *Mycobacterium* indicus pranii Mw in combination with TB drugs. The RUTI vaccine aims to improve treatment outcomes in latent TB infection (LTBI) and active TB disease, with an upcoming phase 2 trial investigating its safety and immunogenicity in MDR-TB cases.[4]

TABLE 1: Various types of TB vaccines in pipeline as of 2024.

	Preclinical	Phase 1	Phase 2a	Phase 2b	Phase 3
Infants and neonates	BCG-ZMP1 University Zurich •				VPM1002 SII, MaxPlank, VPM TBVI •
	BCG-ESX-IMmar, Inst. Pasteur Paris •				MTBVAC, Biofabri, Unizar TBVI •
Adolescents and adults	BCG, ChadOx/ MVA 5Ag Univ. Oxword ▫	Ad5 Ag5A Mc Master, Can Sino ▫	MTBVAC Biofabri TBVI UNIZAR IAVI •	M72 + ASO1 GSK, GMRI ◊	VPM1002 SII, Max Planck, VPM •
	CysVac2/Ad Univ. Sydney ◊	TB/Flu04L RIBSP ▫	ID93/GLA-SE (QTP101) Quratis ◊	DAR-901 Dartmouth University ◦	MIP Immuvac Cadilla Pharma ◦
	BCG-ZMP1 University Zurich •	H107 SSI ◊	AEC/BCO_2 Anhul Zhifei Longcom ◊	BCG Revaccination Gates MRI •	GamTBVac MoH Russia ◊
	BCG:ESX-1Mmar Inst. Pasteur Paris •	BNT164a1 BioNTech/ Gates Foundation ▪	ChadOx1.85A MVA 85A Aerosol/im Univ. Oxford ▫		BCG(Traveler vaccine) HJF •
	TITAN UCT ▪	BNT164b1 Bio Ntech/ Gates foundation ▪			
Therapeutic				Ruti Arhivel Pharma ◦	

Note: ▪: RNA; ▫: Vector; ◊: Subunit; ◦: Whole cell; •: Live.

(BCG: bacille Calmette–Guerin; MTBVAC: *Mycobacterium tuberculosis* vaccine; TBVI: TB vaccine initiative)

Source: Adapted from TB Vaccine Initiative. (2024).[3]

CONCLUSION

Historically, TB control focused on active case finding and treatment. However, to eliminate infectious diseases, prevention is crucial. In cases like MDR-TB, where treatment success rates are low, preventive strategies are more effective. Fortunately, significant research is underway in TB vaccine development, with the MTB VAC phase 3 clinical trial already initiated in India.

REFERENCES

1. WHO. (2023). WHO Global Tuberculosis Report 2023. [online] Available from https://www.who.int/teams/global-tuberculosis-programme/tb-reports/global-tuberculosis-report-2023 [Last accessed September, 2024].
2. World Health Organization. Global Tuberculosis Report 2016. Geneva: WHO Press; 2016.
3. TB Vaccine Initiative. (2024). Pipeline of Vaccines. [online] Available from https://www.tbvi.eu/what-we-do/pipeline-of-vaccines/ [Last accessed September, 2024].
4. Kaufmann SHE, Weiner J, von Reyn CF. Novel approaches to tuberculosis vaccine development. Int J Infect Dis. 2017;56:263-7.

CHAPTER

38

Role of Artificial Intelligence in Tuberculosis

VK Arora, Kamal Chopra, Ankita Anand

Abstract

Artificial intelligence (AI) is poised to revolutionize tuberculosis (TB) management by advancing in diagnosis, treatment, and prevention. AI algorithms can accurately detect TB lesions in chest X-rays and computed tomography (CT) scans, enabling early diagnosis. AI tools enhance diagnostic accuracy and efficiency by interpreting tests such as sputum smear microscopy and molecular tests. Additionally, AI provides decision support by analyzing patient data and diagnostic results, aiding healthcare providers in informed diagnosis and treatment decisions. AI-powered electronic medication monitors and virtual directly observed treatment (VDOT) systems improve treatment adherence through remote supervision and reminders. AI can also analyze genetic data to understand drug resistance mechanisms and develop counter strategies.

Keywords: Artificial intelligence, AI, cough sounds, X-ray, VDOT

INTRODUCTION

John McCarthy coined the term "artificial intelligence (AI)".[1] AI generally refers to computer systems that mimic human-like thinking processes, such as reasoning, understanding, generalizing, or learning from experience, to achieve goals without requiring specific instructions for each action. In healthcare, AI can be utilized in numerous ways:

- AI can aid in the early detection, diagnosis, management, and treatment of medical conditions. Additionally, it has the potential to enhance patient engagement, improve medication adherence, assist the elderly, promote health, provide counselling, streamline administrative tasks, and support the education and training of healthcare professionals.
- AI has been applied to the diagnosis of tuberculosis (TB), with advancements in algorithms enhancing the identification of TB presence or absence. Research is focused on developing strategies to improve the accuracy of TB diagnosis through AI and machine learning. Current TB screening and diagnostic tests can be lengthy and cumbersome, and achieving the desired level of sensitivity continues to be a challenge. Traditional methods for diagnosing TB require significant time and resources, especially in countries where the disease is prevalent and healthcare systems are less developed. In recent decades, the rapid advancement of computer technology has spurred increased interest in AI across various industries, with a notable focus on image

recognition. There has been a significant increase in investment in techniques and technologies for TB treatment, program administration, AI-assisted early diagnosis, surveillance, and patient care.

- In pulmonary TB, coughing is a common and major symptom. Cough characteristics can be clinically assessed throughout the entire continuum of care. For instance, cough sound analysis might be used as a triage tool to prompt further TB testing in patients who show potential symptoms. Additionally, it could be employed to monitor a patient's response to therapy by evaluating changes in cough characteristics over time. This approach helps in both early detection and effective management of TB.

  The Timbre mobile app diagnoses TB by recording a patient's cough. It utilizes AI and machine learning to analyze the cough sounds. This method is easy, noninvasive, affordable, and accessible for TB diagnosis. A medical practitioner or healthcare worker records the patient's cough with a microphone array and gathers additional clinical information, including demographic details, preexisting health conditions, and information about sleep and cough patterns. The recorded cough is then processed in real-time using machine learning to predict whether the patient is positive for TB.[2]
- AI can speed up medical diagnosis by quickly and accurately analyzing medical images, such as chest X-rays (CXRs), in just minutes. For example, AI-based software like qXR rapidly analyzes X-ray scans, detects lung abnormalities, and highlights them directly on the image.[3]
- AI can assist in interpreting the results of the line probe assay (LPA) test to determine drug resistance in TB. Each LPA strip reveals the drug resistance profile of the patient through a series of activated (dark) and inactivated (light) bands, which correspond to different regions of the TB bacterium's genome. AI has great potential in the field of genetics AI improves the accuracy of genome sequencing and allows for the scaling up of sequencing operations.
- AI-enhanced ultrasonography has the potential to significantly accelerate the use of medical ultrasound across various clinical settings. It helps to identify abnormal features in the chest. AI can analyze signals from the ultrasound scan to assist in diagnosing TB and triaging patients more effectively.
- Individuals with latent TB infection (LTBI) usually do not feel unwell and may never show symptoms, which reduce their likelihood of seeking medical care and hence deciding who needs to be tested for LTBI and who should get tuberculosis preventive therapy (TPT) can be difficult at times. AI can assist in pinpointing areas with at-risk populations and those most in need of intervention. It can also forecast the likelihood of LTBI cases advancing to active TB. This insight can enhance the planning and implementation of targeted program strategies.
- AI-assisted analysis of CXRs can help to address the expertise gap by supporting the detection of TB-related abnormalities. This technology supports healthcare providers in identifying which patients should be referred for microbiological testing to confirm a TB diagnosis. For early detection, AI algorithms can analyze CXRs and computed tomography (CT) scans to identify TB lesions with high precision, leading to quicker diagnosis and intervention
- Ensuring medication adherence is a significant challenge for TB patients.[4] Electronic medication monitors that send text messages have proven effective in high-prevalence areas. AI-powered virtual directly observed treatment (VDOT) software detects individual-specific traits, enabling remote monitoring of patients taking medication via smartphones or tablets.[5] AI can significantly improve medication adherence and provide personalized support through:
  - AI-driven chatbots[6] and virtual assistants offer continuous support, information, and address concerns through online platforms (OP) links in Virtual Integrated Networks (VIN) Plus.

- AI increasing efficiency in health system processes, enhancing patient care quality, and reducing healthcare workers' workload
- AI improving clinical decision making

However, AI systems require access to sensitive personal health data, making safeguarding against breaches and misuse crucial. The application of AI in healthcare raises ethical concerns, and developing, integrating, and maintaining AI systems can be costly, potentially leading to unequal access. To address these concerns, it is essential to have:

- Ongoing research
- Transparent practices
- Robust regulatory frameworks
- Careful consideration of AI technology's ethical implications in healthcare

CONCLUSION

Artificial intelligence use can act as triage for early screening of multidrug-resistant tuberculosis (MDR-TB) and can act as early transformative potential in combating MDR-TB in countries with high burden of the disease. AI-assisted analysis enhances detection accuracy, enabling early diagnosis and intervention. AI-powered VDOT improves medication adherence. Benefits include enhanced patient care, reduced healthcare worker workload, and improved clinical decision-making leading to cut in the transmission of the disease.

However, ensuring data security, addressing ethical concerns, and integrating AI into existing systems are crucial. Ongoing research and robust regulatory frameworks are essential. AI can revolutionize MDR-TB management, saving lives and mitigating the global TB burden by improving diagnosis accuracy, patient care, and combating MDR-TB more effectively.

REFERENCES

1. Hayes PJ, Morgenstern L. On John McCarthy's 80th birthday, in honor of his contributions. AI Magazine. 2017;28(4):93.
2. Zimmer AJ, Ugarte-Gil C, Pathri, R, Dewan P, Jaganath D, Cattamanchi A, et al. Making cough count in tuberculosis care. Commun Med. 2022;2:83.
3. qXR. (2022). India Health Fund. [online] Available from https://www.indiahealthfund.org/our portfolio/qxr/ [Last accessed September, 2024].
4. Munro SA, Lewin SA, Smith HJ, Engel ME, Fretheim A, Volmink J. Patient adherence to tuberculosis treatment: A systematic review of qualitative research. PLoS Med. 2007;4:e238.
5. Garfein RS, Collins K, Muñoz F, Moser K, Cerecer-Callu P, Raab F, et al. Feasibility of tuberculosis treatment monitoring by video directly observed therapy: a binational pilot study. Int J Tuberc Lung Dis. 2015;19:1057-64.
6. Kim AJ, Yang J, Jang Y, Baek JS. Acceptance of an Informational Antituberculosis Chatbot Among Korean Adults: Mixed Methods Research. JMIR Mhealth Uhealth. 2021;9(11):e26424.

CHAPTER

39

Artificial Intelligence in Managing Drug Adherence

Sanjay Rajpal, Ankita Anand

Abstract

Partial adherence to tuberculosis (TB) treatment significantly heightens the risk of prolonged culture conversion and ongoing transmission within the community, therapeutic failure, recurrence, and the development or worsening of drug resistance. Artificial intelligence (AI) applications that leverage advanced deep learning techniques can boost the efficiency of monitoring medication adherence through automation. Although AI has not been widely tested for this use in clinical settings, it has the potential to transform healthcare delivery, including in resource-constrained regions like India. These AI tools can be integrated into healthcare to support a variety of functions, including enhancing patient adherence to drug regimens by delivering customized medication reminders, by automatically tracking medication intake, by offering real time insights and feedback to both patients and healthcare providers.

Keywords: Artificial intelligence, medication adherence, tuberculosis, video-based directly observed therapy, chatbot, digital adherence technologies, AI

INTRODUCTION

Tuberculosis (TB) is a major public health issue and adhering to complex TB treatment with multiple medications can be especially difficult because of the extended duration (typically 6 months or longer) with possibility of unpleasant side effects. India bears the highest burden of TB in the world. Nonadherence to TB therapy could adversely impact both clinical and public health outcomes. Medication adherence has a considerable impact on health outcomes for patients and also on system costs for providers. It depends on personal behavior regarding the intake of medication and also corresponds to the agreed recommendations from a healthcare provider.[1] One of the reasons for nonadherence is that patient forgetting if one took a dose, omitted a dose, taking a lower dose than prescribed or stopping the medication altogether. Around 33–50% of patients who start treatment become nonadherent to their prescribed medication regimen,[2] which is associated with emergence of drug resistance, prolonged infectiousness, treatment failure, and death.

Regardless of these challenges, multiple strategies and simple intervention can help support improved medication adherence.

ROLE OF AI IN MEDICATION ADHERENCE

Artificial intelligence (AI) is the future of medication adherence. It has become a central focus and can have a huge impact on patient adherence and personalized support. To support and enhance medication adherence, AI and machine learning technology can be used. Using patient data from these health systems, an AI chatbot[3] can provide the information and motivation to patients to take their medications regularly at the same time every day by giving them a reminder on a timely basis.

National Tuberculosis Elimination Programme (NTEP) has rolled out the TB Aarogya Sathi mobile application to enhance TB control. It helps in raising patient awareness and guaranteeing access to free, high-quality drugs and diagnostic services for all citizens in the country. Additionally, these AI **chatbots** can offer information on the nearest diagnostic and treatment centers and include an assessment tool to evaluate infection risk. They can be equipped with extensive data on thorough treatment management and adherence, and can serve to identify nearby care facilities, issue reminders, and execute patient follow-ups.[3]

Moreover, they can address patient's most frequently posed inquiries. The chatbot can also engage with patients to assess their primary reasons for not taking their medicine and can direct them to different resources for their continuation of treatment. AI can be used to link the electronic medical records to document impact on medication collection, subsequent hospitalizations, and comorbidities that are associated with medication nonadherence. These chatbots can be programmed in regional languages to ensure broader accessibility of information. This approach would alleviate the workload of healthcare professionals and providers, allowing them to allocate additional resources and assistance to high-risk patients.

Artificial intelligence systems have the capability to provide a wealth of crucial data that can support medication adherence efforts. When designed appropriately, AI can boost patient's confidence level and has a positive behavioral impact which will enhance treatment adherence and also give insight to the patients and their health providers about the successful outcomes. AI can be used to identify patient profiles, prescribe effective drugs, save resources, and minimize side effects.

Artificial intelligence-backed telemedicine and digital revolution can easily connect patients with their treatment provider ensuring prompt, quality care, offering timely interventions, promoting transparency, equitable care and bridging healthcare disparities. These features can transgress socioeconomic and geographic challenges also. In India, various Digital Adherence Technologies have been implemented, including the **99DOTS** (Directly Observed Treatment Short Course) system, to monitor patients' adherence to TB treatment.[4] Missed doses trigger SMS notifications to care providers, who subsequently provide personalized follow-up through phone-based counseling. Among other tools, the Medication Event Reminder Monitor **(MERM)** is an advanced digital pillbox designed to provide timely reminders for medication intake and enable remote tracking of adherence.

A physical device **TMEAD**, i.e., Tuberculosis Monitoring Encouragement Adherence Drive, is fitted with an embedded software system and a mobile network system administers reminders, dispenses medication, and monitors patient adherence to the prescribed treatment regimen. This online application provides real-time surveillance with daily updates and patient insights to ancillary health institutions. Furthermore, a mobile application provides real-time updates and a succinct overview for the TB Health Visitor while conducting fieldwork.[4] These technologies provide various methods for monitoring medication adherence, promising high accuracy and greater patient acceptance due to their nonintrusive nature. Nevertheless, documented evidence of their successful clinical implementation remains scarce.

Inefficient supply chain management and instances of shortages or expiry of anti-TB drugs and frequent stockouts of TB medicines lead to delays in treatment initiation, causing treatment interruption, loss of patients, and nonadherence to anti-TB treatment. Such events affect the smooth delivery patient care which will eventually contribute to a heightened risk of infections or the development of drug-resistant strains of *Mycobacterium tuberculosis*, which are more challenging to treat, thereby elevating the risk of mortality. AI can play a crucial role in analyzing data related to drug inventory and provide timely guidance to meet the demand by forecasting the consumption patterns and requirement, minimizing the overstocking and expiry of drugs. The AI solution will streamline decision-making support by meeting demand and supply and direct the program officials to allocate inventory to the store in greatest need, thereby ensuring a continuous and uninterrupted supply of materials. This is being implemented real time by Central TB Division through *Nikshay Aushadhi* program.

In 2017, the World Health Organization endorsed video-based directly observed therapy **(VDOT)** as an alternative to traditional directly observed therapy for monitoring TB treatment. **VDOT** helps overcome geographic barriers by allowing healthcare providers to remotely observe patient's medication intake, even in hard-to-reach areas. This approach provides patients with the flexibility to take their TB medications at times and places that suit them.

Despite its benefits, asynchronous **VDOT** has a major drawback, the repetitive manual task of reviewing and confirming daily adherence, which can result in inaccuracies and fatigue for healthcare providers, particularly with high patient volumes. To improve efficiency and accuracy, automating these routine tasks is a viable solution. By integrating advanced tools such as AI with digital adherence technologies—like medication sleeves, small pill boxes, and video support systems—the adoption and effectiveness of **VDOT** can be significantly enhanced. This would enable patients to take their medications conveniently while remaining connected to their healthcare providers.[5]

In a study published in Malaysia, researchers have developed a mobile phone application called Gamified-Real-Time Video Observed Therapy **(GRVOTS)**[6] that is designed to enhance adherence to TB treatment regimens, the application improves patient tracking and fosters increased engagement between patients and their healthcare providers. Additionally, it offers an interface for supervisors and administrators to actively participate in supporting patient's compliance with their treatment protocols.

However, there are some ethical concerns for AI to be used in the medical field related to confidentiality and security in data management and transmission, along with obtaining informed consent from patient's data safety and data sharing. So, establishing an ethical and regulatory framework is essential before integrating AI into health research and healthcare delivery.

The use of AI offers both opportunities and challenges. While it could enhance adherence rates, its effectiveness may be impacted by technological skill and acceptance. There are serious ethical issues with the use of AI in healthcare. Major concerns include data privacy, ownership, and data protection. There is also lack of standard framework for big data analytics and lack of transparency and accountability in AI-based applications.

When implementing AI solutions, it is crucial to carefully consider infrastructure, training, patient characteristics, and cost-effectiveness. To optimize outcomes, future research should investigate how AI affects various patient populations and focus on developing accessible, patient-centered solutions. Moreover, it should assess the effectiveness, efficiency, and quality of AI applications. Nevertheless, successful adoption of AI requires tackling challenges such as establishing standardized reporting guidelines, resolving implementation issues, creating assessment frameworks for AI technology, and ensuring adequate financial resources.

CONCLUSION

Artificial intelligence offers significant potential to improve TB medication adherence through tools like chatbots, digital adherence technologies, and video-based therapy. These innovations can enhance patient monitoring and timely intervention, especially in resource-limited areas like India. However, challenges such as data privacy, ethical concerns, and infrastructure limitations need to be addressed for effective AI adoption. With proper implementation, AI can streamline healthcare delivery, improve adherence to TB treatments, and help combat drug-resistant TB strains. Future research and investment are essential to optimize these technologies for diverse patient needs.

REFERENCES

1. Babel A, Taneja R, Malvestiti FM, Monaco A, Donde S. Artificial Intelligence Solutions to Increase Medication Adherence in Patients with Non-communicable Diseases. Front Digit Health. 2021;3:669869.
2. Alipanah N, Jarlsberg L, Miller C, Linh NN, Falzon D, Jaramillo E, et al. Adherence interventions and outcomes of tuberculosis treatment: A systematic review and meta-analysis of trials and observational studies. PLoS Med. 2018;15(7):e1002595.
3. Kim AJ, Yang J, Jang Y, Baek JS. Acceptance of an Informational Antituberculosis Chatbot Among Korean Adults: Mixed Methods Research. JMIR Mhealth Uhealth. 2021;9(11):e26424.
4. Saha S, Saxena D, Raval D, Halkarni N, Doshi R, Joshi M, et al. Tuberculosis Monitoring Encouragement Adherence Drive (TMEAD): Toward improving the adherence of the patients with drug-sensitive tuberculosis in Nashik, Maharashtra. Front Public Health. 2022;10:1021427.
5. Sekandi JN, Shi W, Zhu R, Kaggwa P, Mwebaze E, Li S. Application of Artificial Intelligence to the Monitoring of Medication Adherence for Tuberculosis Treatment in Africa: Algorithm Development and Validation. JMIR AI. 2023;2(1):e40167.
6. Abas SA, Ismail N, Zakaria Y, Yasin SM, Ibrahim K, Ismail I, et al. Enhancing tuberculosis treatment adherence and motivation through gamified real-time mobile app utilization: a single-arm intervention study. BMC Public Health. 2024;24(1):249.

CHAPTER

40

Role of DNA Fingerprinting in Multidrug-resistant Tuberculosis

KB Gupta, Rishabh Kacker

Abstract

Multidrug-resistant tuberculosis (MDR-TB) presents a significant global health challenge due to its resistance to key anti-tuberculosis (TB) drugs and the complexities of treatment. DNA fingerprinting, or DNA profiling, has emerged as a pivotal tool in addressing MDR-TB by offering insights into bacterial strain identification, resistance mechanisms, and epidemiological tracking. This technique utilizes molecular typing methods such as Restriction Fragment Length Polymorphism (RFLP), spoligotyping, and Mycobacterial Interspersed Repetitive Unit-Variable Number Tandem Repeat (MIRU-VNTR) to differentiate strains and monitor transmission. It also aids in understanding genetic mutations responsible for drug resistance, informing drug resistance profiles, and enhancing diagnostic accuracy. Additionally, DNA fingerprinting supports outbreak investigations, treatment monitoring, personalized medicine, and vaccine development. While its application offers significant benefits in controlling MDR-TB, ethical concerns regarding patient privacy and practical challenges related to resource constraints must be addressed. Continued advancements and international collaboration are essential to leveraging DNA fingerprinting effectively in the global fight against MDR-TB.

Keywords: DNA fingerprinting, MDR-TB, drug resistance

INTRODUCTION

Multidrug-resistant tuberculosis (MDR-TB) is one of the most important global health issues today. This severe form of tuberculosis (TB) is caused by *Mycobacterium tuberculosis* strains that are resistant to at least two first-line anti-TB drugs—isoniazid and rifampicin. Controlling and treating MDR-TB can be challenging by factors such as protracted treatment times, expensive costs, and the requirement for second-line medications with considerable adverse effects. In these circumstances, DNA fingerprinting has emerged as an important tool in the fight against MDR-TB, providing vital information about disease management, transmission patterns, and treatment methods. DNA fingerprinting, also known as DNA profiling, is a technique for identifying genetic variations between individuals or pathogen strains. In the context of TB, this entails studying the genetic material of *M. tuberculosis* to distinguish between strains and track their spread.[1]

The application of DNA fingerprinting in this context involves the following key aspects:

- *Identification and tracking of MDR-TB strains*:
  - *Molecular typing*: Several approaches are used in the molecular typing of *M. tuberculosis*, including Restriction Fragment Length Polymorphism (RFLP), spoligotyping, and Mycobacterial Interspersed Repetitive Unit-Variable Number Tandem Repeat (MIRU-VNTR).[2] These technologies enable scientists to generate a genetic fingerprint for the bacterial strain. Researchers can use these fingerprints to assess whether different patients are infected with the same strain of *M. tuberculosis*, indicating a common source of infection or ongoing transmission within a population.
  - *Epidemiologic surveillance*: Effective epidemiological surveillance is crucial for preventing the spread of MDR-TB. DNA fingerprinting allows public health officials to track the transmission of MDR-TB strains locally and globally. This surveillance can pinpoint hotspots of transmission, direct targeted treatments, and assess the efficacy of control measures. For example, in areas with a high TB incidence, DNA fingerprinting aids in distinguishing between reactivation of a latent illness and a new infection induced by transmission from another individual.
  - *Outbreak investigation*: In the event of an MDR-TB outbreak, DNA fingerprinting is critical for determining the infection's source and transmission channels. By comparing the DNA profiles of bacteria from different patients, investigators can identify whether they are dealing with a single-source outbreak or numerous distinct instances. This information aids public health initiatives in reducing the spread, such as identifying and treating primary carriers and their contacts.[3]
- *Mechanisms of drug resistance*:
  - *Genetic mutations*: Specific genetic alterations in the bacterial DNA are frequently the cause of TB treatment resistance. For example, mutations in the *katG* gene and the inhA promoter region are frequently associated with isoniazid resistance, whereas changes in the *rpoB* gene provide rifampicin resistance. DNA fingerprinting enables researchers to identify and classify these alterations, so improving our understanding of how resistance arises and spreads. This understanding is crucial for creating new diagnostic tests that can swiftly detect drug-resistant bacteria.
  - *Drug resistance profiles*: Analyzing the genetic profiles of MDR-TB strains provides precise information regarding their resistance to various TB treatments. This data is used for generating drug resistance profiles, which are critical for making treatment decisions. Understanding the exact resistance mechanisms at work allows clinicians to select the most effective drug combinations while avoiding medicines to which the bacteria are resistant, resulting in better treatment outcomes.
- *Clinical and public health applications*:
  - *Diagnostic tests*: Traditional TB diagnostic approaches, such as culture and susceptibility testing, might take weeks to get results. DNA-based diagnostic assays, such as GeneXpert MTB/RIF, deliver results in hours and can detect both TB and resistance to rifampicin, one of the most important medications in TB treatment. Rapid diagnosis is critical for the commencement of appropriate treatment, lowering the risk of transmission, and improving patient outcomes.
  - *Treatment monitoring*: Monitoring the genetic profile of *M. tuberculosis* during therapy aids in recognizing early indicators of treatment failure and growing drug resistance. If a patient's bacterial load does not reduce as expected, or new resistance mutations emerge, clinicians can modify the therapy schedule. This technique improves MDR-TB management and reduces the development of extensively drug-resistant tuberculosis (XDR-TB).
  - *Personalized medicine*: The precise genetic information obtained from DNA fingerprinting facilitates individualized therapy in TB treatment. Healthcare practitioners can enhance treatment success rates by adapting treatment regimens

to the infecting strain's individual resistance profile. Personalized treatment also reduces the likelihood of adverse medication responses and treatment duration, which is especially relevant for MDR-TB patients, who frequently have long and complex treatment regimens.

- *Research and development*:
  - *Vaccine development*: Developing an effective TB vaccine, particularly MDR-TB, is a top concern in global health. DNA fingerprinting contributes to this effort by providing knowledge regarding the genetic diversity and resistance mechanisms of *M. tuberculosis* strains. Understanding these factors can help to design vaccines that are effective against a wide range of strains, including those that are drug-resistant.
  - *Public health policies*: Data from DNA fingerprinting research assist public health initiatives targeted at managing MDR-TB. For example, genetic data on the presence and spread of drug-resistant strains can be used to drive infection control policy in hospital settings, immunization efforts, and antibiotic stewardship initiatives. These strategies are critical to decreasing the burden of MDR-TB and limiting the establishment of new resistant strains.

ETHICAL AND PRACTICAL CONSIDERATIONS

The use of DNA fingerprinting in MDR-TB therapy presents various ethical concerns, including those regarding patient privacy and consent. To protect patient identity, genetic data collection and storage must be kept strictly secret. Informed consent is required, and patients should be aware of how their genetic information will be handled. Furthermore, protections must be put in place to prevent the exploitation of genetic data, such as genetic prejudice. Implementing DNA fingerprinting in resource-constrained environments involves practical hurdles, including the requirement for specialized equipment, qualified workers, and adequate money. Efforts to include DNA fingerprinting into normal TB care must address these issues through capacity building, finance, and partnership with international organizations.[4]

CONCLUSION

DNA fingerprinting has become an essential tool in the fight against MDR-TB. Its ability to detect and track drug-resistant strains, comprehend resistance mechanisms, and guide clinical and public health strategies has greatly improved our ability to manage and control this challenging disease. However, resolving the ethical and practical problems connected with its usage is critical to maximizing its benefits while protecting patient rights. DNA fingerprinting will stay at the vanguard of efforts to eradicate MDR-TB and improve global health outcomes, thanks to ongoing research, innovation, and international collaboration.

REFERENCES

1. McNabb SJ, Braden CR, Navin TR. DNA fingerprinting of Mycobacterium tuberculosis: lessons learned and implications for the future. Emerg Infect Dis. 2002;8:1314-9.
2. de Beer JL, van Soolingen D. DNA Fingerprinting of Mycobacterium TB: A Rich Source of Fundamental and Daily Applicable Knowledge. In: Lu Y, Wang L, Duanmu H, Chanyasulkit C, Strong A, Zhang H (Eds). Handbook of Global Tuberculosis Control. Boston, MA: Springer; 2017.
3. Verma A, Singh S, Kashyap A, Saini R, Dogra R, Sharma A, et al. Mycobacterium tuberculosis and DNA fingerprinting: a vital tool for tracking outbreaks. J Popul Therap Clin Pharmacol. 2023;30:509-20.
4. Khan F, Mer A. The Ethical Considerations of DNA Profiling for Resilience in a Forensic Setting in India: A Comparative Study with International Guidelines. In: Kumar N, Sood K, Özen E, Grima S (Eds). The Framework for Resilient Industry: A Holistic Approach for Developing Economies (Emerald Studies in Finance, Insurance, and Risk Management). Leeds: Emerald Publishing Limited; 2024. pp. 121-34.

CHAPTER

41

Epigenetic Regulation of Drug Resistance in Tuberculosis

SK Katiyar, Arun Sampath

Abstract

Epigenetics is the field of biology that studies chemical modifications of DNA without altering its nucleotide sequence. These modifications alter the chromatin superstructure and DNA-protein interactions, thereby affecting subsequent gene expression, which can result in either overexpression or gene silencing. Key types of epigenetic regulations include histone modifications, DNA methylation, and noncoding RNAs (ncRNA). In prokaryotes, these epigenetic processes enhance virulence and survival in the host environment. *Mycobacterium tuberculosis* (MTB) can develop DNA methylation, acetylation, and phosphorylation modifications, which help the TB bacilli survive in hostile intra- or extracellular environments, evade host immune mechanisms, and contribute to the emergence of drug resistance. Understanding these epigenetic mechanisms can aid in identifying specific genetic targets to develop newer therapeutic drugs for drug-resistant TB.

Keywords: Epigenetics, drug resistance, tuberculosis

INTRODUCTION

Epigenesis refers to changes in genetic expression influenced by environmental factors. According to this theory, development is a process where genetic information is gradually expressed, and the organism's form and structure emerge over time through the interaction of genes with the environment. This process can impact organisms ranging from microorganisms to humans at any point in time. "Epigenetics" is the field of biology dedicated to studying the processes through which chemical modifications of DNA occur without altering the nucleotide sequence. These DNA modifications can induce heritable changes in gene expression, thereby modulating protein production or its activities. The Greek prefix "epi" in epigenetics means "on top of" the regular genetic mechanisms. The term was coined by embryologist Conrad Waddington, who initially defined epigenetics as "the branch of biology which studies the causal interactions between genes and their products, which bring the phenotype into being" and "to describe the impact of the environment on embryonic development." In simpler terms, epigenetics refers to changes in the chromosomal superstructure without affecting the DNA sequence.

BASIC STRUCTURE OF CHROMATIN AND EPIGENETICS

The double helix DNA, composed of nucleotide pairs, is organized by being wrapped around a histone protein octamer, which consists of two pairs each of histones H2A, H2B, H3, and H4. One unit of this histone octamer with a DNA strand is called a nucleosome. Nucleosomes are connected by linker DNA and histone H1 to form chromatin. Chromatin can exist as either loose/open euchromatin, which is transcriptionally active, or dense/closed heterochromatin, which is transcriptionally inactive.

DNA is transcribed into messenger RNA (mRNA), which then initiates the production of individual proteins in cytoplasmic ribosomes based on the specific mRNA code for each protein. Chemical modifications to the histone proteins in euchromatin allow enzymes and transcriptional factors to interact with DNA, facilitating gene expression. Conversely, chemical changes in closed heterochromatin repress gene expression by inhibiting transcription.

These epigenetic regulations modify the chromatin structure and affect subsequent gene coding, turning genes "on" or "off." This can lead to the overproduction or underproduction of proteins in cells and tissues.

Three Important Types of Epigenetic Regulation

1. *Histone modifications*: Histone modifications include several chemical changes that alter DNA-histone interactions within nucleosomes, affecting chromatin structure and gene expression:
   i. *Methylation*: The addition of one to three methyl groups to lysine or one to two methyl groups to arginine. Histone methylation by arginine or lysine methyltransferases can either promote gene expression or lead to gene silencing.
   ii. *Acetylation*: The addition of acetyl groups to lysine residues, which opens the chromatin to promote transcription. Histone acetylation causes an open chromatin conformation, promoting gene transcription, while deacetylation is associated with heterochromatin conformation, suppressing gene expression.
   iii. *Phosphorylation*: The addition of phosphate groups to histone tails, which can modify DNA repair and affect gene expression.
   iv. *Ubiquitination*: The addition of ubiquitin molecules to histones, altering DNA-histone interactions and influencing gene expression.
2. *DNA methylation*: It is catalyzed by DNA methyltransferase enzymes, which add a methyl group directly to a cytosine nucleotide within a cytosine-guanine sequence (CpG). Most CpG islands are located in promoter regions of genes. Methylated cytosines within a promoter region recruit gene suppressor proteins and lead to the formation of heterochromatin, preventing DNA-transcription factor interactions, and resulting in gene silencing. For example, hypermethylation of tumor suppressor genes and demethylation of pro-oncogenes can lead to tumor progression in cancer. Prokaryotes may achieve epigenetic inheritance solely through DNA methylation, forming N6-methyladenine (N6-MdA), N4-methylcytosine (N4-MdC), and 5-methylcytosine (5-MdC).[1]
3. *Noncoding RNA (ncRNA)*: ncRNAs can regulate gene expression by targeting specific gene sequences and transposons:[2]
   i. *miRNA*: MicroRNAs bind to the 3'-untranslated regions of mRNAs, leading to inhibition of protein expression.
   ii. *lncRNA*: Long ncRNAs can interact with transcription factors or modulate chromatin-modifying complexes, thereby suppressing translation.

Unlike genetic mutations, epigenetic changes can be reversible. For instance, DNA methylation can be reversed by DNA demethylation. However, some epigenetic changes can persist through multiple cycles of cell replication and be passed down to subsequent generations.

ROLE OF EPIGENETICS IN PROKARYOTES

The epigenetic changes described above, such as chemical modifications in DNA, can affect chromatin structure, DNA accessibility, and DNA-protein interactions, ultimately altering gene expression. These changes can lead to dysregulation of various critical intracellular signaling pathways. In prokaryotes, such epigenetic modifications are introduced into the target host genes responsible for microbial recognition, clearance, and apoptosis.

By altering these host genes, microorganisms can evade the host's defense mechanisms, providing them with a survival advantage. This evasion can enable microorganisms to become resistant to antimicrobial drugs. Thus, epigenetic modifications play a crucial role in the ability of prokaryotes to adapt to and survive within hostile environments, including the development of drug resistance.

HOW *MYCOBACTERIUM TUBERCULOSIS* BACILLI EVADE OR ADAPT IMMUNE RESPONSE?

The ability of *Mycobacterium* species to adapt and survive in diverse host cellular environments has allowed it to persist for thousands of years. The primary mode of its infection in humans is through inhalation, which initially targets the alveolar macrophages (AM) in the lungs. The *M. tuberculosis* (MTB) can sometimes evade the lysosomal effects of AM and move into the pulmonary interstitium. From there, the bacteria enter dendritic cells and travel to regional lymph nodes, where they stimulate the priming of T-cell lineage.

Within a few weeks, the primed T cells, along with B cells and neutrophils, form granulomas. These granulomas often contain the tubercle bacilli, leading to indolent latent tuberculosis (TB) infection or, in rare instances, complete sterilization of the infection. MTB has the inherent ability to survive even in fibrotic or calcific foci, which can reactivate later if the host's immunity weakens. In about 5–10% of individuals, the initial infection is not controlled, and the immune cells promote a cascade of inflammatory and necrotic responses, leading to progressive pulmonary TB. The outcome of TB infection depends on genetic susceptibility, the host immune system, TB bacilli virulence, and environmental factors. Several molecules, such as toll-like receptors (TLRs), interferon gamma (IFN-γ), tumor necrosis factor alpha/beta (TNF-α/β), interleukins (ILs), early secreted antigenic target-6kDa (ESAT-6), neutrophil extracellular traps (NETs), and reactive oxygen species (ROS), play crucial roles in the pathogenesis of TB.

To survive in the hostile host intra- and extracellular environments, such as hypoxia, low pH, and nutrient scarcity, TB bacilli must modify their gene expression to sustain themselves for long periods. Various research studies have been conducted to understand the complex molecular and genetic pathways through which TB bacilli evade the immune response, but detailed descriptions are beyond the scope of this chapter. Recently, the importance of studying the role of epigenetics in the immune escape mechanism of TB has been emerging. Epigenetic modifications may provide insights into how MTB adapts to and survives within the host, contributing to its persistence and resistance to treatment.

EPIGENETICS IN TUBERCULOSIS AND DRUG RESISTANCE

Tuberculosis bacilli can develop epigenetic changes to adapt to various host environments. These changes can include DNA methylation, phosphorylation, or acetylation.

DNA Methylation

DNA methylation controls both innate and adaptive immune signaling and cell differentiation. In the context of TB, DNA methylation by TB bacilli can enhance its virulence. In a study by Yung Che Chen et al.,[3] TB patients exhibited DNA hypermethylation in *TLR-2* promoter genes. This led to elevated expression of TLR-2 in natural killer (NK) cells and a decline of TLR-2 in monocytes. The methylation of TLR-2 genes was associated with enhanced bacterial growth and impaired immunological function. Interestingly, anti-TB treatment reversed this TLR-2 methylation. Scarlet Shell et al.[4] identified a critical adenine methyltransferase (MamA) in MTB, which created N6-MdA in a specific six-base pair recognition sequence of the MTB genome. Strains lacking MamA could not grow in hypoxic conditions. The deletion of MamA in the Euro-American lineage strain of MTB (H37Rv) affected its survival in hypoxia but not in the Beijing strain (HN878), indicating differential expression of DNA methyltransferases in different strains. Through the TLR-2 signaling pathway, macrophages produce various cytokines such as IL-6, TNF-α, and IL-1β, which further upregulate downstream mediators like IL-10, IL-12, and IL-18 to promote an inflammatory cascade. Zheng L et al.[5] observed that THP-1 derived macrophage cells infected with Beijing/W MTB strains had hypermethylation of the CpG67 region in the *IL6R* promoter gene, leading to altered inflammatory function. Additionally, they found IL-4R and IL-17R hypermethylations in patients with active TB.

The ESAT-6 is an important protein in enhancing MTB virulence and altering immune pathways. It is secreted by ESX-1 (ESAT-6 secretion system-1), which is induced by a genetic locus known as region of difference (RD) 1, a DNA segment encoding nine genes (*Rv3871* to *Rv3879c*). ESAT-6, along with TLR2, induces nitric oxide synthase/NO and ROS, and is associated with the suppression of H3K27 trimethylation in host cells. This leads to hyperexpression of epithelioid macrophage marker molecules (EMMMs), facilitating the transition of bone-derived macrophages to epithelioid macrophages in granuloma formation. Mutant mice lacking TLR2 shows suppression of ESAT-6 modulation, affecting granuloma formation. This epigenetic change could be targeted for new therapies.[6]

Certain DNA methylation patterns are associated with the development of drug resistance in TB. *Methyltransferase genes*: The *Erm(37)* gene encodes a methyltransferase in 23S rRNA, conferring intrinsic resistance to macrolide-lincosamide-streptogramin (MLS) in the MTB complex (MTBC). However, methylation of the A1518 and A1519 regions of 16S ribosomal RNA by the *KsgA* gene confers MTB intrinsic resistance to clarithromycin.[7] Differentially expressed genes leading to either hypermethylation or hypomethylation were documented in INH- or RIF-resistant MTB H37Rv strains.[8] Analyzing various candidate genes, genome-wide DNA methylation, and transcriptome changes in different MTB strains may be a promising area of future research in understanding epigenetics associated with drug resistance. Thus, studying the epigenetic mechanisms in MTB can provide insights into its survival strategies, virulence, and drug resistance, opening avenues for new therapeutic approaches.

Phosphorylation Effects

Post-translational modifications such as protein acetylation and phosphorylation, catalyzed by acetyltransferase and kinase enzymes respectively, play a crucial role in altering chromatin superstructure and DNA-protein interactions. These modified proteins exhibit different functional and catalytic properties, inducing epigenetic changes in host cellular signaling pathways that modulate immune defense, enhance microbial virulence, and contribute to drug resistance.

The MTB employs 11 serine/threonine protein kinases (STPKs) to phosphorylate substrates on aspartate amino acids, generating various phosphorylated products. These modifications enhance MTB dissemination and persistence within host cells by inhibiting the host immune response. In murine models, the antityrosine kinase drug imatinib has been shown to reduce bacterial load and inflammation.[9]

The nucleoprotein RecA is essential for DNA repair in almost all bacteria and plays a central role in the SOS response by homologous pairing of DNA and acting as a coprotease for the LexA repressor, which controls DNA damage through transcriptional repression. Phosphorylation of RecA, specifically at the serine 207 residue (RecA S207) by a serine-threonine protein kinase, inhibits the LexA coprotease function of RecA. This inhibition controls mutagenesis and leads to the emergence of antibacterial drug resistance.

Most antibiotics cause DNA damage, and RecA is crucial for DNA repair. Therefore, phosphorylation of RecA affects its ability to respond to DNA damage, contributing to the development of drug resistance. Inhibitors of RecA could potentially enhance antibiotic potency and prevent drug resistance.[10]

Acetylation Effects

Acetylation, a type of post-translational modification, plays a significant role in bacterial virulence, persistence, and antibiotic resistance. Acetylated protein molecules, such as isocitrate lyase, contribute to these processes. For example, mutations induced at the isocitrate lyase acetylation site have been shown to reduce MTB proliferation, demonstrating the importance of acetylation in bacterial survival.[11]

The MTB can adopt a nonreplicating dormant state in response to hypoxia or nitric oxide in the host cellular/tissue environment. These quiescent bacilli are resistant to conventional anti-TB drugs. Epigenetic processes are thought to play a role in these adaptive mechanisms. The dormancy survival regulator (DosR gene *Rv3133c*) is an operon in MTB that encodes a response regulator, which is upregulated in hypoxic environments, aiding the bacterium's survival within granulomatous lesions typical of TB. This mechanism allows MTB to become nonreplicating dormant bacilli, thus developing resistance to anti-TB drugs.

ROLE OF PROTEIN LYSINE ACETYLTRANSFERASE

The MTB utilizes the enzyme protein lysine acetyltransferase (PAT) (Mt-pat/Rv0998) to alter the carbon flux from oxidative to reductive tricarboxylic acid (TCA) state. This enzyme interacts with malate dehydrogenase (MDH) to regulate the NAD^+/NADH redox reaction. A study by Rittershaus ESC et al.[12] observed that mutation of the gene encoding PAT and genetic/chemical inhibition of MDH loci affected MTB survival under hypoxic conditions in a murine lung model. These pathways present potential targets for new drugs aimed at selectively targeting semidormant or quiescent bacilli.

CONCLUSION

Epigenetic modifications alter the chromatin superstructure, impair DNA accessibility, and regulate DNA-protein interactions and gene expression. DNA methylation, acetylation, and phosphorylation are common epigenetic processes utilized by MTB to enhance its virulence and persistence in the host, reprogram host intracellular signaling systems to escape immune pathways, and develop drug resistance. Understanding these epigenetic mechanisms can aid in identifying specific genetic targets to develop newer therapeutic drugs for drug-resistant TB. Innovative approaches such as CRISPR (clustered regularly interspaced short palindromic repeat), specifically CRISPR-associated protein 9 (Cas9), and RNA interference (RNAi) are being developed to inhibit the expression of virulent genes and prevent the emergence of drug resistance.

REFERENCES

1. Bobetsis YA, Barros SP, Lin DM, Weidman JR, Dolinoy DC, Jirtle RL, et al. Bacterial infection promotes DNA Hypermethylation. J Dent Res. 2007;86:169-74.
2. Holoch D, Moazed, D. RNA-mediated epigenetic regulation of gene expression. Nat Rev Genet. 2015;16:71-84.
3. Chen YC, Hsiao CC, Chen CJ, Chao TY, Leung SY, Liu SF, et al. Aberrant Toll-like receptor 2 promoter methylation in blood cells from patients with pulmonary tuberculosis. J Infect. 2014;69:546-57.
4. Shell SS, Prestwich EG, Baek SH, Shah RR, Sassetti CM, Dedon PC, et al. DNA Methylation Impacts Gene Expression and Ensures Hypoxic Survival of *Mycobacterium tuberculosis*. PLoS Pathog. 2013;9(7):e1003419.
5. Zheng L, Leung ETY, Wong HK, Lui G, Lee N, To KF, et al. Unraveling methylation changes of host macrophages in *Mycobacterium tuberculosis* infection. Tuberculosis (Edinb). 2016;98:139-8.
6. Lin J, Jiang Y, Liu D, Dai X, Wang M, Dai Y. Early secreted antigenic target of 6-kDa of *Mycobacterium tuberculosis* induces transition of macrophages into epithelioid macrophages by downregulating iNOS/NO-mediated H3K27 trimethylation in macrophages. Mol Immunol. 2020;117:189-200.
7. Phunpruch S, Warit S, Suksamran R, Billamas P, Jaitrong S, Palittapongarnpim P, et al. A role for 16S rRNA dimethyltransferase (ksgA) in intrinsic clarithromycin resistance in *Mycobacterium tuberculosis*. Int J Antimicrob Agents. 2013;41:548-51.
8. Chen L, Li H, Chen T, Yu L, Guo H, Chen Y, et al. Genome-wide DNA methylation and transcriptome changes in *Mycobacterium tuberculosis* with rifampicin and isoniazid resistance. Int J Clin Exp Pathol. 2018;11:3036-45.
9. Napier RJ, Rafi W, Cheruvu M, Powell KR, Zaunbrecher MA, Bornmann W, et al. Imatinib-sensitive tyrosine kinases regulate mycobacterial pathogenesis and represent therapeutic targets against tuberculosis. Cell Host Microbe. 2011;10:475-85.
10. Wipperman MF, Heaton BE, Nautiyal A, Adefisayo O, Evans H, Gupta R, et al. Mycobacterial Mutagenesis and drug resistance are controlled by phosphorylation and Cardiolipin-mediated inhibition of the RecA Coprotease. Mol Cell. 2018;72:152.
11. Xie L, Wang X, Zeng J, Zhou M, Duan X, Li Q, et al. Proteome-wide lysine acetylation profiling of the human pathogen *Mycobacterium tuberculosis*. Int J Biochem Cell Biol. 2015;59:193-202.
12. Rittershaus ESC, Baek SH, Krieger IV, Nelson SJ, Cheng YS, Nambi S, et al. A lysine acetyltransferase contributes to the metabolic adaptation to hypoxia in *Mycobacterium tuberculosis*. Cell Chem Biol. 2018;25(12):1495-505.

CHAPTER

42

Functional Analysis of Toxin-antitoxin System in Multidrug-resistant Tuberculosis

Karthikeyan Sundaram, Leela Kagithakara Vajravelu

Abstract

Tuberculosis is a contagious illness caused by the bacteria *Mycobacterium tuberculosis*. The World Health Organization's tuberculosis report has indicated that drug-resistant tuberculosis is a significant global issue. Also, *Mycobacterium tuberculosis* exhibits a particular resistance to commonly used medications such as rifampin and isoniazid, which are associated with the toxin-antitoxin loci expressed genes. Significantly, these genes are strongly connected with the persistence of diseases, as current research has shown that *VapBC* and *MazEF* genes are linked with sig genes and first-line anti-TB drugs. Thus, this chapter provides a concise overview of the role of toxin-antitoxin encoded genes in multidrug-resistant tuberculosis. Also, studying these genes in different strains, we may effectively manage drug-resistant tuberculosis.

Keywords: Tuberculosis, *Mycobacterium tuberculosis*, toxin, antitoxin, disease persistence

INTRODUCTION

Mycobacterium tuberculosis (MTB), a type of acid-fast bacteria with a rod-like shape, causes tuberculosis (TB), an infectious disease. According to the World Health Organization (WHO) Global TB Report 2023, TB affected approximately 10.6 million individuals in 2022, with a 95% uncertainty interval (UI) of 9.9–11.4 million. Furthermore, TB was responsible for an estimated 1.3 million fatalities (with a 95% UI of 1.18–1.43 million) worldwide. In 2022, approximately 410,000 individuals (95% UI: 370,000–450,000 million) acquired either multidrug-resistant (MDR) TB or rifampin-resistant TB, indicating the emergence of drug-resistant (DR) TB. The prevalence of TB in India is significant, at 27%.[1]

Mycobacterium tuberculosis is consisting of several distinctive features that enhance its ability to persist in hosts over extended periods of time. These include a distinct cell wall composition and metabolic processes. The toxin-antitoxin (TA) system is an essential strategy for adapting to and resisting stress in difficult conditions, such as those with inadequate nutrition, oxidative damage, low pH, and hypoxia. The antitoxin can either be a noncoding RNA or a labile protein, whereas the toxin molecule is a stable protein. During times of stress, the antitoxin deteriorates and releases active toxins that interfere with crucial cellular activities. In TA system, classified into seven types; especially, the Type II TA systems specifically consist of protein antitoxins that bind to protein toxins, forming complexes. Crucially, these type II systems do not have equivalents in humans and are prevalent in important bacterial diseases. Notably, VapBC and MazEF are significant in pathogenesis of the disease. However, recent studies evaluated the MazEF functions in DR-TB and drug-susceptible (DS)-TB.[2]

Type II TA System

Multiple TA systems are found in MTB strains, in type II systems, the toxin forms a complex with a protein antitoxin, rendering it inactive. They often inhibit their own transcription automatically.

The VapBC Classes

The VapC toxin, possessing a PilT N-terminal (PIN) domain and exhibiting nuclease activity, is a notable constituent of the VapBC family. The VapB protein acts as an antitoxin, inhibiting the harmful effects of the VapC toxin. Interesting, a recent study has demonstrated that the utilization of cholesterol leads to an elevated occurrence of antibiotic persister synthesis in mycobacteria. This trait was eradicated in an MTB strain lacking the RNase toxin VapC12. This study elucidated the precise method by which the VapC12 RNase toxin interacts with MTB proT tRNA, and examined the impact of toxin-induced alterations in proT tRNA levels on the ability of antibiotics to remain in mycobacteria. In addition, this study demonstrated that the VapC12-null strain's ability to thrive within the host and its impact on disease persistence in a guinea pig model of MTB infection is significantly improved by reducing the occurrence of in vitro antibiotic persisters. Also, these studies shown that the utilization of antibiotics and the duration of the disease, either individually or in conjunction, impact the progression of TB and the efficacy of treatment. These findings align with the recently established definitions and criteria. MTB has undergone coevolution to efficiently utilize lipids, including cholesterol, produced by the host as a primary source of carbon. MTB is capable of acquiring carbon from the host through many mechanisms; however, its long-term viability relies on its capacity to utilize host cholesterol. According to the studies determined that the influence of nutrient-dependent growth modulation on antibiotic resistance and disease duration in MTB infections.[2]

The MazEF Classes

The most well-known of these is MazEF. Under normal conditions, the two components of MazEF, MazE (antitoxin) and MazF (toxin), interact to form a complex. In this system, it is thought that 11 loci in the MTB genome are useful for latency, persistence, cell cycle inhibition, adaptive cell death, and environmental adaptation. MazF3, MazF6, and MazF9 inhibit the development of *Mycobacterium* cells. Furthermore, they have a significant impact on the expression of virulence factors. Thus, MazF6 plays an important role in cellular survival.

However, the results of the study significantly evaluated the MazEF functions in DS and DR-TB compared to the H37Rv standard strain. Remarkably, the expression levels of the *mazE3* and *mazE6* antitoxin genes in DR isolates did not exhibit any substantial differences from those of the normal strain. However, the expression levels of mazF3 and mazF6 were significantly higher than those of the normal strain and the DS isolates. The level of mazF6 over expression was higher than that of mazF3. Previous research has demonstrated a substantial increase in the expression of both toxin genes (*mazF3* and *F6*) and a decrease in the expression of antitoxin-related genes (*mazE3* and *E6*) among DR strains. The presence of mazF3 and mazF6 in DR isolates may be the result of exposure to various antibiotics and other stress-inducing factors. The combined effect of the presence of MazF3 and MazF6 ribonucleases in significant concentrations is to inhibit the development and persistence of MTB, as well as to confer resistance to antimicrobial drugs. Furthermore, these proteins may contribute to the development of chronic infection, enhance MTB's immunity to oxidative stress, elicit nutritional restriction, and improve its ability to survive in macrophages. Similarly, another study results determined the toxin of *MazEF* family genes were up-regulated in DR strain. However, the *mazF3*, F6, and *F9* toxin genes were found to be highly expressed in at least two MDR isolates when they were exposed to rifampicin (RIF) and isoniazid (INH). This is different from the *mazE* antitoxin genes. MDR isolates were more likely to have *mazF* genes turned on by RIF than by INH (72.2% vs. 50%). It was much higher in MDR isolates than in the H37Rv strain and sensitive isolates when mazF3, 6 was activated by RIF and mazF3, 6, and 9 was activated by INH. Still, there was not a clear difference between these groups in the amount of *mazF9* genes that were expressed when INH was added. It was not viable to notify the difference between the MDR and H37Rv strains. But in sensitive isolates, RIF greatly increased the expression levels of mazE3, 6, and INH greatly increased the expression levels of mazE3, 6, and 9. This was not the case in MDR isolates **(Fig. 1)**.[3,4]

DISCUSSION

In this chapter, we analyzed the TA systems genes were associated with DR-TB. However, MTB has high count of VapBC and MazEF loci in its genome, and these TA systems linked with persistence of daughter cells. However, the recent study investigated the relationship between MazF6 and sigma factor-associated genes. It found that over expression of MazF6 led to increased expression of transcriptional regulators such as sigB, sigC, sigD, sigE, virS, and csoR, as well as putative proteins. These changes in expression patterns were likely caused by the over expression of MazF6. Moreover, this study discovered a correlation

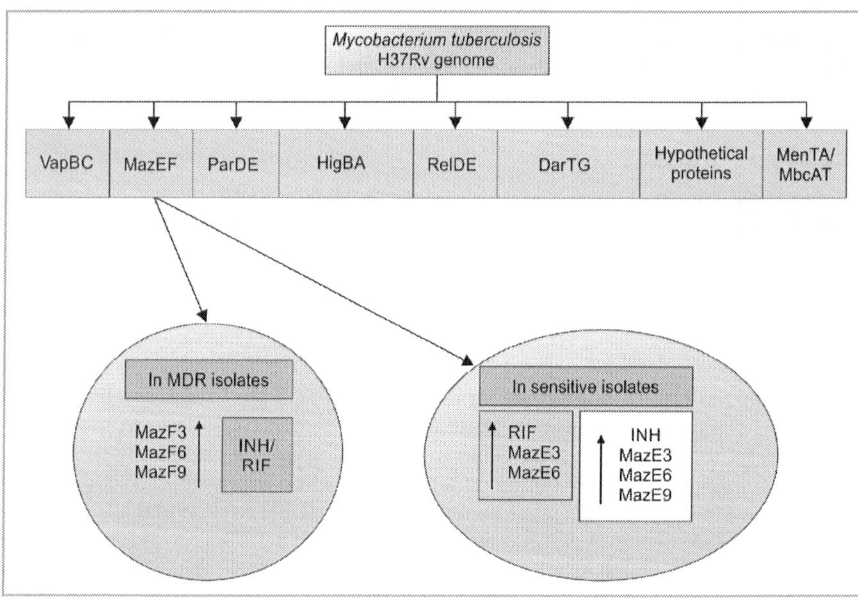

FIG. 1: The different TA system genes, and MazEF actions in drug-resistant TB.

(INH: isoniazid; RIF: rifampicin; TA: toxin-antitoxin; TB: tuberculosis)

between the excessive expression of the transcriptional regulators sigB and virS and the excessive expression of genes associated with virulence, detoxification, and adaptation (hsp, dnaK, and ahpC), intermediate metabolism and respiration (aroG, argC, Rv2672, and pdc), regulatory proteins (clgR), and lipid metabolism (kasA). Thus, the TA system is closely linked with another family of genes in cognate or noncognate partners. So, this vast segment of TA loci will help the fill the gap of the DR-TB strains in future.[4,5]

CONCLUSION

The TA system is a chromosomally encoded genetic element that functions to develop the disease's pathogenesis. However, various studies have demonstrated that TA loci-associated gene links are present in DR-TB. Also, it is closely associated with the first-line TB drugs, INH and RIF. As a result, developing research on these *TA* genes in MTB is critical to determining TB's multidrug resistance.

REFERENCE

1. WHO. Global tuberculosis report 2023. Geneva: World Health Organization; 2023.
2. Kang SM. Focused Overview of *Mycobacterium tuberculosis* VapBC Toxin–Antitoxin Systems Regarding Their Structural and Functional Aspects: Including Insights on Biomimetic Peptides. Biomimetics. 2023;8:412.
3. Kazemian H, Heidari H, Kardan-Yamchi J, Ghafourian S, Pakzad I, Kouhsari E, et al. Comparison of Toxin-Antitoxin Expression among Drug-Susceptible and Drug-Resistant Clinical Isolates of *Mycobacterium Tuberculosis*. Adv Respir Med. 2021;89:110-4.
4. Khosravi AD, Savari M, Khoshnood S, Shahi F, Farshadzadeh Z. Toxin-antitoxin Genes Expression in Multidrug-resistant *Mycobacterium tuberculosis* Isolates under Drug Exposure. Infect Disord Drug Targets. 2023;23(7):66-72.
5. Chattopadhyay G, Bhasin M, Ahmed S, Gosain TP, Ganesan S, Das S, et al. Functional and Biochemical Characterization of the MazEF6 Toxin-Antitoxin System of *Mycobacterium tuberculosis*. J Bacteriol. 2022;204:e0005822.

CHAPTER

43

Phenotypic Drug Resistance: An Update in Pediatric Tuberculosis

Bineeta Kashyap, Rajat Jhamb

Abstract

Despite a significant progress in tuberculosis (TB) control in terms of a substantial decline in mortality in the last few decades, TB still kills one person every 21 seconds. While childhood TB contributes to one-tenth of the global burden of TB, the paucibacillary nature of the disease and lack of standardization in the reliable management make this disease a diagnostic dilemma; despite the availability and access to an effective national prevention program, a treatment regimen and a universal vaccination. Very little is known about the magnitude and pattern of various forms of drug resistance in the pediatric form of TB. Being usually contracted as a direct transmission from the adult form, it becomes an absolute mandate to obtain detailed information on the distribution of pediatric drug-resistant TB in order to move effectively toward the World Health Organization (WHO) end TB strategy.

Keywords: Tuberculosis, pediatric, drug resistance, phenotypic

INTRODUCTION

Even though tuberculosis (TB) is an age-old disease, it affects people of all ages and gender, and continues to remain a significant global public health concern. Several millions of children become exposed to *Mycobacterium tuberculosis* (MTB) each year; TB, thus remaining a leading cause of morbidity and mortality in children all over the world. An estimated 10 million cases of TB disease were reported worldwide by World Health Organization (WHO) in 2021, out of whom approximately 1.2 million were children < 15 years of age. An even bigger proportion of children (14%) accounted for the 1.4 million deaths due to TB disease globally. Most of the childhood disease and the associated deaths have been reported in the low- or middle-income countries of the world.[1] Such reports, despite the availability of an effective TB prevention program, treatment, and access to universal vaccination at birth in endemic countries, send an alarm signal while highlighting the need of that extra effort and increased emphasis on every aspect of childhood TB.

A meagre 3–4% of pediatric drug-resistant (DR) cases are reported to be diagnosed and treated, resulting into deaths in approximately 22% of these infected children. The difficulties of diagnosing pediatric TB remain multifactorial and thus underreporting remains a substantial challenge. The childhood disease has been a diagnostic dilemma and often goes unrecognized due to the diagnostic insufficiencies, the paucibacillary nature of the disease and lack of uniformity or limited access to resistance testing and drug treatment regimens in such cases.[1] Resistance, too, has been reported at higher rates among children with the disease. The varied epidemiology of TB is closely associated with the social determinants of the disease, that influences an individual's vulnerability or resistance to the disease. The need to prioritize pediatric TB as a step to move towards the global strategy to achieve zero TB, is universally recognized.

DRUG RESISTANCE IN PEDIATRIC TB: CURRENT SCENARIO

Drug-resistant TB, especially multidrug-resistant TB (MDR-TB), is a continuing threat to global TB control measures in both children and adults. Pre-extensively drug-resistant TB (pre-XDR-TB) is caused by MTB MDR/RR-TB (rifampicin-resistant) strains that are also resistant to any fluoroquinolone; whereas, XDR-TB is TB caused by MDR/RR MTB strains that are also resistant to any fluoroquinolone and at least one additional group A drug (i.e., bedaquiline or linezolid). These are particularly deadly and difficult to treat strains of TB that impose an elevated risk to children who may have been infected. Literature is not enough on drug resistance patterns in children globally. Roughly more than 58,000, 25,000, and 1,200 children develop RR, MDR, and XDR forms of pediatric TB annually, respectively.

The burden of monoresistance, polyresistance, or multiple drug resistance in pediatric TB is always an underestimate due to the difficulty in bacteriological confirmation of the paucibacillary disease, sampling difficulties and lack of uniformity and standardization in the diagnosis of childhood TB.[2] Literature reports between 25,000 and 32,000 children developing MDR-TB every year. Nodal DR-TB centers report a cumulative prevalence of DR-TB at 16.3% and 18.2% for the year 2018 and 2019, respectively, which reveals an increase of 4.1%; while the prevalence (%) of XDR-TB; MDR-TB; and monoresistant TB for the year 2018, 2019, 2020, and 2021 was (10.9; 88.0; and 1.1), (5.1; 92.8; and 2.1), (3.4; 94.9; and 1.7), and (7.4; 91.6; and 1.0), respectively. The 2020 WHO Global TB Report on MDR-TB in children < 15 years shows that 3,400 and 5,500 children were initiated on second-line treatment in 2018 and 2019, respectively, that indicates 8% of the global target of 1,15,000 in the first 2 years since the UN High Level meeting. For childhood TB, in general, 30% of the 5-year target of 3.5 million has been achieved. In 2019, data from the WHO was used to estimate the prevalence of the incidence of latent TB due to DR-MTB among children < 15 years and it was found to be around 2.9%, which was significantly higher than 1.2% reported in the total population.

Drug-resistant pediatric TB, contrary to the acquired resistant adult form, results mostly from the transmission of DR *Mycobacterium* strains; highlighting even more the need of adequate screening, diagnosis, and management of these cases. Children account for almost 11% of global TB cases, hence, knowing the epidemiology of DR-TB in the pediatric age group will guide timely and appropriate management.

PHENOTYPIC DRUG RESISTANCE IN PEDIATRIC TB

Tuberculosis control program in our country mainly relies on rapid and accurate identification of cases for effective management of the disease, which becomes even more crucial in DR forms. Though the conventional culture-based methods of diagnosis are labor intensive with longer turnaround time, they form the cornerstone of diagnostics. The two currently established testing approaches for DST (drug sensitivity tests) in TB are the proportion method using critical concentration (CC) data and the minimum inhibitory concentration (MIC)-based method. While, the CC is the lowest concentration of the drug that inhibits 99% (90% for pyrazinamide) of wild-type MTB strains, not including clinical strains classified as resistant; MIC is the lowest concentration that completely inhibits MTB growth in vitro.

In a recent study concluded on associated mutations of phenotypic isoniazid resistance in pediatric TB, the authors reported 14% isoniazid resistance in the 71% of the culture positive isolates from clinically suspected cases of pediatric TB, when conventional method of 1% proportion was used.[3] In another follow-up study done in the same setting on pulmonary and extrapulmonary specimens from clinically suspected microbiologically confirmed pediatric TB cases, resistance to the first-line anti-TB drugs by 1% proportion method was reported to be 14%, 11%, 5.5%, and 5.5% each to isoniazid, streptomycin, rifampicin, and ethambutol, respectively. The same study concluded that isoniazid resistance may often go undetected by the existing genotypic methods detecting targeted mutations conferring rifampicin resistance; hence, discrepancies between molecular and conventional phenotypic DST reports should be interpreted with caution in the face of resistance to anti-TB drugs being often encoded by multiple genes that may not be targeted by the currently available molecular tests.[4]

The proportion of MDR-TB among pediatric population is reflective of the proportion of new adult TB patients who have MDR-TB in the same geographical setting, a finding that was later also confirmed by WHO. A 10-year retrospective analysis on culture positive pediatric TB cases, reported a decrease in DR, monoresistant, poly-DR, isoniazid resistant, and RR cases from last 5 years, though the same decrease was not evident in MDR cases. The overall drug resistance in pediatric TB was reported to be 35.16%, while the resistance rates to isoniazid and rifampicin were 13.93% and 13.24%, respectively; MDR reported at 6.39%. The study also compared the rates among different age groups of children and concluded that the children have the same risk of DR-TB between different age groups. The higher resistance to levofloxacin reported in the study, keeping in mind the fact that children mostly get direct transmission of TB from adults; the authors suggested greater need of standardization in the use of the drug to reduce drug resistance in the pediatric age group.[5]

CONCLUSION

The emergence of many different patterns of DR-TB over the past decades has further complicated the use of standardized drug treatment regimens in pediatric TB. WHO recommends rapid diagnostics and universal DST for all people experiencing clinical symptoms of active TB.

REFERENCES

1. Gaensbauer JT, Dash N, Verma S, Hall DJ, Adler-Shohet FC, Li G, et al. Multidrug-resistant tuberculosis in children: A practical update on epidemiology, diagnosis, treatment and prevention. J Clin Tuberc Other Mycobact Dis. 2024;36:100449.
2. Song WM, Li YF, Liu YX, Liu Y, Yu CB, Liu JY, et al. Drug-resistant tuberculosis among children: A systematic review and meta-analysis. Front Public Health. 2021;9:721817.
3. Jhanjhria S, Kashyap B, Gomber S, Gupta N, Hyanki P, Singh NP, et al. Phenotypic isoniazid resistance and associated mutations in pediatric tuberculosis. Indian J Tuberculosis. 2019;66:474-9.
4. Kashyap B, Jhanjharia S, Saha R, Gomber S. Missed phenotypic drug resistance in pediatric tuberculosis: A cause of concern in a resource-limited setting. Indian J Tuberc. 2023;70 Suppl 1: S59-S64.
5. Li M, Deng B, Huang Y, Li Q, Han J, Tang S, et al. Trends and risk factors for drug-resistant tuberculosis among children in Sichuan, China: A 10-year retrospective analysis, 2013–2022. Medicine. 2024;103(15):e37643.

Index

Page numbers followed by *f* refer to figure, *fc* refer to flowchart, and *t* refer to table.

D

E

F

G

H

Q

R

S

T